Thalassemia

Editors

EDWARD J. BENZ JR
VIJAY G. SANKARAN

HEMATOLOGY/ONCOLOGY CLINICS OF NORTH AMERICA

www.hemonc.theclinics.com

Consulting Editors
GEORGE P. CANELLOS
EDWARD J. BENZ JR.

April 2023 • Volume 37 • Number 2

ELSEVIER

1600 John F. Kennedy Boulevard • Suite 1800 • Philadelphia, Pennsylvania, 19103-2899

http://www.theclinics.com

HEMATOLOGY/ONCOLOGY CLINICS OF NORTH AMERICA Volume 37, Number 2
April 2023 ISSN 0889-8588, ISBN 13: 978-0-443-18320-1

Editor: Stacy Eastman
Developmental Editor: Ann Gielou M. Posedio

Hematology/Oncology Clinics (ISSN 0889-8588) is published bimonthly by Elsevier Inc., 360 Park Avenue South, New York, NY 10010-1710. Months of issue are February, April, June, August, October, and December. Business and Editorial Offices: 1600 John F. Kennedy Blvd., Ste. 1800, Philadelphia, PA 19103–2899. Customer Service Office: 3251 Riverport Lane, Maryland Heights, MO 63043. Periodicals postage paid at New York, NY and at additional mailing offices. Subscription prices are $470.00 per year (domestic individuals), $1190.00 per year (domestic institutions), $100.00 per year (domestic students/residents), $495.00 per year (Canadian individuals), $100.00 per year (Canadian students/residents), $1232.00 per year (Canadian institutions) $563.00 per year (international individuals), $1232.00 per year (international institutions), and $255.00 per year (international students/residents). International air speed delivery is included in all *Clinics* subscription prices. All prices are subject to change without notice. **POSTMASTER:** Send address changes to *Hematology/Oncology Clinics of North America*, Elsevier Health Sciences Division, Subscription Customer Service, 3251 Riverport Lane, Maryland Heights, MO 63043. Customer Service (orders, claims, online, change of address): Elsevier Health Sciences Division, Subscription **Customer Service, 3251 Riverport Lane, Maryland Heights, MO 63043. Tel: 1-800-654-2452 (U.S. and Canada); 314-447-8871 (outside U.S. and Canada). Fax: 314-447-8029. E-mail: journalscustomerservice-usa@elsevier.com (for print support); journalsonlinesupport-usa@elsevier.com (for online support)**.

Reprints. For copies of 100 or more, of articles in this publication, please contact the Commercial Reprints Department, Elsevier Inc., 360 Park Avenue South, New York, New York 10010-1710; Tel.: 212-633-3874, Fax: 212-633-3820, E-mail: reprints@elsevier.com.

Hematology/Oncology Clinics of North America is covered in *MEDLINE/PubMed (Index Medicus), EMBASE/ Excerpta Medica, and BIOSIS.*

Contributors

CONSULTING EDITORS

GEORGE P. CANELLOS, MD
William Rosenberg Professor of Medicine, Department of Medical Oncology, Dana-Farber Cancer Institute, Boston, Massachusetts, USA

EDWARD J. BENZ Jr, MD
President and CEO Emeritus, Dana Farber Cancer Institute, Director Emeritus, Dana-Farber/Harvard Cancer Center, Richard and Susan Smith Distinguished Professor of Medicine, Professor of Pediatrics, Professor of Genetics, Harvard Medical School, Boston, Massachusetts

EDITORS

EDWARD J. BENZ Jr, MD
President and CEO Emeritus, Dana Farber Cancer Institute, Director Emeritus, Dana-Farber/Harvard Cancer Center, Richard and Susan Smith Distinguished Professor of Medicine, Professor of Pediatrics, Professor of Genetics, Harvard Medical School, Boston, Massachusetts, USA

VIJAY G. SANKARAN, MD, PhD
Jan Ellen Paradise, MD Associate Professor of Pediatrics, Harvard Medical School and Lodish Family Chair, Division of Hematology/Oncology, Boston Children's Hospital, Boston, Massachusetts, USA

AUTHORS

MATTIA ALGERI, MD
Department of Hematology/Oncology, Cell and Gene Therapy – IRCCS, Bambino Gesù Children's Hospital, Rome, Italy

MICHAEL ANGASTINIOTIS, MD
Thalassameia International Federation, Nicosia, Cyprus

DANIEL BAUER, MD, PhD
Division of Hematology/Oncology, Boston Children's Hospital, Department of Pediatric Oncology, Dana-Farber Cancer Institute, Department of Pediatrics, Harvard Stem Cell Institute, Broad Institute, Harvard Medical School, Boston, Massachusetts, USA

EDWARD J. BENZ Jr, MD
President and CEO Emeritus, Dana Farber Cancer Institute, Director Emeritus, Dana-Farber/Harvard Cancer Center, Richard and Susan Smith Distinguished Professor of Medicine, Professor of Pediatrics, Professor of Genetics, Harvard Medical School, Boston, Massachusetts, USA

RAYAN BOU-FAKHREDIN, MSC
Department of Clinical Sciences and Community Health, University of Milan, Milan, Italy

MARIA DOMENICA CAPPELLINI, MD, PhD
Department of Clinical Sciences and Community Health, University of Milan, UOC General Medicine, Fondazione IRCCS Ca' Granda Ospedale Maggiore Policlinico, Milan, Italy

KATIE T. CARLBERG, MD
Division of Hematology/Oncology, UCSF Benioff Children's Hospital, Oakland, California, USA

GEORGIOS E. CHRISTAKOPOULOS, MD
Department of Oncology, St. Jude Children's Research Hospital, Memphis, Tennessee, USA

ANDROULLA ELEFTHERIOU, PhD
Thalassameia International Federation, Nicosia, Cyprus

DIMITRIOS FARMAKIS, MD
Associate Professor, University of Cyprus Medical School, Nicosia, Cyprus

TOMAS GANZ, PhD, MD
Distinguished Professor of Medicine and Pathology, Department of Medicine, David Geffen School of Medicine at UCLA, Los Angeles, California, USA

KEVIN H.M. KUO, MD, MSC
Division of Hematology, University of Toronto, Toronto, Ontario, Canada

JANET L. KWIATKOWSKI, MD, MSCE
Director, Thalassemia Program, Division of Hematology, Children's Hospital of Philadelphia and Professor of Pediatrics, Department of Pediatrics, Perelman School of Medicine, University of Pennsylvania, Philadelphia, Pennsylvania, USA

ASHUTOSH LAL, MD
Professor of Clinical Pediatrics, UCSF School of Medicine, UCSF Benioff Children's Hospital, Oakland, California, USA

FRANCO LOCATELLI, MD, PhD
Department of Hematology/Oncology, Cell and Gene Therapy – IRCCS, Bambino Gesù Children's Hospital, Department of Life Sciences and Public Health, Catholic University of the Sacred Heart, Rome, Italy

MARIACHIARA LODI, MD
Department of Hematology/Oncology, Cell and Gene Therapy – IRCCS, Bambino Gesù Children's Hospital, Rome, Italy

HENRY Y. LU, PhD
Division of Hematology/Oncology, Department of Pediatric Oncology, Dana-Farber Cancer Institute, Harvard Medical School, Broad Institute of Massachusetts Institute of Technology (MIT) and Harvard, Karp Family Research Laboratories, Boston Children's Hospital, Boston, Massachusetts, USA

AURELIO MAGGIO, MD
Professor, Campus of Haematology Franco and Piera Cutino, AOR Villa Sofia-V, Cervello, Palermo, Italy

IRENE MOTTA, MD
Department of Clinical Sciences and Community Health, University of Milan, UOC General Medicine, Fondazione IRCCS Ca' Granda Ospedale Maggiore Policlinico, Milan, Italy

ELIZABETA NEMETH, PhD
Professor, Department of Medicine, David Geffen School of Medicine at UCLA, Los Angeles, California, USA

STUART H. ORKIN, MD
Division of Hematology/Oncology, Department of Pediatric Oncology, Dana-Farber Cancer Institute, Harvard Medical School, Karp Family Research Laboratories, Boston Children's Hospital, Boston, Massachusetts, USA; Howard Hughes Medical Institute, Chevy Chase, Maryland, USA; Harvard Stem Cell Institute, Cambridge, Massachusetts, USA

MORGAN PINES, MD
Post-Doctoral Fellow, Division of Pediatric Hematology Oncology, Department of Pediatrics, Weill Cornell Medicine, Department of Pediatrics, Memorial Sloan Kettering Cancer Center, New York, New York, USA

STEFANO RIVELLA, PhD
Division of Hematology, Department of Pediatrics, Children's Hospital of Philadelphia, Philadelphia, Pennsylvania, USA

VIJAY G. SANKARAN, MD, PhD
Jan Ellen Paradise, MD Associate Professor of Pediatrics, Harvard Medical School and Lodish Family Chair, Division of Hematology/Oncology, Boston Children's Hospital, Boston, Massachusetts, USA

FARZANA A. SAYANI, MD
Division of Hematology/Oncology, Hospital of the University of Pennsylvania, Perelman School of Medicine, Philadelphia, Pennsylvania, USA

SUJIT SHETH, MD
Professor and Chief, Division of Pediatric Hematology Oncology, Department of Pediatrics, Weill Cornell Medicine, New York, New York, USA

SYLVIA T. SINGER, MD
Division of Hematology/Oncology, UCSF Benioff Children's Hospital, Oakland, California, USA

SOTERIS SOTERIADES, PhD
Department of Anaesthesiology and Intensive Care, AHEPA University General Hospital of Thessaloniki, Thessaloniki, Greece

ALI T. TAHER, MD, PhD
Division of Hematology-Oncology, Department of Internal Medicine, American University of Beirut Medical Center, Beirut, Lebanon

RAHUL TELANGE, MS
Department of Hematology, St. Jude Children's Research Hospital, Memphis, Tennessee, USA

NICOLÒ TESIO
Department of Clinical and Biological Sciences, University of Torino, Torino, Italy

ELLIOTT P. VICHINSKY, MD
Professor of Pediatrics and UCSF Endowed Physician, UCSF School of Medicine, Division of Hematology/Oncology, UCSF Benioff Children's Hospital, Oakland, California, USA

MITCHELL J. WEISS, MD, PhD
Department of Hematology, St. Jude Children's Research Hospital, Memphis, Tennessee, USA

JONATHAN YEN, PhD
Department of Hematology, St. Jude Children's Research Hospital, Memphis, Tennessee, USA

Contents

Thalassemia is a heterogeneous group of inherited anemias having in common defective biosynthesis of one or more of the globin chain subunits of human hemoglobin. Their origins lie in inherited mutations that impair the expression of the affected globin genes. Their pathophysiology arises from the consequent insufficiency of hemoglobin production and the imbalance in the production of globin chains resulting in the accumulation of insoluble unpaired chains. These precipitate and damage or destroy developing erythroblasts and erythrocytes producing ineffective erythropoiesis and hemolytic anemia. Treatment of severe cases requires lifelong transfusion support with iron chelation therapy.

Epidemiology is the practical tool to provide information on which policy makers should base planning of services. Epidemiological data for thalassemia is based on inaccurate and often conflicting measurements. This study attempts to demonstrate with examples the sources of inaccuracy and confusion. The Thalassemia International Foundation (TIF) suggests that congenital disorders, for which increasing complications and premature death are avoidable through appropriate treatment and follow-up, should be given priority based on accurate data and patient registries. Moreover, only accurate information about this issue, especially for developing countries, will move national health resources in the right direction.

Thalassemia syndromes are common monogenic disorders and represent a significant health issue worldwide. In this review, the authors elaborate on fundamental genetic knowledge about thalassemias, including the structure and location of globin genes, the production of hemoglobin during development, the molecular lesions causing α-, β-, and other thalassemia syndromes, the genotype-phenotype correlation, and the genetic modifiers of these conditions. In addition, they briefly discuss the molecular techniques applied for diagnosis and innovative cell and gene therapy strategies to cure these conditions.

stimulates a state of stress that leads to the ineffective production of RBCs. We herein describe the main features of erythropoiesis and its regulation in addition to the mechanisms behind ineffective erythropoiesis development in β-thalassemia. Finally, we review the pathophysiology of hypercoagulability and vascular disease development in β-thalassemia and the currently available prevention and treatment modalities.

Allogeneic hematopoietic stem cell transplantation (allo-HSCT) is the only consolidated, potentially curative treatment for patients with transfusion-dependent thalassemia major. In the past few decades, several new approaches have reduced the toxicity of conditioning regimens and decreased the incidence of graft-versus-host disease, improving patients' outcomes and quality of life. In addition, the progressive availability of alternative stem cell sources from unrelated or haploidentical donors or umbilical cord blood has made HSCT a feasible option for an increasing number of subjects lacking an human leukocyte antigen (HLA)-identical sibling. This review provides an overview of allogeneic hematopoietic stem cell transplantation in thalassemia, reassesses current clinical results, and discusses future perspectives.

After many years of intensive research, emerging data from clinical trials indicate that gene therapy for transfusion-dependent β-thalassemia is now possible. Strategies for therapeutic manipulation of patient hematopoietic stem cells include lentiviral transduction of a functional erythroid-expressed β-globin gene and genome editing to activate fetal hemoglobin production in patient red blood cells. Gene therapy for β-thalassemia and other blood disorders will invariably improve as experience accumulates over time. The best overall approaches are not known and perhaps not yet established. Gene therapy comes at a high cost, and collaboration between multiple stakeholders is required to ensure that these new medicines are administered equitably.

Advances in understanding the underlying pathophysiology of β-thalassemia have enabled efforts toward the development of novel therapeutic modalities. These can be classified into three major categories based on their ability to target different features of the underlying disease pathophysiology: correction of the α/β globin chain imbalance, targeting ineffective erythropoiesis, and targeting iron dysregulation. This article provides an overview of these different emerging therapies that are currently in development for β-thalassemia.

HEMATOLOGY/ONCOLOGY CLINICS OF NORTH AMERICA

SERIES OF RELATED INTEREST

Surgical Oncology Clinics
https://www.surgonc.theclinics.com/
Advances in Oncology
https://www.advances-oncology.com/

THE CLINICS ARE AVAILABLE ONLINE!
Access your subscription at:
www.theclinics.com

Preface

Thalassemia

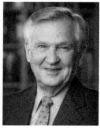 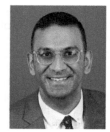

Edward J. Benz Jr, MD   Vijay G. Sankaran, MD, PhD
Editors

The thalassemia syndromes are inherited disorders of hemoglobin synthesis associated with heterogeneous clinical manifestations ranging from barely detectable microcytosis to profound transfusion-dependent anemia associated with severe stigmata of hemolysis and ineffective erythropoiesis. Taken as a group, the thalassemias are likely the single most common inherited disorders in the world. Indeed, in some populous Southeastern Asian regions, gene frequencies for certain thalassemia alleles can range as high as 30% to 40%, comparable to the frequency of blood group A+ in the United States. In these and several other areas of the world, the serious forms of thalassemia thus represent significant public health issues and, importantly, are a major cause of human suffering.

The vast majority of individuals heterozygous for thalassemia ("thalassemia trait" or "thalassemia minor") exhibit only mild hematologic laboratory abnormalities and no or minimal symptoms. In areas of the world where malaria is endemic, they appear to have a selective advantage by being at least partially protected from its most severe manifestations. Individuals homozygous for thalassemia alleles, or compound heterozygous for a thalassemia allele and an allele for another hemoglobinopathy, such as hemoglobin E or sickle hemoglobin, exhibit varying degrees of hemolytic anemia and deficient production of mature red cells due to ineffective erythropoiesis. The genetic, molecular, and pathophysiologic basis for these hematologic abnormalities and clinical manifestations has been characterized in considerably greater detail, perhaps, than for almost any other human illnesses. After many years during which red cell transfusions and the use of iron-chelating agents to mitigate consequent hemosiderosis were the only therapeutic options available to these more severely afflicted patients, a number of exciting new disease-modifying and even curative options are either available or on the horizon. Thus, for hematologists and oncologists, it is mandatory to develop a thorough understanding of the thalassemias, their clinical variability, and the standard and emerging therapeutic strategies available to individual patients.

Hematol Oncol Clin N Am 37 (2023) xiii–xv
https://doi.org/10.1016/j.hoc.2023.01.001
0889-8588/23/© 2023 Published by Elsevier Inc.

hemonc.theclinics.com

In addition to their clinical and public health importance, the thalassemias are also extraordinarily important as "molecular medicine's index case." As outlined in the article entitled, "Introduction to the Thalassemias, Molecular Medicine's Index Case" in this issue, these disorders were the first to be delineated as arising from deficient *biosynthesis* of the specific protein products of specific genes, namely the genes encoding the individual globin subunits of hemoglobin. Delineation of their molecular pathophysiology constituted the first demonstration of the clinical consequences not only of deficient production of a specific protein but also of the imbalanced accumulation of the components of multimeric proteins. Studies of the molecular genetics of the thalassemias led to the first demonstration of messenger RNA defects and specific gene deletions responsible for human disease, the first isolation of an individual messenger RNA product of a human gene, the first cloning of human cDNAs and genomic loci, the first DNA-based techniques for antenatal diagnosis of inherited disorders, and numerous other initial breakthroughs that inspired the incursion of molecular biology into the study of clinical medicine. The study of these syndromes set the paradigm for investigating and illuminating the pathway that connected specific mutations with their consequences on the expression of the affected gene, and the cellular, organismic, and homeostatic consequences of altered expression of the affected gene or genes. This approach has been adopted to the study of many inherited and acquired disorders. More recently, these disorders have been targeted for the first application of CRISPR/Cas9 genome editing in the clinic. Some familiarity with the molecular pathology and pathophysiology of the thalassemia syndromes thus remains important for students of hematology, oncology, and, indeed, most medical specialties.

The editors and authors of this issue dedicate it to the memory of Sir David Weatherall. He more than any other single individual codified the thalassemia syndromes as specific disorders impairing the expression of specific genes that are needed to produce an essential life-sustaining protein, namely, hemoglobin. His contributions over the span of his career can quite literally be credited with opening the doors of medicine to the transformative strategies and techniques that we now call precision molecular medicine. The article in this issue entitled, "Remembering the Contributions of David Weatherall," provides a remembrance and appreciation for the positive impact he made on this field, on hematology, and on global health.

We, the guest editors, attempted to organize this issue in a manner that offers an interrelated array of articles covering the distinct and most important features of the thalassemias, both clinically and scientifically. We hope that they will provide the reader a richer level of understanding and insight into the complex yet elegantly defined pathophysiology and clinical features of these numerous but interrelated syndromes. We also feel that this update is timely. Earlier this year, the Food and Drug Administration approved the first gene replacement therapy for the treatment of transfusion-dependent forms of these illnesses. In addition, the past two to three years have witnessed the introduction and expanded use of disease-modifying drugs that, in properly selected patients, ameliorate many of the more severe manifestations of the disease. These agents are based on emerging insights into the complex derangements of the bone marrow microenvironment, hematopoietic stem cell function, and inflammation that occur as the result of defects in globin gene expression. We thus hope that the material included in this issue will be useful to the reader, both as a practical clinical update about the prevention, diagnosis, and treatment of patients with these conditions and as an important heuristic lesson for understanding the flood of information emerging daily about the molecular genetic abnormalities associated with myriad disorders, particularly hematologic neoplasms.

Edward J. Benz Jr, MD
Dana-Farber Cancer Institute
Dana-Farber/Harvard Cancer Center
Harvard Medical School
Boston, MA 02215, USA

Vijay G. Sankaran, MD, PhD
Boston Children's Hospital
1 Blackfan Street
Karp Family Research Building, Room 7211
Boston, MA 02115, USA

E-mail addresses:
edward_benz@dfci.harvard.edu (E.J. Benz)
sankaran@broadinstitute.org (V.G. Sankaran)

Dedication

Remembering the Contributions of Professor David J. Weatherall

We dedicate this issue of the *Hematology/Oncology Clinics of North America* to the memory of Professor Sir David J. Weatherall (**Fig. 1**). The field of thalassemia research has, for the past 75 years, been marked by seminal discoveries that laid the foundation for molecular medicine. It has been populated by many of the world's most outstanding scientists. Among these, David Weatherall stands out, universally acknowledged as the individual who contributed more than anyone. He provided foundational insights into the mechanisms underlying these severe inherited anemias and advanced an entire field through his laboratory and clinical research, his writings, and his advocacy. His leadership inspired generations of world-class investigators to make truly breakthrough discoveries in ways that have improved the outlook for many patients afflicted with these inherited disorders.

Sir David's career was embedded in his deep compassionate concern for the plight of the first patient with thalassemia that he encountered. Driven to understand the causes of her symptoms, he pursued decades of groundbreaking research that codified their nosology, genetics, ontogeny, hematology, biochemical and molecular pathology, and fundamental strategies for their diagnosis and therapy. This attracted many talented investigators to study the globin genes, causing them to be the first human genes characterized, isolated, and expressed in model systems. By so doing, Weatherall's contribution to science and medicine transcended even his profound impact on the thalassemia field. As discussed in the article in this issue by Edward J. Benz Jr entitled, "Introduction to the Thalassemias, Molecular Medicine's Index Case," these studies of hemoglobinopathies demonstrated the feasibility of applying the emerging techniques and strategies of molecular genetics to the study of human diseases. Indeed, the globin genes remain the best (though incompletely) understood in terms relating their structure and function to the development of complex phenotypes expressed in embryonic, fetal, and postnatal life.

Professor Sir David John Weatherall was born March 9, 1933, in Liverpool, United Kingdom, where he spent his childhood and youth, ultimately graduating in Medicine from Liverpool University in 1956. While serving his military duty he was assigned to a military hospital in Singapore. Having had no specialty training in Pediatrics, he encountered a young girl, named Jaspir Thapa, who, since the age of 3 months, had been severely anemic and kept alive only by repeated blood transfusions.[1] Exhibiting the relentless commitment to the care of his patients that marked his entire career, Weatherall did extensive research to try to find the cause of her anemia and, perhaps, a more effective treatment. This yielded no fruit until a chance meeting with a Maltese biochemist named Frank Vella, who was on the faculty at the University of Singapore. Hearing the description of Ms Thapa's anemia and transfusion dependency, he pointed Weatherall to a paper that had been published a few years earlier describing a patient with "Mediterranean anemia" (ie, thalassemia) in

Hematol Oncol Clin N Am 37 (2023) xvii–xxi
https://doi.org/10.1016/j.hoc.2022.11.002
0889-8588/23/© 2022 Published by Elsevier Inc.

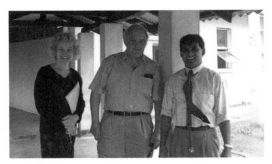

Fig. 1. Professor Sir David Weatherall (*center*) with Dr Nancy Olivieri (*left*) with whom he founded the nonprofit advocacy group, Hemaglobal, and pediatrician Dr Mahinda Arambepola (*right*), during a consulting visit a local clinic to Sri Lanka. (*Courtesy of* Dr Nancy Olivieri, see Ref. 3.)

Thailand. This paper pointed out that there were patients in southeast Asia whose clinical features strongly resembled thalassemia, a condition that at that time was thought to be common only in the Mediterranean region.

In the mid-1950s, techniques to characterize, separate, and quantitate human hemoglobins were just emerging. Lacking access to state-of-the-art scientific resources, Weatherall adapted a new method called starch gel electrophoresis to analyze Ms Thapa's blood. He improvised, using filter paper as his matrix and automobile batteries as his power source. He was able to confirm that Jaspir did indeed suffer from thalassemia. Weatherall and Bella published a paper in the *British Medical Journal* entitled "Thalassemia in a Gurkha family."[2] In his book, "Thalassemia: the Biography,"[1] Weatherall wryly noted that this was an inauspicious start to his career in academic hematology, because he was nearly court-martialed for publishing a paper without permission, and especially, for reporting that the family of elite Gurkha officers had "bad genes."[1] This vignette, well known to almost everyone who is a student of the thalassemia syndromes, marked the beginning of a career that would lead David to preeminence in advancing our understanding, diagnosis, and treatment of the thalassemias.

Upon completing his military service, Weatherall undertook a Fellowship in Hematology at Johns Hopkins, where he mastered the specialty under the tutelage of C. Lockhart Conley and began his lifelong study of hemoglobinopathies. He returned to Liverpool from 1965 until 1974, when he was recruited to Oxford University as the Nuffield Professor. He founded Oxford's Institute for Molecular Medicine in 1989 (renamed the Weatherall Institute for Molecular Medicine in 2000 by Oxford University in recognition of his profound influence on the founding the field of molecular medicine). In 1992, he was appointed Regius Professor, the most prestigious professorial appointment in the United Kingdom.[1,3,4]

Throughout his incredibly productive career, Sir David made many contributions to hematology, particularly the hemoglobinopathies. He contributed nearly 600 papers to the literature, many books and monographs, and communications for the lay press outlining the basic understanding of molecular biology and its relevance to clinical medicine. During those early years at Johns Hopkins and Liverpool, he made some of his most seminal contributions.

By the late 1950s and early 1960s, it was well established that the various hemoglobins consisted of tetramer of globin peptides, each bound to the heme group consisting of a protoporphyrin IX moiety within which was coordinated an ion of reduced iron

(Fe^{++}) (see the article in this issue by Edward J. Benz Jr entitled, "Introduction to the Thalassemias, Molecular Medicine's Index Case"). It was also clear that there were several forms of thalassemia. By far, the most common forms were the alpha-thalassemias, due to reduced or absent accumulation of alpha-globin chain and beta-thalassemia, reflecting deficient accumulation of the beta-globin chains. What was not clear was the mechanism by which these globin chains failed to accumulate. Most investigators believed that the underlying cause was defective biosynthesis; others believed that posttranslational instability was responsible. Unfortunately, there were no methods available for measuring the biosynthesis of the individual globin chains, until, in 1965, Weatherall and his colleagues made perhaps the most pivotal advance in our understanding of the cause of the thalassemias by demonstrating unequivocally that the reduced accumulation of globin chains was due to reduced biosynthesis.[5]

A major problem impeding the analysis of the individual globin chains is that they are both resistant to dissociation and highly insoluble in aqueous solutions. Solutions containing 8-molar urea dissociated the individual globins, but the chains aggregated, prohibiting further analysis. Weatherall and his colleagues J.B. Clegg and M.A. Naughton discovered that adding 2-mercaptoethanol alleviated the aggregation. They then demonstrated that the soluble disaggregated chains could be cleanly separated by ion exchange chromatography on columns comprising carboxy-methylcellulose resin. Exploiting the new availability of C-14–labeled amino acids, coupled with the observations of others that circulating reticulocytes retain the protein synthetic machinery, Weatherall and Clegg were able to compare the biosynthesis of alpha- and beta-chains by normal and thalassemic reticulocytes. These studies demonstrated definitively that the defect responsible for reduced globin *accumulation* in thalassemia was due to defects in the primary biosynthesis of the affected globin chain.[5]

As described in the article in this issue by Edward J. Benz Jr entitled, "Introduction to the Thalassemias, Molecular Medicine's Index Case," this development opened the doors to the studies by several groups of the underlying defects in the protein biosynthetic apparatus responsible for the defective production of the affected globin chains. Neinhuis and Anderson[6] and Benz and Forget[7] ultimately utilized "Clegg columns" to measure the synthesis of globin chains in cell-free systems primed with mRNA from nonthalassemic and thalassemic reticulocytes. Their results proved that the defects leading to reduced biosynthesis were due to defective amounts or translatability of globin mRNA. These breakthroughs demonstrated that the early methods of molecular biology could be used to study human diseases. They were possible only because of the availability of the Clegg columns and the Weatherall group's proof that thalassemias arose from defective biosynthesis of the affected globin.

Throughout his career, Weatherall had a genius for collaborations and for attracting distinguished investigators into the study of the thalassemias. Douglas Higgs, John B. Clegg, Bill Woods, John Pritchard, Swee Lay Thien, among numerous others, emerged as key contributors. Their work helped to advance the field. Sir David also collaborated with laboratory investigators around the world, and with clinicians in the regions most affected by the thalassemias (see the article in this issue by Aurelio Maggio entitled, "The Epidemiology of the Thalassemia Syndromes").

In 1965, Weatherall and Clegg[8] published a monograph entitled simply "The thalassemia syndromes." This monograph was equally pivotal in advancing the field. It synthesized massive amounts of loosely connected reports into a coherent picture of what was then known about the globin gene system, and their abnormalities in the thalassemias. To this day, his nosology of the thalassemias remains the guide for diagnosing these illnesses. This monograph, throughout several subsequent editions, continues to be universally regarded as the "Bible" for students of thalassemia. Each succeeding edition elegantly incorporated disparate advances in the field into a coherent whole that guided further advances in their study.

Sir David's passion for studying the thalassemia syndromes was rooted in his concerns for patients around the world, many in the most socioeconomically deprived areas. He constantly pointed out to those of us in the field that thalassemia, while fascinating scientifically, is a massive public health concern in many areas of the world where access to the resources needed to provide the most advanced life-prolonging therapies is limited or nonexistent. He wrote and lectured extensively about these global health issues, pointing out that, as these economies began to emerge and develop the public health measures that prevent many of the childhood infectious diseases that previously carried these debilitated patients away, the need for basic infrastructure and resources, such as a blood supply, access to iron chelating medicines, and so forth, would present an enormous social, moral, and economic burden on the countries most affected. Subsequent events proved him right.

Sir David did not merely write and speak about these issues. He invested substantial amounts of his time throughout his career, even while holding the prestigious Regius Professorship and the Directorships of the Institute for Molecular Medicine at Oxford. He worked with collaborators in the field and at the bedside, fully engaged and enhancing patient care and onsite research. He advocated tirelessly for the provision of adequate support that could provide for the diagnostic and therapeutic resources needed for optimal care of these patients. He guided where feasible the development of clinical trials' infrastructure that made patients eligible to participate in studies of emerging therapies. His devotion to this cause was such that it eventually led to a life-altering injury. He suffered a fall in Sri Lanka that tore both of his quadriceps. The fall occurred in a temple, prompting Sir David, in keeping with his legendary wry British wit, to observe that he "should have known better than to go into a place of worship."[3]

Sir David was uncomfortable about having attention focused on him. Weatherall was so unassuming that it was sometimes possible to overlook how truly brilliant he was. At many meetings, we observed him sit quietly throughout heated debates about this or that scientific point, and then politely ask a question or make a comment that pulled all of the contending points together into a synthetic conclusion or hypothesis that was illuminating. Yet, it was inevitable that he would be repeatedly honored for his many contributions.[3,4] He was elected a Fellow of the Royal Society in 1977, knighted by the British Empire in 1987, was elected to the American Philosophical Society in 2005, and received the Lasker Award, the "American Nobel Prize," in 2010. Among many other prestigious awards and recognitions included selection as one of the few foreign members of the US National Academy of Sciences and appointment as Knight Grand Cross of the Order of the British Empire in 2017.

For those of us who knew him and were blessed to be numbered among his friends as well as colleagues, David will be most fondly remembered and missed for who he was even more than what he accomplished. He was an unassuming individual whose wit was often self-deprecatingly directed at himself, or, affectionately, at his long-time, very close friend, Professor David G. Nathan, of Harvard Medical School, Children's Hospital of Boston, and the Dana-Farber Cancer Institute. Indeed, the "two Davids" constantly exchanged affectionately barbed correspondence for decades. Nathan chided Sir David for his failure to obtain an invitation for Nathan to have tea with the Queen, while Weatherall would constantly grouse about the many times he had to cross the pond to attend fests for Nathan as he retired from one position after another. He was a wonderful house guest, being completely undemanding except for his need to "smoke me pipe." In fact, one of the few things he ever groused about in the United

States was the increasingly stringent limitation on where one could smoke at meetings, conferences, in hotels, and so forth. Indeed, the best way to have an informal chat with David during his later years was in an outdoor space near the auditorium or lecture hall, in any weather, at any temperature, where he could puff on his beloved pipe.

For his brilliant contributions as a scientist, his compassionate care and concern of many, many patients with hemoglobinopathies and other blood disorders, his uncanny ability to integrate the most advanced biological sciences, clinical medicine, epidemiology, public health, and clinical research into a coherent picture of one of the world's most common inherited disorders, for his authenticity, genuine warmth, and the integrity with which he carried out his professional and academic life, we are deeply honored as editors of this issue to dedicate it to Professor Sir David John Weatherall.

Edward J. Benz Jr, MD
Dana-Farber Cancer Institute
Dana-Farber/Harvard Cancer Center
Harvard Medical School
Room D1644a
Dana Building
450 Brookline Avenue
Boston, MA 02215, USA

E-mail address:
edward_benz@dfci.harvard.edu

REFERENCES

1. Weatherall DJ. Thalassaemia: the biography. Oxford (United Kingdom): Oxford University Press; 2010.
2. Weatherall DJ, Vella F. Thalassemia in a Gurkha family. Br Med J 1960;1:1711–3.
3. Richmond C., Sir David Weatherall obituary, The Guardian, 2018, London, UK. Available at: http://www.theguardian.com/science/2018/dec/16/sir-david-weatherall-obituary.
4. Nathan DG. A life-long quest to understand and treat genetic blood disorders. Cell 2010;143:17–20.
5. Weatherall DJ, Clegg JB, Naughton MA. Globin synthesis in thalassaemia: an in vitro study. Nature 1965;208:1061–5.
6. Neinhuis AW, Anderson WF. Isolation and translation of hemoglobin messenger RNA from thalassemia, sickle cell anemia, and normal human reticulocytes. J Clin Invest 1971;50:2460–6.
7. Benz EJ Jr, Forget BG. Defect in messenger RNA for human hemoglobin in beta thalassemia. J Clin Invest 1971;50:2755–61.
8. Weatherall DJ, Clegg JB. The thalassaemia syndromes. Oxford (United Kingdom): Oxford University Press; 1965.

Introduction to the Thalassemia Syndromes
Molecular Medicine's Index Case

Edward J. Benz Jr, MD

KEYWORDS

- Beta thalassemia • Alpha thalassemia • Molecular medicine • Globin chain synthesis
- Globin chain imbalance

KEY POINTS

- The thalassemia syndromes are inherited anemias due to deficient biosynthesis of one or more of the globin chain subunit f human hemoglobins.
- The thalassemias arise mostly from mutations in the globin gene clusters that impair the expression of specific globin gene(s).
- The clinical features of the thalassemias are due not only to deficient production of hemoglobin, but also to the imbalance in globin chain accumulation.
- The hemoglobins, the genes encoding them, and the derangement in them producing thalassemia were the first to be analyzed by the emerging tools of molecular genetics. Thalassemias are the prototype for the application of molecular genetic approaches to study human diseases.

INTRODUCTION

A proper understanding of the thalassemia syndromes must be grounded in a basic familiarity with the pathobiology of the human hemoglobins produced during embryonic, fetal, and adult life. The mutations responsible for the various forms of thalassemia affect the accumulation of these hemoglobins within the developing and circulating erythrocytes in specific ways that illuminate the phenotypic features of these forms, but only if understood in the context of that pathobiology. This article attempts to review the anatomy and physiology of normal hemoglobin production in sufficient detail to provide the necessary knowledge base for understanding the more detailed descriptions, outlined in subsequent chapters, of the various thalassemia syndromes. In addition, an introduction to the clinical features and treatment of these disorders is included. Finally, it is instructive to reflect on the ways in which the regulated expression of the globin genes and the delineation of derangements causing

Dana Farber Cancer Institute, Dana Farber/Harvard Cancer Center, Harvard Medical School, Room D 1644a, Dana Building, 450 Brookline Avenue, Boston, MA 02215, USA
E-mail address: edward_benz@dfci.harvard.edu

Hematol Oncol Clin N Am 37 (2023) 245–259
https://doi.org/10.1016/j.hoc.2022.11.001
0889-8588/23/© 2022 Elsevier Inc. All rights reserved.

hemonc.theclinics.com

various forms of thalassemia truly served as "molecular medicines index case." These disorders were the first to be dissected by molecular genetics strategies at the level of the basic processes of gene expression in differentiating human cells. This article will provide thoughts on this aspect on the central importance of thalassemia to progress in present-day precision medicine.

Relevant Features of the Human Hemoglobins

Normal human hemoglobins are complex tetrameric globular proteins (**Fig. 1**) essential for acquiring inspired oxygen in the lungs, transporting it through the circulation, and delivering it to the tissues for oxidative metabolism (Reference[1] serves as the source material for this section). They are biochemically and biophysically proteins adapted to bind oxygen at the ambient partial pressure of oxygen in the lungs, and to release it at the lower partial pressure of oxygen extant in the tissues. They are also remarkably soluble proteins in their tetrameric form. This allows them to accumulate within erythrocytes to extraordinary concentrations of 33 to 38 g of protein per 100 mL of erythrocyte cytoplasm. Because circulating hemoglobin molecules are rapidly catabolized or excreted through the kidneys, hemoglobins must be packaged within erythrocytes to survive in the bloodstream for extended periods of time. The erythrocyte's maintenance of such high concentrations of hemoglobin in soluble form throughout its 120-day lifespan is essential for providing sufficient oxygen transport capacity to sustain life. These two features of the hemoglobins: their high solubility in tetrameric form, and their reversible oxygen acquisition and release properties, are highly relevant to the pathophysiology of different forms of thalassemia.

Each hemoglobin tetramer consists of a pair of "α-like" chains and a pair of "non-α" chains (see **Fig. 1**). The tetramers consist of paired dimers. Each dimer contains an alpha-like and a non-alpha chain. Each globin monomer is a highly helical polypeptide that enfolds a single heme moiety. Heme, in turn, consists of a ferrous (Fe^{++}) iron ion complexed within a protoporphyrin IX molecule. An important feature relevant to the pathophysiology of the thalassemias is that the individual globin chains, in contrast to the high solubility of tetrameric hemoglobins, are highly or completely insoluble in physiologic fluids.

The α-like chains are ζ, produced only during embryonic life when hematopoiesis occurs in the yolk sac, and α, produced throughout the remainder of fetal and adult life (**Fig. 2**). The non-α chains are ε, produced only during embryonic life; γ, which predominates during fetal life when hematopoiesis occurs primarily in the fetal liver; β, the predominant non-α-chain produced in post-natal life, when hematopoiesis transfers almost exclusively to the bone marrow; and δ, a chain highly homologous to β, but expressed only at very low levels and only in adult life. The human hemoglobins differ from one another by their compositions of α and non-α chains **Fig. 2** lists the various human hemoglobins produced during different life stages. The predominant hemoglobin produced throughout gestation is thus fetal hemoglobin, hemoglobin F (HbF: $\alpha_2\gamma_2$), whereas Hemoglobin A (HbA: $\alpha_2\beta_2$) constitutes approximately 97% to 98% of normal adult hemoglobin. Hemoglobin A2 (HbA2: $\alpha_2\delta_2$) is a minor hemoglobin constituting 1.5% to 2.5% of adult hemoglobin.

The globin chains are encoded by two gene clusters (**Fig. 3**). The α and ζ globin genes are located on chromosome 16, and the "non-α globin genes" (β, γ, δ, and ε) are present on chromosome 11; the γ globin genes are duplicated, whereas the β and δ genes are present as single copies. Located upstream of both structural gene clusters are regions that control the expression of these gene clusters called Locus Control Regions, or "LCRs." For present purposes, the LCRs can be thought of as "master switches," which open the regions of chromatin containing the structural genes and their local controlling

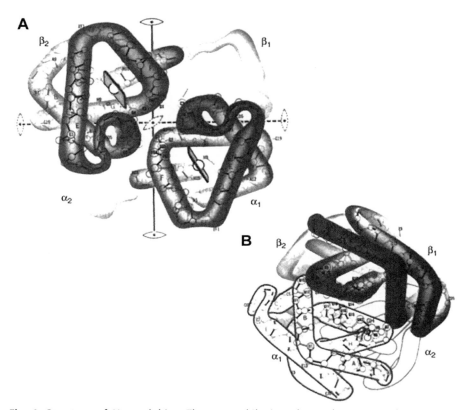

Fig. 1. Structure of Hemoglobins: The upper (*A*) view shows the contacts between the darker alpha chains and the fainter beta chains from a "front view the heme groups with a central iron atom are visible in the pocket of each alpha chain but cannot be seen in the beta chains in this view. The lower (*B*) view shows a "side view, showing additional contacts holding the tetramer together. (*From* Chapter 33, in Hoffman, R., Benz, E.J., Jr, Silberstein, L.E., Heslop, H.E., Weitz, J.I., Anastasi, J., Salama, M.E., and Abutalib, S.A., eds., Hematology: Principles and Practice, Elsevier, 7th ed. Philadelphia, PA., page 452 (Reference 1); (Figure 33.4 in original).)

sequences (enhancers, promoters, and silencers) to allow their interaction with transcription factors. These in turn promote the transcription of the appropriate globin genes at each developmental stage into messenger RNA. The discovery, characterization, and experimental manipulation of the LCR sequences has made it possible to replicate the very high rates of tightly regulated expression characteristic of the expression of the globin genes during normal erythropoiesis in experimental cell systems, animal models, and now, gene therapy platforms.

Each globin gene consists of three protein-coding sequences (exons) interrupted by two introns (**Fig. 4**). The introns are cleanly spliced out from the pre-messenger RNA post-transcriptionally; in contrast to many other genes, there are no normal alternative splicing pathways involved in the production of the globin polypeptides. However, many forms of thalassemia have been shown to arise from mutations in or near the introns that create alternative splice sites. They promote pathologic alternative splicing with consequent disruption of mRNA translation and stability, thereby leading to deficits in the production of that affected globin mRNA.

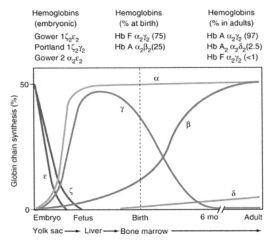

Fig. 2. Ontogeny of hemoglobin synthesis. The upper table provides the globin chain composition of each hemoglobin produced during embryonic, fetal, and adult life. The graph depicts the relative changes in biosynthesis of each globin chain as a function of time during development. The bottom line indicates the corresponding changes in the primary sites of erythropoiesis during gestation. (*From* Steinberg MH: Hemoglobinopathies and thalassemias. In Stein JH, editors: Internal medicine, ed 4, St. Louis, 1994, Mosby-Year Book, p. 852.)

The α-like globins are 141 amino acids long and the non-α, 146 amino acids long. Including the initiator methionine codon, and the terminator or "stop" ("nonsense") codon signaling the beginning and end of translation, the coding sequences of these mRNA's are thus 429 and 444 nucleotides, respectively. However, the mature messenger RNAs that is transported to the cytoplasm for translation on ribosomes are approximately 650 nucleotides in length. This is due to the presence of additional

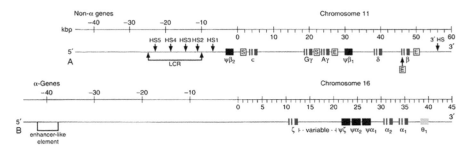

Fig. 3. Globin gene clusters: The relative positions and intergenic distances are shown, for the non-alpha genes on Chromosome 11, and the alpha-like globin genes on Chromosome 16. Each gene cluster includes primordial "pseudo genes" (ψ) that have been inactivated by mutation. The "master switch" LCR regions for the non-alpha cluster, and "enhancer-like regions" for the alpha-like cluster are also shown. The exons of the globin genes are indicated in red. E, enhancer sequences; S, silencer sequences. HS = DNA'ase "Hypersensitive Site", a sequence region indicating an "open" or "active region of chromatin. (*From*: Chapter 33, in Hoffman, R., Benz, E.J., Jr, Silberstein, L.E., Heslop, H.E., Weitz, J.I., Anastasi, J., Salama, M.E., and Abutalib, S.A., eds., Hematology: Principles and Practice, Elsevier, 7th ed. Philadelphia, PA., page 453 (Reference 1); (Figure 33.6 in original).)

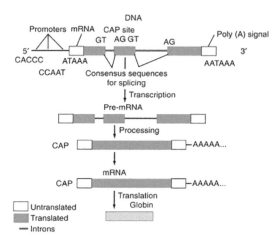

Fig. 4. Globin gene expression: See text for details. The "CAP" at the 5' end of the mRNA and the "Poly-(A) tail" at the 3' end confer stability and transportability to the cytoplasm on the mRNA. (*From* Steinberg MH: Hemoglobinopathies and thalassemias. In Stein JH, editors: Internal medicine, ed 4, St. Louis, 1994, Mosby-Year Book, p. 852.)

nucleotides at the 5' and 3' extremities of the mRNA's, called the 5' and 3' untranslated sequences (UTRs). The UTRs contain sequence motifs that influence the translational efficiency and stability of each mRNA species. As described in later chapters, mutations affecting virtually every structural component of these mRNAs, including the UTRs, have been found to produce thalassemia through a variety of mutations that derange mRNA metabolism, translation, and stability.

The "hemoglobin switches" during embryonic to fetal to adult life occur exclusively at the transcriptional level. The fetal to adult hemoglobin switch has been the most thoroughly studied, and the key steps have only recently begun to be delineated. During fetal life, as shown in **Fig. 4**, the γ globin genes are expressed at very high rates; their expression begins to decline precipitously just before birth. Conversely, β globin gene expression occurs at very low levels throughout gestation but begins to rise precipitously just before birth. This results in a switch from hemoglobin F production (composed of two α- and two γ globin chains) to hemoglobin A (composed of two α- and two β globin chains) production in the perinatal period. The switch appears to be irreversible under physiologic conditions.

Even though the switch in globin *biosynthesis* occurs largely *in utero,* the *composition* of hemoglobins in the peripheral blood switches mostly after birth because of the persistence in the circulation of HbF-containing red cells produced before the transcriptional switch occurs. This feature explains why infants inheriting severe forms of β-chain hemoglobinopathies are born healthy, protected by the residual dominance of HbF for the first few months of life. Infants inheriting α-chain hemoglobinopathies, however, are symptomatic *in utero* are and at birth because α-chain expression is required throughout fetal and adult life.

The control of the fetal hemoglobin switch depends on the interaction of DNA binding factors with sequences upstream and downstream of the various globin genes that are called enhancers. When bound to their cognate DNA-binding proteins, these enhancer sequences promote or repress the formation of transcriptional complexes on the relevant genes. The existence of these sequences had been known for decades because of patients expressing higher than normal levels of fetal hemoglobin in adult

life ("Hereditary Persistence of Fetal Hemoglobin"). They were found to have mutations within these sequence regions that enhance their interaction with positive transcription activators. More recently, as outlined in Henry Y. Lu and colleagues' article,
"Fetal Hemoglobin Regulation in Beta-Thalassemia," in this issue, the protein factor
BCL11 A was identified as a major regulator of this switch. When BCL11 A binds
particular regulatory sequences near the γ globin genes, expression is repressed. Inhibition of the binding of BCL11 A experimentally has been shown to be compatible
with high levels of the fetal hemoglobin expression during adult life in experimental animal models, and, more recently, in patients undergoing gene therapy with vectors
designed to inhibit this interaction or via genome editing approaches (see Henry Y.
Lu and colleagues' article, "Fetal Hemoglobin Regulation in Beta-Thalassemia," in
this issue). For hemoglobinopathies involving mutations in the β globin gene, this is
a promising therapeutic strategy.

THE THALASSEMIA SYNDROMES: THE CONSEQUENCES OF UNBALANCED EXPRESSION OF THE INDIVIDUAL GLOBIN GENES

For the purposes of this volume, we shall be considering only thalassemias involving
the α, β, and δ globin genes. The thalassemia syndromes are a heterogenous group of
inherited anemias characterized by reduced or absent biosynthesis of one or more
globin chains (The source material for this section can be found in References[2]
and[3]). Reduced or absent β globin synthesis causes the β thalassemias, whereas
reduced or absent α globin synthesis causes α thalassemia. There are uncommon
forms of thalassemia in which both δ and β globin synthesis or, rarely, γ, δ, and β globin
synthesis are all impaired. These are mentioned in the appropriate chapters in this
volume.

The β thalassemia syndromes: introduction and overview

The most common forms of β Thalassemia arise from mutations within or near the β
globin structural gene. Most are point mutations or short deletions or insertions that
disrupt the transcription, post-transcriptional pre-messenger RNA splicing, translatability, and/or stability of globin messenger RNA. Rare patients have also been
described who suffer from mutations elsewhere in the genome that affect the interaction of transcription factors with key regulatory sequences surrounding the β globin
genes. A detailed summary of the primary types of mutations causing the β thalassemias can be found in Nicolò Tesio and Daniel Bauer's article, "Molecular Basis and
Genetic Modifiers of Thalassemia," in this issue.

The net result of each of these mutations in individual patients is to cause a reduction (β^+ thalassemia) or total absence (β^0 thalassemia) of β globin synthesis generated
from the affected allele. Patients inheriting a β^0 thalassemia allele from each parent are
said to have β^0 thalassemia. Patients inheriting a β^+ thalassemia allele from each
parent or a β^+ thalassemia allele from one parent and β^0 thalassemia from the other
are said to have β^+ thalassemia. Heterozygous thalassemia, or β thalassemia trait, results when the individual inherits one β thalassemia allele from one parent and a
normal β globin allele from the other.

The consequences of reduced or absent β globin gene production during erythropoiesis are, first, that inadequate amounts of intact hemoglobin tetramers are formed.
This results in the production of hypochromic microcytic red cells, superficially resem-
bling iron deficiency anemia, a condition that also causes inadequate production of
hemoglobin. In contrast to iron deficiency anemia, however, the failure to produce β
globin chains results in an imbalance in the accumulation of globin subunits. During

normal erythropoiesis, the assimilation of iron and its incorporation into heme and the production of α and β globin subunits all occur in and exquisitely coordinated and balanced manner, promoting the production of large amounts of soluble hemoglobin tetramers, without accumulating insoluble precursors. In β thalassemic erythroblasts α globin synthesis continues at normal rates despite having no β globin with which to partner. The nearly completely insoluble unpaired α globin chains accumulate, aggregate, and precipitate forming intracellular inclusions. Proteolytic elements within the developing erythroblasts attempt to degrade these inclusions.

In heterozygous thalassemia, the burden of unpaired α chains is less, so that proteolysis clears these chains, and inclusion bodies rarely form. β thalassemia trait is thus marked by significant hypochromia and microcytosis, minimal anemia and, in most cases, few or no stigmata of hemolytic anemia. In moderate to severe cases of homozygous β thalassemia, the burden of unpaired α chains overwhelms the proteolytic clearance mechanisms available and inclusion bodies accumulate. These tend to be catabolized into "hemi-pyrroles" containing heme and iron. They create oxidative stress within the erythrocyte. Through a variety of biochemical mechanisms described in Rayan Bou-Fakhredin and colleagues' article, "Pathogenic Mechanisms in Thalassemia I: Ineffective Erythropoiesis & Hypercoagulability," in this issue, these inclusion bodies and their byproducts damage intracellular and plasma membranes, disrupt mitochondrial function, damage nuclear function, and provoke premature programmed erythroblast cell death (apoptosis), resulting in massive destruction of most developing erythroblasts before they are able to mature to the reticulocyte stage for release into the circulation. In symptomatic forms of β thalassemia it is this "ineffective erythropoiesis" that dominates the pathophysiology and clinical features seen in these patients. Moreover, the few red cells that do reach the circulation carry inclusions as well as severe membrane defects and thus have a shortened survival in the blood stream, adding a significant component of hemolytic anemia. Finally, of course, the cells that remain in the circulation contain little or no adult hemoglobin, thus further compromising the oxygen transport capacity available to these patients.

Patients destined to suffer from severe thalassemia are well at birth, because of the predominance of fetal hemoglobin during gestation and the first few post-natal months. After that, infants with β thalassemia become progressively anemic and develop the stigmata of hemolytic anemia including jaundice, inanition, growth retardation, and metabolic and endocrine deficiencies, described in more detail in Rayan Bou-Fakhredin and colleagues' article, "Pathogenic Mechanisms in Thalassemia I: Ineffective Erythropoiesis & Hypercoagulability"; and Rayan Bou-Fakhredin and colleagues' article, "Clinical Complications and Their Management," in this issue.

The most profound symptomatology results from the massive ineffective erythropoiesis. Severe anemia stimulates high levels of erythropoietin which in turn drives the commitment and early maturation of many erythroid progenitors (erythroid hyperplasia) in the bone marrow. However, as already mentioned, very few of these developing erythroblasts are able to survive beyond the metachromatophilic stage of erythroblast maturation. The anemia thus persists and the erythropoietic drive is sustained, causing further useless hyperproliferation of early erythroid progenitors that divert caloric resources and triggers inflammatory responses to the high rate of cell turnover.

Ineffective erythropoiesis a potentially lethal dimension to the anemia of β thalassemia that is not encountered in most other forms of hemolytic anemia. The erythropoietic drive fills marrow cavities of bones not usually used for normal hematopoiesis. That drive is often so intense that early erythroblasts sometimes invade the bony cortex and can even break through the bone setting up masses of extra-medullary hematopoiesis, potentially causing pathologic fractures. These pathologic effects on bony development and structure cause abnormal skeletal development, including facial deformities in some patients, producing a characteristic "thalassemic facies." More importantly, the massive diversion of caloric resources to the production of useless early erythroid progenitors deprives the patient of calories needed for growth and development. Untreated infants with severe thalassemia exhibit failure to thrive, growth retardation, susceptibility to infection, and many other downstream sequela. The excessive demands on the circulation in the face of inadequate oxygen transport capacity cause high-output cardiac failure. The high rates of red cell turnover and overstimulation of erythropoiesis can lead to iron overload even in the absence of transfusions because of stimulation of the hepcidin circuit (Rayan Bou-Fakhredin and colleagues' article, "Pathogenic Mechanisms in Thalassemia I: Ineffective Erythropoiesis & Hypercoagulability," in this issue). For the most severely affected patients, death is common within the first decade of life without treatment.

The situation just described represents the most extreme end of the clinical spectrum. Clinical severity of patients with homozygous or compound heterozygous β thalassemia syndromes is highly variable. Some patients have mild to moderate hemolytic anemia with minimal to moderate signs of ineffective erythropoiesis. Most patients exhibit some stigmata of all three of the clinical components producing symptomology: hyperchromic microcytic anemia, ineffective erythropoiesis, and hemolytic anemia.

As discussed in Rayan Bou-Fakhredin and colleagues' article, "Clinical Complications and Their Management"; and John Brooke Porter's article, "Iron Chelation in Thalassemia"; and Janet L. Kwiatkowski's article, "Clinical Challenges with Iron Chelation in Beta Thalassemia," in this issue, all three components of the clinical picture in moderate to severe β thalassemia can be addressed by a regular regimen of red blood cell transfusions, administered at intervals designed to maintain hemoglobin levels in the range of 9.5 to 10.5 g per deciliter This hypertransfusion approach provides survivable oxygen transport capacity, suppresses ineffective erythropoiesis, and reduces stigmata of hemolytic anemia by reducing the percentage of circulating red cells that are thalassemic. These regimens are effective, but carry with them the risks of prolonged transfusion therapy, especially transfusional hemosiderosis.

Fortunately, there are now effective iron-chelating agents available that have greatly mitigated this risk, as discussed in John Brooke Porter's article, "Iron Chelation in Thalassemia"; and Janet L. Kwiatkowski's article, "Clinical Challenges with Iron Chelation in Beta Thalassemia," in this issue. Although these regimens have significantly increased the lifespan of moderately to severely affected thalassemic patients, they are cumbersome, expensive, and widely available only in regions having reasonably sophisticated and well resources health care systems (Janet L. Kwiatkowski's article, "Clinical Challenges with Iron Chelation in Beta Thalassemia," in this issue). This is not the case in many areas of the world where these conditions are encountered the most frequently. Thus, the search continues for effective, inexpensive, and readily deliverable therapies that address the root cause of the illness, namely, the inadequate production of non-α globin chains.

A curative therapy does exist for individuals inheriting the severe forms of thalassemia: allogeneic hematopoietic stem cell transplantation (Mattia Algeri and colleagues' article, "Hematopoietic Stem Cell Transplantation in Thalassemia," in this issue). Several patients have been successfully treated in this manner. Mortality, due largely to immunosuppression and graft versus host disease, is lower than encountered with transplantation for many other indications if the procedure is done at an early age before iron overload becomes severe. One form of gene replacement therapy has recently been approved in both the United States and Europe, with promising initial results (Georgios E. Christakopoulos and colleagues' article, "Gene Therapy and Gene Editing for β Thalassemia," in this issue), and promising medical therapies targeting ineffective erythropoiesis are emerging (Rayan Bou-Fakhredin and colleagues' article, "Emerging Therapies in β-Thalassemia," in this issue). Unfortunately, lack of access to the necessary resources in the regions where the disease is most prevalent is limiting the global impact of these advances.

Henry Y. Lu and colleagues' article, "Fetal Hemoglobin Regulation in Beta-Thalassemia," in this issue discusses the role played by partial persistence of fetal hemoglobin in mitigating some of the symptomatology of β thalassemia, and the efforts inspired by these observations to manipulate therapeutically the switch from fetal to adult hemoglobin. Indeed, patients with a rare condition called hereditary persistence of fetal hemoglobin have undergone complete deletion of the β and δ globin loci, but, for complex molecular reasons, are able to produce very high levels of γ globin in adult life. They are clinically well, demonstrating that it is possible to survive an adult life solely with hemoglobin F.

The α thalassemia syndromes: introduction and overview

The most common forms of α-thalassemia arise from deletions involving 1, 2, 3, or all 4 of the α globin loci present in the diploid erythroid cell (the Source for this sectional can be found in References[2] and[3]). However, "non-deletion" forms of α-thalassemia have been described. These typically arise from point mutations in an α-globin allele that code for hemoglobins that are highly unstable because of the mutant α-chain. Examples include Hb Heraklion.[4] These hemoglobins are so highly unstable that they fail to accumulate, producing the thalassemia phenotype. There is also a highly instructive form of α-thalassemia, Hemoglobin Constant Spring,[5] that arises from a point mutation converting the normal translation stop codon at position 142 into a codon specifying the incorporation of 31 additional amino acids. As a result, ribosomes translating this α-globin mRNA "read through" the stop codon until encountering another in frame stop codon about 94 bases downstream. This elongated hemoglobin is somewhat unstable, and its α-globin mRNA is highly unstable, because the readthrough interferes with the binding of an α-globin mRNA stabilizing factor to cognate sequences in the 3' untranslated regions of the mRNA. As a result, the mutant globin mRNA is rapidly degraded, and α-globin encoded from it is produced at only 1% the normal rate regardless of the mutational mechanism involved, the net output of α-globin chains in all these non-deletion forms is only about 1% to 5% of normal.

"α-Thal-2 trait" results from the deletion or mutation of only 1 α-globin allele. It is clinically silent, and barely or not at all detectable as mild microcytosis. It is a "silent carrier type" in the sense that α-thal-2 individuals appear to be clinically normal but, when producing offspring with individuals carrying other α-thalassemia genes are at risk for transmitting more severe forms of α-thalassemia. "α-Thal-1 trait" results from the deletion or malfunctioning of 2 α-globin alleles. Individuals inheriting α-thal-1 trait are generally well, exhibiting microcytosis and no or mild anemia. Exceptions can occur in some individuals inheriting two α^{cs} constant spring alleles who also exhibit mild hemolytic anemia with some stigmata of ineffective erythropoiesis.

The two symptomatic forms of α-thalassemia are Hemoglobin H disease" and "Hemoglobin Barts with hydrops fetalis." The former results from deletion or malfunction of 3 of the 4 α-globin alleles. This results in a severe underproduction (20%–30%) of α-globin chains and consequent accumulation of unpaired β-chains. Free β-chains are insoluble, but not as highly insoluble as unpaired α-globin. Consequently, they form β_4 homotetramers, consisting only of β-chains (known as hemoglobin H or

HbH). This hemoglobin has an extremely high oxygen affinity, failing to effectively deliver oxygen to tissues so that it is a useless pigment. Moreover, it is moderately unstable in circulating red blood cells. In typical patients with hemoglobin H disease, ineffective erythropoiesis is significant, but not as pronounced as in severe β-thalassemia. A higher, though inadequate, percentage of erythroblasts survive erythropoiesis and release red cells into the circulation. HbH precipitates over time in the peripheral blood, producing inclusion bodies and a hemolytic anemia. Individuals inheriting hemoglobin H disease in which one or more alleles encode the HbCS allele or one of the highly unstable alpha chain variants tend, for incompletely understood reasons, to exhibit more severe disease with a higher degree of ineffective erythropoiesis.

Hemoglobin Barts with hydrops fetalis is the most severe form of α-thalassemia, and it occurs when all 4 of the α-globin genes are deleted or malfunctioning. Since α-globin gene expression is required *in utero*, the consequences are experienced early in gestation once the embryonic phase erythropoiesis ceases. In the absence of any α-globin chains, unpaired γ-globin accumulates. These form $γ_4$ homotetramers called Hemoglobin Barts. In addition to being moderately unstable, Hb Barts has an extremely high binding affinity for oxygen, it fails to release oxygen to the tissues. These fetuses thus suffer profound tissue hypoxia and develop cardiac failure producing hydropic edema. Most hemoglobin Barts patients die in utero. More recently, some have survived until birth by being provided with intrauterine transfusions or resuscitative red cell transfusions in the peri-natal period. A few have become transfusion independent after undergoing allogeneic bone marrow transplantation.[6]

α-thalassemias are extraordinarily common in several ethnic groups. Like β-thalassemia, they are prevalent in the Mediterranean basin, southern Asia, including India, and the Polynesian Islands. They also reach gene frequencies of 5% to 15% in individuals of African origin. However, in contrast to Asians and individuals of Mediterranean origin, African individuals rarely get hemoglobin-H disease and almost never inherit Hb Barts with hydrops fetalis. The reasons for this are genetically complex, as discussed in Ashutosh Lal and Elliott Vichinsky's article, "The Clinical Phenotypes of Alpha Thalassemia," in this issue.

The clinical features, diagnosis, and treatment of the α-thalassemias is discussed in detail in Ashutosh Lal and Elliott Vichinsky's article, "The Clinical Phenotypes of Alpha Thalassemia," in this issue. The basic approach for most symptomatic patients is similar to that for β-thalassemia, namely, management with blood transfusions where needed to sustain life, with consequent management of iron overload. Patients with hemoglobin-H disease, because they carry a burden of the unstable hemoglobin-H, must be monitored for infections, and treated promptly as well as avoiding the same kinds of exposure to oxidant food stuffs or drugs that one would use for patients with unstable hemoglobins or G6PD deficiency. Some patients have been treated with stem cell transplantation, but gene therapy agent for severe alpha thalassemia has not yet been developed.

THE THALASSEMIAS AS MOLECULAR MEDICINE'S INDEX CASE

We live in a time where it is possible to sequence whole genomes at will, and to clone, manipulate or even use as therapeutic agents to target almost any individual gene one chooses. It is routine to design, synthesize, and used therapeutically or experimentally almost any desired DNA, RNA, or amino acid sequence. Investigators can readily design monoclonal antibodies and engineered cells and organoids to suit most experimental or clinical purposes. Most of this technology is possible only because of advances made in the 1950s-70s. Before then it was not possible to isolate most individual proteins, let alone specific DNA or RNA sequences. Attempts to elucidate the basic primary, secondary, tertiary, and quaternary structures of proteins thus focused on naturally occurring situations in which a single protein predominated in a readily obtainable and isolatable state. Because of their accessibility by simple venipuncture and the fact that 95% of the protein within them was hemoglobin, it is not surprising that red cells and hemoglobin became objects for the application of each new technique to study of their properties. Moreover, these new methods could be applied readily to patients afflicted with disorders of the red cell because their blood was accessible for repeated sampling. Basic scientists from many disciplines, as well as hematologists, thus became students of the red cell and its hemoglobins. As a result hemoglobin and hemoglobinopathies were widely adopted as models for the study of life's macromolecules.

Sickle cell anemia is properly regarded as the first "molecular" disease. It can be so regarded because it was the first inherited human disorder that could be traced to a specific protein, the β-globin subunit of adult hemoglobin. The sickle (βˢ) globin chain has a mutation substituting the normal glutamic acid at position 6 with valine, thus altering its net electrostatic charge. This charge difference allowed it to be as a distinct abnormal hemoglobin variant seen only in these patients using the then-primitive techniques of protein electrophoresis. This monumental discovery, culminating with the work of Linus Pauling, Harvey Itano, and Vernon Ingram,[7] who applied emerging methods of protein sequencing to the identify the abnormal amino acid, showed, for the first time, that a human disease with a profound and protean symptomatology could result from a single amino acid change within a single protein.

Although sickle cell anemia is the first molecular disease, it is entirely correct to argue that the thalassemia syndromes represent the "prototype" or "index case" of the discipline that we now practice in many forms called "molecular medicine." The seminal contribution of Weatherall, Clegg, and Naughton[8] described in Edward J. Benz's article, "Remembering the Contributions of Professor David J. Weatherall," in this issue provided definitive proof that the thalassemias were due to defective biosynthesis of globin polypeptide chains rather than other mechanisms impeding accumulation, such as proteolysis. Because they were found to arise from defects in protein synthesis, the thalassemias were the first human diseases to be probed for abnormalities in the actual processes by which genes are expressed.

The recognition that thalassemias had in common reduced or absent globin synthesis occurred only a few years after the discovery of the existence of messenger RNA and the delineation of the basic mechanisms of mRNA translation. The thalassemias per force had to be caused by the derangements in one or more steps in the basic mechanism by which genes were expressed. They were thus the very first human diseases to be scrutinized by the emerging, now largely obsolete, technologies of an embryonic discipline called "molecular biology." Understanding the root causes of these disorders would require the ability to dissect the actual mechanisms of transcription, mRNA metabolism, and translation into globin. Conversely, identification of the defects in these processes would delineate ways in which mutations could disrupt gene expression.

Numerous experiments (see Reference[2]) performed during the mid to late-1960s attempted to identify defects in ribosomes, transfer RNAs, initiation in elongation factors, etc., that could account for specific reductions in only one globin chain while permitting full expression of the others. A fruitful byproduct of these experiments was the development of cell-free systems that could sustain protein synthesis tracked with radioactive amino acids. None of these results could account for the specificity of the defect in the biosynthesis of a single polypeptide chain in β-thalassemia or α-thalassemia. By process of elimination, therefore, attention was focused on the primary product of gene expression, messenger RNA. However, methods for isolating individual messenger RNAs did not exist at the time.

As already noted, a major advantage of studying hemoglobin is its ready accessibility by venipuncture. In patients with hemolytic anemias, a further advantage is that these patients have elevated reticulocyte counts. Reticulocytes have lost the nucleus but retain the components necessary for the translation of messenger RNA. Indeed, upwards of 5% of an erythrocyte's total hemoglobin content is synthesized during the 24 to 48-h period when reticulocytes circulate in the peripheral blood.[2] Fortuitously, even though the initial predictions of the size of globin messenger RNAs were a 50% under-estimate, its predicted size would place it considerably larger than transfer RNA, and considerably smaller than 18S and 28S ribosomal RNA. Two groups, Nienhuis and Anderson at the National Institutes of Health[9] and Benz and Forget at the Boston Children's Hospital and Harvard[10] separated total RNA preparations from reticulocytes by sucrose density gradient centrifugation and translated each fraction in cell-free lysates engineered to contain no other source of translatable mRNA. They were able to show that a predicted "9S-10S" sized RNA fraction, accounted for essentially all the ability of reticulocyte RNA to promote globin synthesis in the cell-free system. Partially purifying this fraction allowed comparison of the ability messenger RNA from normal reticulocytes to messenger RNA from thalassemic reticulocytes to stimulate globin chain synthesis. Both groups were able to show definitively that the defect in globin synthesis in thalassemic reticulocytes was due to a deficiency in the quantity or the translational capability of β-globin mRNA. These experiments also represented the first at least partial purification of a human messenger RNA molecule, and the first proof that the origins of a human disease could be discerned by direct analysis of specific mRNAs.

Subsequent experiments by documented mRNA deficiencies in multiple forms of thalassemia.[2,3] The question remained whether the messenger RNA in thalassemia was present in normal amounts but unable to be translated efficiently, or whether there were true quantitative deficiencies. As another indication that the thalassemias were molecular medicine's index case, it was possible to exploit, for the first time a recently discovered RNA-dependent DNA polymerase (reverse transcriptase) to synthesize, for the first time, specific radiolabeled DNA probes able to detect and quantitate a specific human gene in a complex mixture. These synthetic DNA copies of m RNA are known as complementary DNAs (cDNAs). Using these, Housman and colleagues[11] and Kacian and colleagues[12] were able to document unequivocally that the deficiency in mRNA in various forms of β-thalassemia were quantitative defects in the absolute amounts of the messenger RNA rather than qualitative defects in translatability (For common forms of thalassemia, the conclusion that mRNA levels were reduced, while correct, was incomplete. Later work showed that non-translatable mRNAs were catabolized, thus reducing their amount).[12]

The ability to synthesize cDNA probes against specific individual globin mRNAs allowed many investigators to take advantage of emerging technologies by which DNA fragments prepared from cDNAs or isolated directly from genomic DNA could be packaged into bacteriophage or bacterial plasmids, and isolated in pure form (cloned) from individual bacterial colonies, each expressing a specific DNA fragment by using these cDNAs.[13] The globin genes were the first genes to be purified by molecular cloning; the human globin genes were the first human genes to be isolated by molecular cloning. These advances occurred in the mid-1970s and led to many further advances. In quick succession, the entire α and β-globin gene clusters were characterized, localized to chromosomes 16 and 11, respectively, and inserted into model cell systems and even transgenic mice, where their expression could be analyzed in vivo. All these accomplishments, now routinely used to study many human diseases, were first achieved in the human globin system. Many of these efforts were motivated by the quest to analyze thalassemia mutations and their consequences on hemoglobin production.

The human globin genomic loci were also the first to be isolated and characterized and the first in which it was recognized that most eukaryotic genes do not exist as a single continuous protein coding sequence, but rather as tandem arrays of protein-coding sequences (exons) interrupted by non-coding intervening sequences or introns. These were also the first human genes in which the sequences marking the boundaries between introns and exon that served as the signals for excising the introns during post-transcriptional mRNA processing were identified. Moreover, the recognition that most eukaryotic mRNAs have UTRs at their 5′ and 3′ extremities and are elongated at their 3′ ends by a "poly (A) tail" were all documented for the first time in the globin gene system.

The rapid uptake and improvements in early methodologies of molecular biology, coupled with the huge advance of the development of the polymerase chain reaction, allowed many investigators to identify literally dozens of mutations causing thalassemia. Thus, there are now over 100 known mutations or other alterations (short deletions or insertions of nucleotides) that can cause different forms of thalassemia.

Ironically, although the defects in globin production are invariably due to significant quantitative deficiencies in the encoding mRNAs, many of the mutations responsible for the most common forms of thalassemia are not those that alter the actual transcription of the gene. Rather, some common mutations alter splicing, creating mis-spliced mRNAs, whereas others are single base changes that alter a sense codon into a "nonsense" or translation stop codon. In both cases, the ultimate failure to produce intact globin chains actually resides at the translational level. Several investigators documented that quantitative deficiencies in the messenger RNA were present even though the primary mutations were those that blocked translation.

The pioneering studies of Maquat and colleagues[14] showed that globin mRNA that cannot be translated is rapidly degraded. The intracellular mechanisms responsible for recognizing translational failure and catabolizing the defective mRNAs were first fully characterized using studies of globin messenger RNA. These processes, now named "Nonsense Mediated Decay" (NMD) are now widely recognized as essential "housecleaning" mechanisms that preempt the accumulation of pathologically misfolded or malfunctioning truncated proteins encoded by mRNAs bearing the relevant mutations. These systems exist in almost all complex organisms.

Many of the mutational mechanisms identified first in the study of thalassemia systems, such as the fusion of two genes (eg, Hb Lepore, α_2 ($\delta\beta$), a fusion of the δ and β globin genes, but now under the control of the nearly inactive δ globin gene promoter), and hemoglobin E, due to a splicing mutation that creates use of an alternative splice site about 50% of the time, so that 50% of the resulting mature RNAs are mis-spliced and non-translatable while the remaining 50% are properly spliced and encode an amino acid substitution at the site where the mutation not only alters protein coding properties but also creates and alternative splice site, and hemoglobin constant spring, mentioned above, are prototypes of these pleiomorphic mutations that create structurally abnormal proteins as well as altered patterns of gene expression. These are models for complex mutations, such as that producing the BCR-ABL fusion protein driving the proliferative phenotype of chronic myelogenous leukemia, which is due to an unequal crossover and recombination event at the whole chromosome level not unlike the one creating hemoglobin Lepore. Thus, the study of the globin genes, driven initially and for decades thereafter by the quest to characterize the molecular origins and potential treatment of the thalassemia syndromes truly led the way in bringing each successive advance in applied molecular biology to bear on the study of many human diseases. Among many examples is the fact that the first DNA-based antenatal diagnosis of a congenital disease was accomplished using molecular probes for sickle cell disease and thalassemia.

In carrying on the tradition of these pioneering advances in molecular biology, as more sophisticated genome engineering tools have been recently identified, including the discovery of CRISPR/Cas9, this has led to rapid therapeutic advances in the hemoglobin disorders, including for individuals with β-thalassemia, as discussed in Henry Y. Lu and colleagues' article, "Fetal Hemoglobin Regulation in Beta-Thalassemia," in this issue.

These selected examples make clear that breakthroughs in the study of the thalassemias that were also breakthroughs in the application of emerging technologies of molecular genetics to the study of specific human diseases. Insights into the mechanisms by which thalassemia mutations altered globin gene expression served were prototypes for the often pleomorphic effects of mutations later identified as causative of other disease states. The thalassemia syndromes thus truly are molecular medicines index case and continue to be a key target for emerging molecular approaches.

CLINICS CARE POINT

- The mainstay of therapy for patients with severe thalassemia (symptomatic anemia or significant stigmata) of hemolysis and/or ineffective erythropoiesis is regular transfusions with well-matched red cells to maintain a Hgb. level of 9 to 10.5 g/dL, combined with an iron chelation regimen.

DISCLOSURE

The author serves on the Boards of Directors of Deciphera Pharmaceuticals, Candel Therapeutics, F-Star Therapeutics, and Renovacor, and the Scientific or Clinical Advisory Boards of Autoimmunity Biologic Solutions, Kernal Therapeutics, and Riverside Partners None of these have commercial or competitive interest with the subject matter of this article.

REFERENCES

1. Steinberg MH, Benz EJ Jr, Adewoye AH, et al. Pathobiology of the Human Erythrocyte and its Hemoglobins, Chapter 33. In: Hoffman R, Benz EJ Jr, Silberstein LE, et al, editors. Hematology: Principles and practice. 7th edition. Philadelphia, PA: Elsevier; 2018. p. 447–57.
2. Benz EJ Jr, Forget BG. The Molecular Genetics of the Thalassemia syndromes. In: Brown EB, editor. Prog Hematol 1975;9:107–55.
3. Chapin J, Giardina PJ. Thalassemia syndromes, Chapter 40. In: Hoffman R, Benz EJ Jr, Silberstein LE, et al, editors. Hematology: principles and practice. 7th edition. Philadelphia: Elsevier; 2016. p. 546–70.
4. Traeger Synodinos J, Papassotiriou I, Metaxatou-Maurommati A, et al. Distinct phenotypic expression associated with a new hyper-unstable alpha globin variant

α1cd37(C2) Pro>0: Comparison to other α thalassemic hemoglobinopathies. Blood Cells Mol Dis 2000;4:276–84.

5. Clegg JB, Weatherall DJ, Milner PF. Haemoglobin constant spring: an alpha chain termination mutant? Nature 1971;5328:337–40.

6. Chan WYK, Lee PPW, Lee V, et al. Outcomes of allogeneic transplantation for hemoglobin barts hydrops fetalis syndrome in Hong Kong. Pediatr Transplant 2021; 25:e14037.

7. Ingram V. Sickle Cell Anemia: The Molecular Biology of the First "Molecular Disease". The Crucial Importance of Serendipity. Genetics 2004;167:1–7.

8. Weatherall DJ, Clegg JB, Naughton MA. Globin synthesis in Thalassaemia: an *in vitro* Study. Nature 1965;208:1061–5.

9. Neinhuis AW, Anderson WF. Isolation and Translation of Hemoglobin Messenger RNA from Thalassemia, sickle cell anemia, and normal human reticulocytes. J Clin Invest 1971;50:2460–6.

10. Benz EJ Jr, Forget BG. Defect in messenger RNA for human hemoglobin in beta thalassemia. J Clin Inves. 1971;50:2755–61.

11. Housman D, Skoultchi A, Forget BG, et al. Quantitative deficiency of chain specific globin messenger ribonucleic acids in the thalassemia syndromes. Proc Natl Acad Sci, USA 1973;70:1809–13.

12. Kacian DL, Gambino R, Dow LW, et al. Decreased globin messenger RNA in thalassemia detected by molecular hybridization. Proc Natl Acad Sci, USA 1973;70: 1886–90.

13. Steinberg MH, Forget BG, Higgs DR, et al. Disorders of human hemoglobin. 1st edition. New York: Cambridge University Press; 2000.

14. Maquat LE, Kinniburgh AJ, Rachmilewitz EA, et al. Unstable beta globin mRNA in mRNA deficient beta zero thalassemia. Cell 1981;27(3 Pt 2):543–5.

The Need for Translational Epidemiology in Beta Thalassemia Syndromes
A Thalassemia International Federation Perspective

Soteris Soteriades, PhD[a], Michael Angastiniotis, MD[b],
Dimitrios Farmakis, MD[c], Androulla Eleftheriou, PhD[b],
Aurelio Maggio, MD[d],*

KEYWORDS

- Thalassemia • Sickle cell disease • Epidemiology • Hemoglobinopathies
- Health care

INTRODUCTION

According to Lilienfeld,[1] epidemiology is the study of the distribution of a disease or a physiological condition in the human population and the factors that influence this distribution. An inherited disorder, β-thalassemia has its own distinct geographical distribution, affecting certain populations more than others. This is the result of an interaction of genetic and environmental factors with other confounding factors, such as customary consanguineous marriages, population migrations, and to a lesser extent other human interventions including a reduction in crude birth rate and programs to limit birth incidence. Such factors have influenced the prevalence of both carriers and those clinically affected globally.

The most important environmental factor that has affected thalassemia epidemiology is the protective effect of the carriers when infected by *Plasmodium falciparum*.[2,3] This selective advantage has contributed to the survival of carriers with the mutated β globin gene, allowing them to increase in numbers in areas where the malarial parasite is or was most active. This correlation has been more strongly supported where the sickle cell and alpha (α)-thalassemia genes are concerned; however, the geographical coexistence between β-thalassemia and the malaria belt seems to

[a] Laboratory of Hygiene and Epidemiology, Faculty of Medicine, University of Thessaly, Larissa, Greece; [b] Thalassaemia International Federation, Nicosia, Cyprus; [c] University of Cyprus Medical School, Nicosia, Cyprus; [d] Campus of Haematology Franco and Piera Cutino, AOR Villa Sofia-V, Cervello, Palermo, Italy
* Corresponding author.
E-mail address: md.amaggio@gmail.com

hemonc.theclinics.com

confirm the same relationship. The well-known thalassemia belt has been mapped through epidemiological studies.

It has been estimated that 5% to 7% of the world's population carries a mutated gene affecting the production or function of the hemoglobin molecule.[4] About 56,000 new individuals affected by beta thalassemia syndromes are born annually. These numbers, and country-specific figures, are based on data collected by individuals and groups who maintain databases based on literature reports, such as Modell's Hemoglobinopathologist's Almanac (www.Modell-Almanac.net) and the IthaMaps database maintained by the Ithanet project (www.ithanet.eu) ithamaps). The Thalassaemia International Federation (TIF) keeps its own database, based not only on published surveys but also on information gathered through its global network, country visits, and discussion with local experts. Their data are consisted with this estimate.

The importance of collecting data and supporting databases lies in the need for accurate epidemiological parameters, such as the number of patients needing treatment, births adding to patient numbers, deaths, the proportion of carriers in the population, and how these facts affect the development of health policies. Some of these facts are not be static but change from year to year and so must be carefully assessed and interpreted. Epidemiology is the basis of public health and policymaking. The eminent epidemiologist and ex-director of the Centre of Disease Control, William H Foege[5,6] noted that "epidemiology is no better than the information on which it is based."

Complex chronic disorders, such as β-thalassemia, require policies and strategies that provide a strong diagnostic infrastructure, day clinic transfusion services, multidisciplinary care, cost-effective treatment modalities, centers of expertise, and provision of accurate and understanding information about the personal and social implications of screening services that offer the possibility of preventing affected births.[7] In view of the economic pressures that such policies imply, providing policymakers with convincing information is a major element needed to advocate for policy changes and service improvement for the benefit of the patient. In addition, such data can enable further understanding of the social implications of disease. Epidemiological data thus provide invaluable information for the monitoring and evaluation of policies, as well as for the study of the natural history and prognosis of syndromes. In addition, this information is crucial for the accurate evaluation of the influence of high-cost innovative treatments, compared with current conventional treatments. Accurate information about this issue, especially for developing counties is indispensable if national health resources are to be directed toward the right interventions.

The collection of accurate figures (using surveys and registries) is imperative, as is their correct interpretation (using probability and other statistical methods). However, the data collected by various databases is not always of the quality that can assure accuracy or even approximation in many locations. Additionally, patient registries that are regularly updated are scarce.[8,9] Survey data are often based on small projects, which cannot be representative of the whole population. Consequently, approximations have become an accepted norm since. These approximations are often challenged as to whether they are an adequate basis on which to establish a health policy and plan adequate quality services.

EPIDEMIOLOGY-BASED PLANNING OF SERVICES

TIF is concerned with service provision because it relates to patient survival and well-being. Accurate epidemiological data must be the basis of rational planning of health-care services. Haphazard development is uneconomical and will not serve the purpose of equity of care. High-quality epidemiology therefore is required to influence policy and planning, to "translate" data into actions and interventions. It is from this that the term "translational epidemiology" is derived.[10]

Basic data resources required include the following:

- Prevalence and country distribution of hemoglobin disorders; these pieces of evidence will determine the needs for dedicated services, including blood supplies and medications, expert manpower, reference centers, and related resources.
- Carrier rate, number of at-risk couples in need of counselling and annual number of new affected births, so that planning for future expansion may be facilitated.
- Cultural information, for example, whether consanguineous marriage is a preference of the population, and the impact of these practices and how this affects birth rates of affected individuals.
- Other factors that may affect the size of the patient population such as migrations.

For the basic necessary information, only simple descriptive epidemiology is needed. However, the reliable information about the distribution of patients and carriers within a population is also needed in a micromapping exercise, in order to capture population subgroups, geographical variations, and possible changes over time in the present era of population movements. Clusters of the population may be identified toward whom services need to be directed. The evidence pointing to such clusters will determine the method of data collection.

METHODOLOGY AND SOURCES OF DATA COLLECTED BY THALASSAEMIA INTERNATIONAL FEDERATION

The main pieces of data collected by TIF through published studies, country visits, and local experts included carrier rates of the major β-thalassemia and sickle cell disease genes, consanguinity index, calculation of the expected annual births of children with major syndrome, based on the Hardy-Weinberg equilibrium, and total annual expected births based on the actual birth or calculated from the crude birth rate of each population. The total number of patients known to a region or country was also recorded.

A survey of published literature was conducted during the last decade (2009–2019), with the aim to establish the prevalence and incidence of patients with symptomatic thalassemia and of thalassemia-related genes around the world. A relate aim was to assess the quality of data reported. Three research databases were searched: PubMed, Scopus and Web of Science for studies whose methodology involved sampling and screening of the following conditions: any thalassemia syndrome, α-thalassemia trait (α+-thalassemia and α0-thalassemia), Haemoglobin H disease, Hb Barts hydrops fetalis, β-thalassemia heterozygotes, and β-thalassemia homozygotes.

A total of 6373 research articles were identified by the initial search and screened; 432 articles containing relevant information were selected. These were subjected a more thorough process of evaluation in order to compose a final list. On this basis, 116 studies from 31 countries were determined to have fulfilled the above criteria. However, about two-thirds of these studies were conducted from only 4 countries: China, India, Thailand, and Turkey. Only 3 studies were nationwide: Brazil, Malawi, and Saudi Arabia.

EPIDEMIOLOGY OF BETA THALASSEMIA
Carrier Rates

For thalassemia, relatively simple techniques, suitable for testing large numbers of individuals exist. These have been used extensively in screening programs as well as in surveys.[11]

Diagnostic methods: Extensive heterogeneity existed among the studies about the way in which carriers or cases were ascertained. For example, in the case of β-thalassemia minor, the commonest diagnostic method was measuring the levels of HbA2. However, different thresholds were applied. Although most studies used greater than 3.5%, some studies used 3.4%, 3.6%, 3.9%, or 4.0% as the cutoff point. Furthermore, some studies used the naked-eye single-tube red-cell osmotic fragility test, others used capillary electrophoresis to measure HbA2, whereas others still used high-performance liquid chromatography or reverse dot-blot hybridization.

Other studies checked for specific β-globin gene mutations using DNA sequencing. Some studies had 2 stages of screening, in which they would check the levels of HbA2 and then perform DNA sequencing on those who were positive in the first stage. This diversity of methodology is understandable since each diagnostic test has a different cost and each research team has its own amounts of funding or resources available to them. This precludes a total comparison of different studies to one another, and requires cautious interpretation of any attempted comparisons.

Sampling methods: The way population samples were selected was variable, using a variety of methodologies. The vast majority were cross-sectional (over a period of a few months) or prospective studies (lasting more than 1 year). Recurring themes included (1) screening camps in specific rural/tribal communities, (2) screening of blood donors, (3) screening of pregnant women visiting antenatal clinics, (4) screening of couples seeking premarital screening (mandatory or voluntary), (5) screening healthy subjects receiving routine health checks, (6) newborn screening, and (7) screening students in selected schools. Very few studies applied multistage clustered or stratified sampling, which would be the most reliable way to minimize the risk of bias. Furthermore, it was not always clear in some studies as to how they selected their participants and the sampling methodology was only implied or omitted completely. This means that an assessment of the risk of bias cannot be made with confidence and thus there is significant uncertainty about the external validity (generalizability) of the results.

It is important to mention that studies were excluded if they involved participants who were referred for thalassemia screening specifically because of anemia or clinical suspicion of thalassemia or known family history. Such a sample would be heavily biased and would not allow for an estimation of thalassemia prevalence that is representative of the general population.

Statistical analysis: In this recent review of the literature, the most striking finding was that only 3 studies reported 95% confidence intervals along with their point estimates. Another observation was that since most samples were nonprobabilistic, weighting could not be applied to the individual measurements. In the case of probabilistic sampling, it was not always clear if and how weighting was applied.

Micromapping: The importance of micromapping cannot be over emphasized because even in relatively small countries, the distribution of thalassemia is uneven, with some areas or tribal groups being more affected than others. This observation was recognized many years ago and has been attributed to a possible relationship with historical malaria prevalence in a specified region.[12] For a more accurate estimate of the number of carriers, the number of at-risk couples and the need for service planning, the local data for a country are good indicators of where to locate services and the size of services to meet real needs. Micromapping is an essential exercise[13] that is rarely found in practice. Examples of such efforts are given below, including those of Iran and Azerbaijan. Micromapping provides information about geographic variations and should provide more accurate prevalence data on which to base calculations concerning birth incidence and other indicators of the burden of disease.

Sample size: In the literature review, the sample size varied from 120 participants to 4.6 million. The median sample size was 1272 participants.

We have examined the data on carrier frequencies, mostly published but in some cases according to local reports, and attempted to judge accuracy. Accuracy is based on sample size and whether the sample was random and could represent the entire population.

Forty-four countries were studied with the following observations:

In 17 (38.6%), the carrier rate was based on adequate data, and in 27 (61.4%), the data were inadequate. Dividing according to region:

- In the European countries, 5 out of 12 had acceptable data but, if UK and France, which have a largely migrant carrier population, are removed, then 50% of countries have acceptable data.
- In the 15 countries of the East Mediterranean region, 10 countries had acceptable data (66.7%).
- From the 14 Asian countries only 2 based their carrier rate on acceptable data.
- In the 3 remaining countries of the African and American regions, none had accurate data.

Fifteen out of 44 countries attempted to provide regional data, in a geographical micromapping exercise. Three of the countries are too small to need micromapping (Cyprus, Brunei, and Trinidad) and thus 36.6% of countries have made this attempt.

Because carrier frequencies are the basis for calculating expected birth incidence, then the accuracy of any attempt predict annual births is in doubt. This is especially so when other parameters such geographical variations, ethnic or other population subgroups, and a changing crude birth rate are not being considered.

Consanguineous marriage is considered a significant factor in such a calculation. However, this is a changing variable in several populations. For example, in Bahrain the total consanguinity rate and the first cousin marriages rate in 1990 were 39% and 24%, respectively, whereas the rate was reduced to 11% and 7%, respectively, in 2009, denoting a 66% decline.[14] Similar changes have been described in other Arab urban populations.[15–17] Such a reduction is expected as a consequence of urbanization and social changes. Nevertheless, marriage between close relatives is still common particularly in the Middle East, where thalassemia is also common. In these populations, cousin marriage is a factor that must be considered but updated consanguinity index is required to enter the calculation.

Patient numbers

Accurate numbers of β-thalassemia patients are available exclusively when a national registry is kept and updated. With few exceptions, regular data are also obtained by health authorities from reports from treatment centers, even though this would miss patients not on blood transfusions or rarely transfused.

From information collected for the TIF database, 12 out of 44 (27.3%) of countries can state the number of patients without counting on a rough estimate. However, only 7 maintain a patient register at national level[8] and are able to publish information based on national data, the other 5 seem to gather annual information from treatment centers. Even of the 7 countries that seem to have a national registry, there is doubt if this includes all patients in the country. Moreover, any numbers reflect the patients at the year in which they were reported and fluctuations due to births and deaths and migrations are examined only over time.

In the absence of registry-based data, TIF has resorted to collecting information from collaborators, health officials, and organizations. Based on this collection, which is probably a minimal estimate, there are 486,353 patients with a beta thalasemia syndrome (TDT and NTDT) in the 44 countries that are part of this study. They are distributed, according to WHO regions as follows:

- European region: 21,270;
- East Mediterranean region: 116,118;
- South East Asia region: 316,327;
- West Pacific region: 28,438 (without counting China and Cambodia for which we have no approximation but probably 200,000 together);
- African region: 3200;
- Americas: 1000.

In addition to these countries, there is an estimate for the rest of the world, again according to official and unofficial country reports, which reaches a minimum of 29,710. The total living global patient population with beta thalassemia syndromes is 519,063 at least.

Of these patients:

- 19,530 (4%) live in very high Human Development Index (HDI) countries,
- 130,326 (26.8%) live in high HDI countries (excluding China),
- 316,086(65%) live in medium/low HDI countries (excluding Cambodia).

New affected births each year

Unless all new cases are registered, the new births are calculated from the carrier rate (with all its limited accuracy described above) based on the Hardy-Weinberg equilibrium (ref). This has to consider additional factors such as the effect of consanguineous couplings (nonrandom mating), and the interaction of hemoglobin variants with β-thalassemia trait, which may lead to symptomatic thalassemia syndromes. The most common is HbE, which in a double heterozygosity with β-thalassemia, will result in a thalassemia syndrome of variable severity. These factors are considered in all calculations. In TIF database, β-thalassemia homozygosity and HbE/thalassemia are reported both separately and as a total of beta thalassemia syndromes.

Our effort to estimate birth incidence is hampered by contradictory published information.

Some striking examples are as follows:

- *Azerbaijan:* carrier rates have variously been reported as 4% to 8.6%,[14] mean of 8.7%,[15] 3.71%,[18] and 5.4% quoted by the Modell Global Database for Congenital Disorders (https://discovery.ucl.ac.uk/1532179/27/TA05-Hb-Disorders-WHO-2017-04.xlsx)[19]. One has to choose which of these very different results is nearest to the truth. TIF has chosen the 3.71% because it is based on a very large (430,668 individuals) sample of the population, with broad coverage. It seems unselected because it is derived from a premarital screening program. If one accepts these data as the basis for calculation, the birth rate of homozygous β-thalassemia is expected to be 0.3344/1000 livebirths. If the 5.4% carrier rate is the basis of the calculation then 1.04/1000 affected births may be expected. Both results point to a need for an efficient prevention program. However, more information is needed to implement specific services. Open questions include: What is the total incidence of thalassemic births in each region? What reasons account for local fluctuations? Is awareness of the issue adequate to predict success of proposed interventions? What increase in staff and total budget will be required and over what time frame?

- *Kingdom of Saudi Arabia:* The premarital screening program reported, as of 2015, a β-thalassemia carrier rate of 1.36%, among 1,230.582 individuals tested.[20] The overall annual birth rate based on this large sample is 0.044/1000 live births, which increases to 0.1/1000 when the HbE carriers are included. Other databases[19] quote a figure of 6.7% carriers and so 1.4/1000 thalassemia births per year. In an older study from the national screening program from 488,315 individuals screened, 3.22% had thalassemia trait.[21]

The discrepancies noted in Saudi Arabia were also encountered when different authors researched similar populations. Some examples from China include the following:

- In Meizhou city (Guangdong province), there were 2 published surveys—one study of 15,229 residents identified 4.13% carriers of β-thalassemia and 0.12% carriers of HbE.[22] A second study in the same city reported a much higher rate of the carriers:11.6% (sample size 14,524).[23]
- In Baise city (Guangxi province), one study of 47,500 inhabitants indicated a carrier rate 8.72%,[24] whereas another of 12,900 reported 4.8%.[25] In yet another publication of 57,229 samples, the carrier rate was found to be 5.49%.[26]
- In Nanning (capital of Guangxi province), 5.56%[27] and 7.62%[28] were reported again in large samples.

The samples from these Chinese cities may be small compared with the whole city population but compared with sample size reported by many other countries, they are mostly in line with expected results.

DISCUSSION

In this report, we attempt to demonstrate the large variations reported even in the same populations, making epidemiology at best an approximate tool for policy making about thalassemia. Gross inequalities in health outcomes are well established. Looking at survival data and the age distribution of patients (**Table 1**) confirms what is already known. The challenge is whether the thalassemias are avoidable causes of premature death on a population wide basis through public policy interventions.

According to public health philosophy, a community faced with limited resources should prioritize spending to address health threats that affect the majority, thus safeguarding an adequate level of community well-being. This logical approach has been the basis of the investment in primary care, of aiming for "maximum health gain for the money spent,"[39] which has led to the Alma Ata declaration of 1978 by the WHO. This approach has had a positive impact on health services globally. It is the philosophy on which cost–benefit has become the motto of health planners. It has established the application of evidence-based costing as a prime guide to policymaking.

Although the comparison of cost to the benefits gained is a pragmatic approach to macro health economic thinking, the assessing benefit becomes less clear when the outcomes of service interventions are examined more closely for specific maladies. The efficient application of resources to less common illnesses, especially their prevention or early intervention, can have outsized impacts on community health, especially in regions where higher prevalence might be clustered. Congenital lethal disorders that are treatable require a different approach, if avoidance of disability and premature death are the outcomes for which services are truly aiming. The focus of health systems must also consider the individual and not just the overall benefit of the majority. Health planning must thus assess the investment in congenital diseases with a more precise mindset. In terms of the burden of disease, congenital disorders

Table 1
Survival of patients with β-thalassemia

Country	Date	Age Peak/Range	Comments	References
Turkey	2017	10–20 y	72% of patients <20 y	Aydinok Y et al,[29] 2018
Maldives	2014	13–15 y		WHO report
Sri Lanka	2019	Mean 13.2 y (SD 12.9)	Includes HbE/thalassemia and some SCD	Premawardhana AP et al,[30] 2019
Malaysia	2020	10–14 y TM 15020 Y HbE/T		Mohd Ibrahim H et al,[31] 2020
Spain	2017	Median 8.9 y (0.2–33.7)	Includes SCD	Cela E et al,[32] 2017
Taiwan	2011	Median 17.2 y (0.1–48)	58% younger than 20 y	Wu HP et al,[33] 2017
France	2019	Median 23 y		Agouti et al,[34] 2019
Iran	2018	23.8 ± 11.3 y	Combined data from 5 locations	Ansari et al,[35] 2018
Italy	2020	35–50 y Peak	68% ≥ 35 y 11% ≤ 18 y	Longo F et al,[36] 2020
Greece	2019	41–45 TM 46–55 TI (peak)		Voskaridou E et al,[38] 2019
Cyprus	2020	Mean 42.3 y Median 44 y		Telfer P et al,[37] 2019

cannot be "lumped" in the same category as more common but often less correctable maladies. For example, numbers of patients and the number of deaths each year, are used to derive measures such as years of life lost (YLLs) or disability adjusted life years (DALYs) in the Global Burden of Disease (GBD) project.[40] Accurate survival data that lead to such scaling have not yet been collected. Hemoglobin disorders are treated as causes of global DALUs only in children of the 0 to 9-year age group. Because they are not mentioned in other age groups, they are incorrectly presumed to be a low cause of death or disability. This erroneous information may provide health authorities in some settings with a reason to move on to "other priorities."

If the total number of patients and the actual number of deaths are not known because of the absence of registries, then the disease-specific YLLs can only be based on estimates of challengeable accuracy or value.

In addition, if the number of cases added each year by new affected births (because this number is calculated from the carrier rate if there are no registry data), then the annual estimates are also estimates of unknown accuracy. If the evaluation is based on a representative sample of the population, then more needs to be known about the selected sample. What is the level of care that the sample has benefited from—or not?

It is known that untreated patients with transfusion-dependent thalassemia (about 75% of the total number of patients) will die before reaching the age of 5 years. It is hoped that this situation is the experience of a diminishing minority, whereas a growing majority receive treatment that allows them to live another 20+ years on average, according to the age distribution of patients in countries where data are available. An even smaller minority of patients, living mostly in high-income countries, are now reaching the age 50 to 60 years (see **Table 1**). Yet even these have a deficit of life expectancy compared with the general population.[41] Survival is directly related to the quality of care, mainly associated with effective iron chelation. Experience has shown that in thalassemia greatly reduced mortality is attainable. For the foreseeable future, progress in this regard will only partially be related to the emergence of innovative therapies.

The greatest immediate impact on mortality and morbidity will be achieved by improving the availability and accessibility of best existing clinical practices (as defined by evidence-based guidelines), the supply of essentials (blood and chelation), and patient adherence; which in turn is related to the quality of patient support. Different levels of health care are prevalent in different countries. This variation is reflected in the age distribution of patients. For these reasons, the concept of "avoidable mortality" is an accepted measure to monitor the quality of health-care services in thalassemia, and we suggest that further research is needed to validate the measure in different geographical settings and time trends.

Based on limited data, the 2016 GBD report lists 6300 thalassemia deaths, 493.3 thousand YLL for all ages (about 8 times less than sickle cell disease for which even fewer global data are available). Premature death alone cannot reflect the overall burden of disease, which is assessed using the DALY, a time-based measure that combines YLLs due to premature mortality (YLLs) and YLLs due to time lived in states of less than full health, or years of healthy life lost due to disability (YLDs). One DALY represents the loss of the equivalent of 1 year of full health. DALYs for a specific cause are calculated as the sum of the YLLs from that cause and the YLDs for people living in states of less than good health resulting from the specific cause. What should be incorporated into the DALY summary measure has been decided by a panel of philosophers, ethicists, and economists. However, a combined disability weight is required to account for individuals with more than one condition, and thalassemia is one such condition due to the protean manifestations of the disease and the morbidity inherent in transfusion therapy that is incomplete or administered in the absence of effective iron chelation. In thalassemia, multiorgan complications accumulate over time. In addition to severe anaemia, common downstream morbidities arise from chronic hemolysis and profound ineffective erythropoiesis in severely affected individuals. Common stigmata include disfigurement, varying degrees of heart failure, infertility, and other endocrine disorders such as hypothyroidism, and diabetes, back pain, dental caries, and the need for daily medication.

To calculate a combined disability weight, the health loss associated with 2 disability weights are multiplied together, and then a weighted average of each constituent disability weight is calculated. Such complication is additive as the thalassemia patient ages and variable as to the ages at which they emerge. Because the well-treated population increases in median age, an increasing rate of complications is to be expected. For this reason, it is questionable whether "disability" burden is actually increased on a years lived basis relative to a population in which younger ages at death are more common. When the majority dies in adolescence or early adulthood, the YLD value cannot be improving even if the morbidity occurs a few years later in life.

The main point of this discussion is not to dispute the data that the GBD program has gathered. Despite recognized discrepancies, these are likely to be the best available figures. The issue is that chronic, potentially lethal conditions, where the threat of premature death is ever present, and in which over time brings new complications even in well-treated patients, the position of these disorders in the order of policy makers attention, cannot be homogenized with other noncommunicable diseases. Interventions are needed both to reduce incidence and to ensure quality care throughout the patients' lives.

A further question is whether the gross global inequalities in patient care are addressed or can be. Inequalities are to some extent linked to health policy and the selection of investments in service provision and service improvements. In low-income countries, the challenges of communicable diseases will necessarily compete for resources leaving chronic conditions a secondary concern. There are, however, several other social factors that must be considered such as community awareness and understanding of hereditary conditions, parental education, the availability of universal health coverage and the level of out of pocket expenses that must be incurred, immigrant status and above all patient lifelong adherence without which the door for organ damage becomes wide open. In rare and chronic diseases, physician unawareness or inexperience is also a factor. Finally, an accurate information on translation epidemiology, especially for a developing country, may drive national health resources toward the right direction.

CLINICS CARE POINTS

- Optimal clinical care allows thalassaemia patients to survive to the 6th decade and longer with a good qualoty of life.
- Optimal care requires resources which can only be be offered by policies and actions based on acurate epidemilogical data.
- Epidemiology will allow health planners to prioratise these chronic conditions.
- Priotitisation will reduce inequity in service provision.

REFERENCES

1. Lilienfeld AM. Lilienfeld's Foundations of Epidemiology. In: Schneider D, Lilienfeld DE, editors. 4th edition. Oxford University Press; 2015.
2. Haldane JBS. The rate of mutation of human genes. Hereditas 1949;35(S1): 267–73.
3. Weatherall DJ. Thalassaemia and malaria, revisited. Ann Trop Med Parasitol 1997;91(7):885–90.
4. Modell B, Darlison M. Global epidemiology of haemoglobin disorders and derived service indicators. Bull World Health Organ 2008;86(6):480–7.
5. IthaMaps – IthaNet, Available at: https://www.ithanet.eu. Accessed October 26, 2022. ithamaps.
6. Foege WH. Uses of epidemiology in the development of health policy. Public Health Rep 1984;99(3):233–6.
7. Taher AT, Weatherall DJ, Cappellini MD. Thalassaemia. Lancet 2018;391(10116): 155–67.
8. Farmakis D, Angastiniotis M, El Ghoul MM, et al. Thalassaemia registries: a call for action. a position statement from the Thalassaemia International Federation. Hemoglobin 2022;46(4):225–32.
9. Noori T, Ghazisaeedi M, Aliabad GM, et al. International comparison of thalassemia registries: challenges and opportunities. Acta Inform Med 2019;27(1): 58–63.
10. Windle M, Lee HD, Cherng ST, et al. From epidemiologic knowledge to improved health: a vision for translational epidemiology. Am J Epidemiol 2019;188(12): 2049–60.

11. Brancaleoni V, Di Pierro E, Motta I, et al. Laboratory diagnosis of thalassemia. Int J Lab Hematol 2016;1(38 Suppl):32–40.

12. Stamatoyannopoulos G, Fessas Ph. Thalassaemia, glucose-6-phosphate dehydrogenase deficiency, sickling and malaria endemicity in greece: a study in five areas. Br Med J 1964;1:875–9.

13. Weatherall DJ. The importance of micromapping the gene frequencies for the common inherited disorders of haemoglobin. Br J Haematol 2010;49(5):635–7.

14. Al-Arrayed S, Hamamy H. The changing profile of consanguinity rates in Bahrain, 1990-2009. J Biosoc Sci 2012;44(3):313–9.

15. Hamamy H, Jamhawi L, Al-Darawsheh J, et al. Consanguineous marriages in Jordan: why is the rate changing with time? Clin Genet 2005;67(6):511–6.

16. Aliyeva G, Asadov C, Mammadova T, et al. Molecular and geographical heterogeneity of hemoglobinopathy mutations in Azerbaijanian populations. Ann Hum Genet 2020;84(3):249–58.

17. Rustamov RSh, Gaibov NT, Akhmedova Alu, et al. Rasprostranenie nasledstvennykh gemoglobinopatiĭ v Azerbaĭdzhanie [Incidence of hereditary hemoglobinopathies in Azerbaijan]. Probl Gematol Pereliv Krovi 1981;26(9):12–6.

18. Asadov C, Aliyeva G, Mikayilzadeh A, et al. Thalasaemia preventionin Azerbaijan: what have we achieved so far. Abstract of the IXth International Eurasian Hematology Oncology Congresss. Leuk Res 2018;73S1:S1–570.

19. Available at: https://discovery.ucl.ac.uk/1532179/27/TA05-Hb-Disorders-WHO-2017-04.xlsx. TA05. Accessed November 2, 2022.

20. Alsaeed ES, Farhat GN, Assiri AM, et al. Distribution of hemoglobinopathy disorders in Saudi Arabia based on data from the premarital screening and genetic counseling program, 2011-2015. J Epidemiol Glob Health 2018;(Suppl 1):S41–7.

21. Alhamdan NA, Almazrou YY, Alswaidi FM, et al. Premarital screening for thalassemia and sickle cell disease in Saudi Arabia. Genet Med 2007;9(6):372–7.

22. Lin M, Wen YF, Wu JR, et al. Hemoglobinopathy: molecular epidemiological characteristics and health effects on Hakka people in the Meizhou region, southern China. PLoS One 2013;8(2):e55024.

23. Zhao P, Wu H, Weng R. Molecular analysis of hemoglobinopathies in a large ethnic Hakka population in southern China. Medicine (Baltimore) 2018;97(45): e13034.

24. He S, Qin Q, Yi S, et al. Prevalence and genetic analysis of α- and β-thalassemia in Baise region, a multi-ethnic region in southern China. Gene 2017;619:71–5.

25. Pan HF, Long GF, Li Q, et al. Current status of thalassemia in minority populations in Guangxi, China. Clin Genet 2007;71(5):419–26.

26. Munkongdee T, Chen P, Winichagoon P, et al. Update in Laboratory Diagnosis of Thalassemia. Front Mol Biosci 2020;7:74.

27. Chen Ping, Guangxi Key Laboratory of Thalassemia Research, Guangxi Medical University, Nanning. Presentation at the 2012 TIF Pan-Asian Conference

28. Zhang XH, Zhou YJ, Luo RG. [Thalassemia screening in 4976 pairs rural couples of child bearing age in Nanning Guangxi and follow-up of high-risk pregnant women]. Zhonghua Liu Xing Bing Xue Za Zhi 2009;30(3):311–2. Chinese.

29. Aydınok Y, Oymak Y, Atabay B, et al. A National Registry of Thalassemia in Turkey: Demographic and Disease Characteristics of Patients, Achievements, and Challenges in Prevention. Turk J Haematol 2018;35(1):12–8.

30. Premawardhana AP, Mudiyanse R, De Silva ST, et al. A nationwide survey of hospital- based thalassemia patients and standards of care and a preliminary assessment of the national prevention program in Sri Lanka. PLoS One 2019; 14(8):e0220852.

31. Mohd Ibrahim H, Muda Z, Othman IS, et al. Che Mohd Razali CH, Din ND, Abdul Latiff Z, Jamal R, Mohamad N, Mohd Ariffin H, Alias H. Observational study on the current status of thalassaemia in Malaysia: a report from the Malaysian Thalassaemia Registry. BMJ Open 2020;10(6):e037974.

32. Cela E, Bellón JM, de la Cruz M, et al. SEHOP- Hemoglobinopathies Study Group (Sociedad Española de Hematología y Oncología Pediátricas). National registry of hemoglobinopathies in Spain (REPHem). Pediatr Blood Cancer 2017;64(7). https://doi.org/10.1002/pbc.26322.

33. Wu HP, Lin CL, Chang YC, et al. Survival and complication rates in patients with thalassemia major in Taiwan. Pediatr Blood Cancer 2017;64(1):135–8.

34. Agouti I, Thuret I, Bernit E, et al. Data from the French registry for beta- thalassemia patients, *EHA Learn Cent Badens C*, 2019, 266587. Available at: https://library.ehaweb.org/eha/2019/24th/266587/catherine.badens.data.from.the.french.registry.for.beta-thalassemia.patients.html. Accessed October 2022.

35. Ansari-Moghaddam A, Adineh HA, Zareban I, et al. The survival rate of patients with beta-thalassemia major and intermedia and its trends in recent years in Iran. Epidemiol Health 2018;40:e2018048.

36. Longo F, Corrieri P, Origa R, et al. Changing patterns of thalassaemia in Italy: a WebThal perspective. Blood Transfus 2020. https://doi.org/10.2450/2020.0143-20.

37. Paul Telfer, Petros Kountouris, Soteroula Christou, Michael Hadjigavriel, Maria Sitarou, Anita Kolnagou, Marina Kleanthous. Changing causes of mortality in TDT during the era of oral chelation therapy from 2000 to 2018, *EHA Learn Cent*, 2019, 266584. Available at: https://library.ehaweb.org/eha/2019/24th/266587/catherine.badens.data.from.the.french.registry.for.beta-thalassemia.patients.html. Accessed October 2022.

38. Voskaridou E, Kattamis A, Fragodimitri C, et al. National registry of hemoglobinopathies in Greece: updated demographics, current trends in affected births, and causes of mortality. Ann Hematol 2019;98(1):55–66.

39. World Development Report 1993: Investing in Health, Available at: https://openknowledge.worldbank.org/handle/10986/5976. World bank. Accessed November 2, 2022.

40. GBD 2019 Diseases and Injuries Collaborators. Global burden of 369 diseases and injuries in 204 countries and territories, 1990-2019: a systematic analysis for the Global Burden of Disease Study 2019. Lancet 2020 Oct 17;396(10258):1204–22 [Erratum in: Lancet. 2020 Nov 14;396(10262):1562].

41. Ladis V, Chouliaras G, Berdoukas V, et al. Survival in a large cohort of Greek patients with transfusion- dependent beta thalassaemia and mortality ratios compared to the general population. Eur J Haematol 2011 Apr;86(4):332–8.

Molecular Basis and Genetic Modifiers of Thalassemia

Nicolò Tesio[a], Daniel E. Bauer, MD, PhD[b,c,d],*

KEYWORDS

- Thalassemia • Molecular genetics • Globin genes • Hemoglobin
- Hemoglobin switch • Genotype-phenotype • Genetic modifiers

KEY POINTS

- The regulated developmental and lineage-restricted expression of α-like and β-like globin genes assure the balance between α-like and β-like globin chains and the production of stage-specific hemoglobin.
- Deletional and nondeletional mutations in the α-globin genes and their regulatory elements impair α-globin synthesis and cause α-thalassemia of varying severity, according to the number of unaffected α-globin genes.
- Mutations that affect β-globin gene expression cause β-thalassemia, whose clinical presentation depends primarily on the type of causative mutation and is ameliorated by genetic factors that increase fetal hemoglobin synthesis and by the coinheritance of α-thalassemia.
- The comprehensive understanding of the molecular basis of thalassemias is key to provide accurate diagnosis through molecular analysis and enables development of cell and gene therapies for the prevention, treatment, and cure of these diseases.

INTRODUCTION

Thalassemia syndromes are recessively inherited hemoglobinopathies in which the reduced or absent synthesis of hemoglobin chains results in chronic anemia of varying severity.[1] With an estimated 1% to 5% of the global population carrying a mutation, thalassemia is one of the most common monogenic disorders worldwide. Nearly 70,000 children affected by various forms of thalassemia are born each year.[2]

During human evolution, globin gene mutations have been selected to high frequencies in malaria endemic regions, as many globin mutations in the heterozygous

[a] Department of Clinical and Biological Sciences, San Luigi Gonzaga University Hospital, University of Torino, Regione Gonzole, 10, 10043 Orbassano, Turin, Italy; [b] Division of Hematology/Oncology, Boston Children's Hospital, Boston, MA, USA; [c] Department of Pediatric Oncology, Dana-Farber Cancer Institute, Boston, MA, USA; [d] Department of Pediatrics, Harvard Stem Cell Institute, Broad Institute, Harvard Medical School, Boston, MA, USA
* Corresponding author. Division of Hematology/Oncology, Boston Children's Hospital, Karp RB 8215, 300 Longwood Avenue, Boston, MA 02115.
E-mail address: bauer@bloodgroup.tch.harvard.edu
Twitter: @nicolotesio (N.T.); @danielevanbauer (D.E.B.)

Hematol Oncol Clin N Am 37 (2023) 273–299
https://doi.org/10.1016/j.hoc.2022.12.001
0889-8588/23/© 2022 Elsevier Inc. All rights reserved.

state provide modest protection against malaria.[3] For this reason, most of the patients with thalassemia live in a tropical/subtropical belt extending from the Atlantic to Pacific Oceans, including parts of sub-Saharan Africa, the Mediterranean, the Middle East, South Asia, Southeast Asia, and East Asia. Because of population migrations, improvements in patient care, and prevention and screening programs, the epidemiology of thalassemia is dynamic, with increasing prevalence in North America and Northern Europe.[4,5]

The study of globin genes and hemoglobin has long been at the forefront of biomedical research. Globin genes were indeed the first genes to be cloned, hemoglobin was the first complex protein to have its tertiary and quaternary structure solved, and sickle cell disease was the first disease to be characterized at a molecular level.[6–9] Moreover, the β-globin gene promoter and its locus control region were among the first proximal and distal regulatory elements to be extensively characterized.[10,11] Currently, numerous gene and cell therapy approaches are being tested in β-thalassemia and sickle cell disease, demonstrating that the hemoglobin disorders remain at the vanguard of molecular medicine.

The α and β Globin Gene Loci

Human hemoglobin is a tetramer assembled of 2 homodimers of α and β globular subunits, each composed of a globin chain tightly conjugated with a prosthetic heme moiety. Human hemoglobin synthesis is directed by α and β gene clusters, which diverged about 500 million years ago.[12] The α-globin gene cluster is located around the tip of the short arm of chromosome 16 (16p13.3), in a genomic region that includes housekeeping genes that are transcriptionally active in most cells. The α-globin gene cluster consists of the embryonic ζ (HBZ) gene and the fetal/adult α_1 (HBA1) and α_2 (HBA2) genes. In addition, 2 pseudogenes ($\Psi\zeta_1$/HBZP1 and $\Psi\alpha_1$/HBAP1) and 2 genes of uncertain function (μ/HBM and θ/HBQ1) are found within the gene cluster.[13,14]

The β-globin gene cluster is located on the short arm of chromosome 11 (11p15.4) in a genomic region that is tightly condensed and transcriptionally silent in nonerythroid cells and contains the embryonic ε (HBE1), the fetal $^{G}\gamma$ (HBG2) and $^{A}\gamma$ (HBG1) and adult δ (HBD) and β (HBB) genes, and a pseudogene ($\Psi\beta$/HBBP1). Within both clusters, globin genes are arrayed 5' to 3' in the order of developmental expression, and from each of the two clusters one globin chain is synthesized in a coordinated way at high level during erythroid differentiation (**Fig. 1A**). Although segregated on different chromosomes and in different genetic environments, gene expression from these clusters is regulated to balance production of α- and β-globin chains for hemoglobin assembly.

Expression of α-globin genes is controlled by 4 enhancers located 10 to 48 kb upstream of the α-globin genes in sequences overlapping introns of the widely expressed NPRL3 gene. These cis-acting elements are highly conserved, demonstrate DNAse I hypersensitivity, and are referred as multispecies conserved sequences (MCS) R1-R4.[15] The 4 enhancers vary in their capacity to enhance α-globin expression, and MCS-R2 (previously known as HS-40) seems to be the strongest and most critical regulatory element for α gene expression.[16] Similarly, expression of β-globin genes is regulated by upstream cis-acting regulatory elements located within the β locus control region (β-LCR). The β-LCR acts as the major enhancer of the β globin locus and is responsible for the lineage-specific expression of β-globin genes. It is composed of 5 DNAse I hypersensitivity sites located 6 to 20 kb upstream of the β-globin genes.[17,18] During erythroid differentiation, erythroid transcription factors bind to these enhancer sites and form transcriptional complexes,

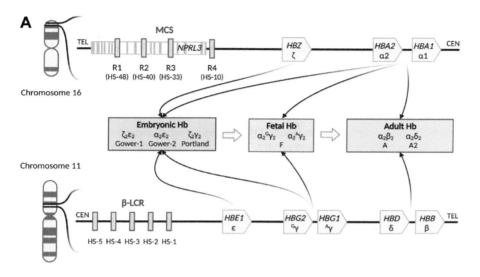

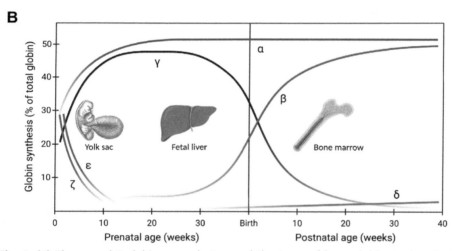

Fig. 1. (*A*) The α- and β-globin gene clusters and the types of hemoglobin produced at different developmental stages. For simplicity, pseudogenes are not shown, and the β-globin gene cluster is shown in reverse orientation with respect to conventional genomic coordinates. Regulatory elements are shown in orange and globin genes in blue, with resultant hemoglobin tetramers shown in boxes. (*B*) Developmental stage–specific globin gene expression and site of erythropoiesis. (Created with BioRender.com.)

which promote interactions with the promoters of the downstream gene clusters, driving their lineage and developmental stage appropriate expression.[19–25]

Hemoglobin Production During Development

Throughout human development, the sites of erythropoiesis change along with the types of hemoglobin produced (**Fig. 1**B). During embryonic development following gastrulation, primitive erythroid cells are first transiently produced within blood islands of the yolk sac. At this early embryonic stage, hemoglobins Gower-I ($\zeta_2\varepsilon_2$), Gower-II

($\alpha_2\epsilon_2$), and Portland ($\zeta_2\gamma_2$) are produced. Midway through the first trimester of gestation, definitive hematopoietic stem cells (HSCs) emerge from the ventral wall of the dorsal aorta and populate the fetal liver, which represents the main site of hematopoiesis during fetal life. This transition coincides with the switch to the production of fetal hemoglobin (HbF, $\alpha_2\gamma_2$). Finally, around the perinatal period, HSCs migrate to the bone marrow, where in physiologic conditions hematopoiesis will take place for the rest of life, and adult hemoglobin A (HbA, $\alpha_2\beta_2$) and A2 (HbA2, $\alpha_2\delta_2$) start to be produced in place of HbF.[26]

Hemoglobin switching is the result of tightly regulated changes in transcription programs taking place during development. The β-globin gene cluster represents a paradigm for tissue- and developmental stage–specific gene regulation.

Fetal-to-Adult Hemoglobin Switch

The understanding of hemoglobin switching has important clinical and therapeutic implications. Genetic, biochemical, and clinical observations suggest a beneficial role for HbF in the major β-globin disorders β-thalassemia and sickle cell disease. Partially reversing the γ- to β-globin switch is a major therapeutic strategy for both diseases.[27] Although the detailed mechanisms of the fetal to adult hemoglobin switch are still being investigated, a broad model has emerged centered on several major transcription factors and chromatin complexes that orchestrate developmental gene regulation at the β-globin gene cluster (**Fig. 2**). GWAS studies identified 3 loci associated with HbF level and β-globin disorder severity across various ancestral backgrounds: the β-globin cluster on chromosome 11, the *HBS1L-MYB* intergenic interval on chromosome 6, and *BCL11A* on chromosome 2.[28–30]

The B-cell lymphoma/leukemia 11A (BCL11A) DNA-binding protein is a major repressor of γ-globin. In erythroid precursors, BCL11A is found within multiprotein transcriptional complexes, which include numerous erythroid transcription factors (such as GATA1 and TAL1) but also chromatin regulators (such as the nucleosome remodeling and deacetylase [NuRD] complex) and additional transcriptional corepressors.[31] BCL11A binds and recruits NuRD to the γ-globin promoters and favors interactions between the β-LCR and the β-promoter at the expense of the γ-promoters.[32–35] Common genetic variants associated with HbF level at the *BCL11A* locus overlap enhancers necessary and sufficient for *BCL11A* expression specifically in adult erythroid precursors.[36] Rare haploinsufficiency of *BCL11A* is associated with hereditary persistence fetal hemoglobin (HPFH), albeit also with impaired neurodevelopment.[37]

In the fetal stage, the evolutionarily conserved repressor HIC2 binds to erythroid *BCL11A* enhancers to reduce chromatin accessibility and binding of transcription factor GATA1, suppressing BCL11A expression.[38] In addition, in the fetal stage, activators such as GATA1 and NF-Y bind and activate expression of the γ-globin genes.[35,39]

The transcription factor ZBTB7A, otherwise known as leukemia/lymphoma-related factor (LRF), also plays a role in γ-globin gene silencing through the BCL11A-independent recruitment of the NuRD complex to the γ-globin promoters.[34,40] Both BCL11A and ZBTB7A interact with components of the NuRD complex, which has a critical role in restraining globin gene transcription and may represent a common pathway through which γ-globin silencers act.[41–43] Moreover, the DNA-binding transcription factor ZNF410 represses HbF indirectly through activating the expression of *CHD4*, which encodes a key component of the NuRD complex.[44,45] The erythroid transcription factor Kruppel-like factor 1 (KLF1) is involved in globin switching by specifically interacting with the β-promoter as well as by activating the expression of BCL11A.[46–49] The hematopoietic transcription factor MYB indirectly represses γ-

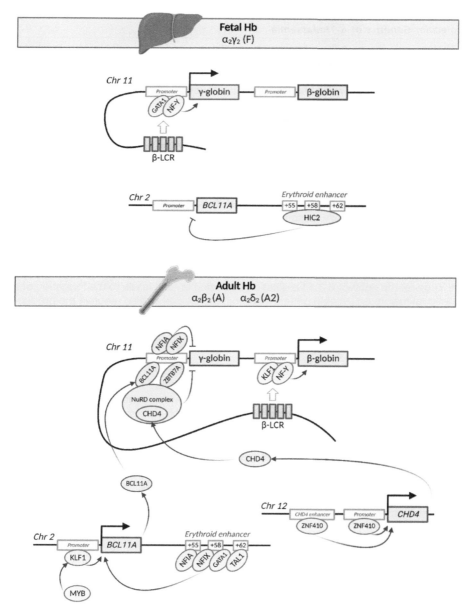

Fig. 2. Molecular machinery involved in fetal-to-adult hemoglobin switch. Displayed are some of the transcription factors, chromatin complexes, and loci involved in developmental regulation of the β-globin gene cluster. (Created with BioRender.com.)

globin gene transcription by activating KLF1.[50–52] Furthermore, the transcription factors NFIA and NFIX function cooperatively to repress γ-globin by stimulating the expression of BCL11A and directly repressing γ-globin gene expression.[53] Notably, all these factors function within large multiprotein complexes with chromatin-modifying activity able to influence the epigenetic state of the globin cluster.[25]

α-THALASSEMIA
Molecular Genetics of α-Thalassemia

α-Thalassemia is a hereditary hemoglobinopathy caused by genetic lesions involving the α-globin genes that impair α-globin synthesis.[54] More than 120 disease-causing mutations have been described (**Table 1**; for a comprehensive list see http://globin.cse.psu.edu/or https://www.ithanet.eu/db/ithagenes).

The predominant types of α-thalassemia mutations are deletions of variable length. α-globin genes are duplicated (α_1 and α_2) and localized into 2 highly homologous units on chromosome 16. Unequal crossing over between these units during meiosis is likely to be the underlying mechanism of gene deletion and triplication. Deletions are classified as α^+ deletions (-α/or α-/), which remove only one α-globin gene, and α^0 deletions (–/), which remove both α-globin genes. α^0 deletions completely abolish α-globin expression from a single chromosome.[55,56] In physiologic conditions, two-thirds of the α-globin synthesis comes from the α_2 gene, so mutations that affect the α_2 gene are typically associated with a more severe reduction of α-globin synthesis.

The most common α^+-thalassemia deletions are $-\alpha^{3.7}$ and $-\alpha^{4.2}$ that result from unequal crossing-over due to recombination between misaligned highly homologous regions (Z or X boxes). Although the leftward 4.2 kb deletion causing $-\alpha^{4.2}$ only involves the α_2 gene, the rightward 3.7 kb deletion occurring in $-\alpha^{3.7}$ leads to the formation of a functional fusion $\alpha_2\alpha_1$-globin gene. Recombinational events also result in the production of chromosomes containing 3 α-globin genes.[55] Particular deletions may be concentrated within specific ancestral populations, with the single gene deletion $-\alpha^{3.7}$ being especially frequent in Africa, whereas α^0 deletions such as $-^{SEA}$ are most common in Southeast Asia.[54]

Rarely, α-thalassemia can be caused by deletions involving the upstream enhancer elements ([αα]^T) and not α-globin genes. Although variable in length and embracing different combinations of enhancer elements, all such deletions seem to include the critical MCS-R2 enhancer. Enhancer deletions profoundly reduce expression of both α-globin genes in cis, but usually do not completely abolish it, resulting in milder phenotypes.[57–60]

Nondeletional mutations causing α-thalassemia are rarer and include both point mutations and oligonucleotide deletions/insertions (indels) ($\alpha^T\alpha$/or $\alpha\alpha^T$/), which affect different stages of gene expression, such as mRNA transcription, mRNA processing,

Table 1
Molecular genetics of α-thalassemia

Type of Mutation	Genotype	Examples (Including Relative Geographic Concentration)
Deletions		
Restricted to a single α-globin gene	-α or α- (α^+)	$-\alpha^{3.7}$ (Africa), $-\alpha^{4.2}$
Involving both α-globin genes	– (α^0)	$-^{SEA}$ (Southeast Asia), $-^{MED}$ (Mediterranean), ATR16 syndrome
Involving upstream regulatory elements (MCS-R2)	[αα]^T	(αα)^{RA}
Nondeletional mutations	$\alpha^T\alpha$ (α_2) or $\alpha\alpha^T$ (α_1)	Hb Constant Spring (Southeast Asia), $\alpha^{IVS1(5nt)}\alpha$ (Mediterranean)
Trans-acting mutations	[αα]^T	ATRX syndrome

mRNA translation, and protein stability.[61] Although these mutations are usually confined to a single α-globin gene, the magnitude of α-globin reduction in nondeletional $α^+$-thalassemia is often greater than in deletional $α^+$-thalassemia.[61] This effect may be partially explained by lack of compensatory increase of expression of the remaining functional gene when one gene is inactivated by a nondeletional mutation or by the high instability of some mutated α-globin variants.[62] The most common nondeletional α-thalassemia variant is Hb Constant Spring, which results from a single base substitution at the stop codon of the $α_2$-globin gene leading to the production of an abnormally long α chain, with 31 terminal amino acids in excess. Because of the disruption of the 3'-untranslated region of normal alpha globin mRNA, which is critical for mRNA stability, only 1% to 5% of the normal $α_2$-globin output is produced. Moreover, the elongated α-globin polypeptide ($α^{CS}$) is unstable and causes a significant reduction of erythrocyte lifespan.[63–65]

In rare instances, α-thalassemia can be caused by trans-acting mutations in genes outside the α-globin cluster. Mutations in the *ATRX* gene located on chromosome X cause α-thalassemia in association with neurodevelopmental delay, facial dysmorphisms, and genital abnormalities in men (ATRX syndrome).[66] The specificity of the chromatin remodeling protein ATRX for α-globin gene regulation is not completely understood but may relate to its G4 quadruplex forming sequence binding function.[67,68] Another syndromic presentation of α-thalassemia associated with intellectual disability, neurodevelopmental delay, and variable nonspecific dysmorphisms may arise from large deletions in 16p13.3, removing the α-globin genes plus additional adjacent genes (ATR16 syndrome).[69,70]

Genotype-Phenotype Correlation of α-Thalassemia

The number of functional α-globin genes is the main determinant of the clinical severity of α-thalassemia (**Fig. 3**).[54] Normal individuals carry 4 α-globin genes (αα/αα). Silent carriers of α-thalassemia have 3 functional α-globin genes and manifest with very mild hematological changes.

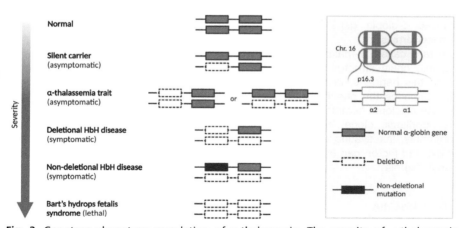

Fig. 3. Genotype-phenotype correlation of α-thalassemia. The severity of α-thalassemia widely ranges from the silent carrier with a single gene deletion, α-thalassemia trait with 2 genes deleted in trans (*left*) or in cis (*right*), 3 genes deleted (deletional HbH disease), and 2 genes deleted plus 1 nondeletional mutation (nondeletional HbH disease), up to the most severe form with all 4 genes deleted (Bart's hydrops fetalis syndrome). (Created with BioRender.com.)

Carrying 2 functional α-globin genes ($-/\alpha\alpha$ or $-\alpha/-\alpha$) results in asymptomatic microcytic hypochromic anemia and is referred to as the α-thalassemia trait. Although clinically mild, molecular diagnosis may be relevant when considering a differential diagnosis for iron deficiency or β-thalassemia trait and in the context of reproductive counseling, where heterozygous α^0-thalassemia ($-/\alpha\alpha$) has much greater risk of severely affected reproductive outcomes as compared with homozygous α^+-thalassemia ($-\alpha/-\alpha$).

The inheritance of a single functional α-globin gene causes hemoglobin H disease ($-/-\alpha$). Hemoglobin H (HbH) is produced when excess β chains form β_4 tetramers characterized by very high oxygen affinity and instability. HbH disease is often a disorder of intermediate severity, which manifests clinically as nontransfusion-dependent thalassemia, with moderate anemia and splenomegaly demanding infrequent intermittent transfusions. However, more severe phenotypes may sometimes be observed, including patients requiring regular blood transfusions and iron chelation.[71] HbH disease tends to be especially severe when caused by nondeletional α-globin mutations together with α^0-thalassemia deletions ($\alpha\alpha^T/-$) such as hemoglobin H-Constant Spring disease.[72]

The complete absence of functional α-globin genes ($-/-$) results in Bart's hydrops fetalis syndrome (BHFS), which is usually lethal in utero or soon after birth due to severe hypoxia.[54] Most prevalent in Southeast Asia, BHFS cases have been increasingly observed in Europe and North America due to the changing epidemiology of thalassemias.[2] The clinical features of BHFS are intrauterine anemia, marked hepatosplenomegaly, cardiovascular deformities associated with signs of cardiac failure, skeletal deformities, retardation in brain growth, and edema. Advancements in fetal medicine and neonatal care have enabled the survival of a limited number of affected children who require lifelong blood transfusions and often have associated congenital abnormalities, such as urogenital defects, limb deformities, and atrial septal defects, and present with somatic and neurodevelopmental delay.[72,73] In the context of BHFS, embryonic globins may represent a diagnostic, predictive, and therapeutic opportunity.[75] When deletions leave the ζ-globin gene intact, a low level of ζ-globin gene expression is maintained, and the small amount of functional Hb Portland ($\zeta_2\gamma_2$) produced allows the fetus to survive up to the second or third trimester.[74] Moreover, reactivation of the silenced ζ-globin gene could represent a treatment strategy for the various α-thalassemias.[76,77]

In rare cases, α-thalassemia mutations can be inherited in heterozygosity with α-globin chain structural variants, such as the Hb G Philadelphia ($\alpha68$Asn-Lys). When this happens, increased incorporation of the variant chains to hemoglobin may influence the phenotype.[78] Acquired α-thalassemia can develop as a consequence of clonal hematological disorders, such as myelodysplastic syndrome.[79] In the neoplastic clone, acquired deletion of the α-globin gene cluster or, more commonly, inactivating mutations of *ATRX*, encoding the trans-acting chromatin-associated factor, can downregulate α-globin gene expression and lead to acquired α-thalassemia.

β-THALASSEMIA
Molecular Genetics of β-Thalassemia

β-thalassemia is caused by mutations that affect the production of the β-globin chains.[80] More than 400 causative mutations have been described (**Table 2**; for a comprehensive list see http://globin.cse.psu.edu/or https://www.ithanet.eu/db/ithagenes). In contrast to α-thalassemia, which is primarily caused by longer deletions, most of the β-thalassemia causing variants are short mutations, including mainly

Table 2
Molecular genetics of β-thalassemia

Type of Mutation	Phenotype	Examples (Including Relative Geographic Concentration)
Point Mutations		
Transcriptional mutations		
Promoter regulatory elements	β^+ or β^{++}	−101 (C > T) (Mediterranean)
5′ UTR	β^+ or β^{++}	CAP +22 (G > A) (Mediterranean)
Mutations affecting RNA processing		
Splice junction	β^0	IVS1-1 (G > T) (Asia)
Consensus splice sites	β^0 or β^+	IVS1-5 (G>C) (Asia)
Cryptic splice sites	β^0 or β^+	IVS1-116 (T>G) (Mediterranean), IVS1-110 (G>A) (Mediterranean), CD26 (GAG>AAG) (HbE) (Southeast Asia)
RNA cleavage—Poly A signal	β^+ or β^{++}	AATAAA > AATGAA (Mediterranean)
3′ UTR	β^{++}	Term CD 16, C > G (Greece)
Mutations affecting RNA translation		
Initiation codon	β^0	ATG > ATA (Italy)
Nonsense codons	β^0	CD39 (CAG > TAG) (Mediterranean)
Frameshift	β^0	CD41/42 (-TTCT) (Asia)
Deletions		
Restricted to β-globin gene	β^0	−619 bp deletion (Asia)
Extending to other globin genes and/or involving the β-LCR	β^0	$\delta\beta$-thalassemia, $\gamma\delta\beta$-thalassemia, $\varepsilon\gamma\delta\beta$-thalassemia
Trans-acting mutations identified in *TFIIH, GATA1, KLF1, SUPT5H*		

single nucleotide substitutions and some indels leading to frameshift. Any stage of gene expression from gene transcription, through mRNA processing, to mRNA translation and protein stability can be affected by mutations causing β-thalassemia.[81] Mutations are broadly categorized according to the residual β-globin chain production. Mutations are described as β^{++} (silent) or β^+ when they cause respectively mild or moderate-to-severe reduction in β-globin chain synthesis and β^0 when they lead to its complete absence. β^{++} or β^+ mutations involve the β-globin gene promoter (CACCC or TATA box), the polyadenylation signal, and the 5' and 3' untranslated regions or compromise RNA splicing. β^0 mutations include initiation codon mutations, nonsense mutations, frameshifts, and mutations involving essential RNA splicing and processing elements.[82] Mutations of the β-globin gene promoter tend to manifest with higher HbF levels with respect to other β-thalassemia mutations, presumably due to a shift in the competition between the β-globin and γ-globin promoters for interactions with the β-LCR regulatory elements.[83,84]

The prevalence of variants differs by region. For example, IVS1-110 (G>A) and CD39 (CAG>TAG) are common mutations in the Mediterranean and Middle East, CD41/42 (-TTCT) and IVSII-654 (C>T) common in Southeast and East Asia, and IVS1-5 (G>C) common in South Asia.[85] The CD26 (GAG>AAG) mutation, which is common throughout Asia, especially Southeast Asia, results in the activation of a cryptic splicing site, which results both in the reduced production of a translatable β^E-globin mRNA and the synthesis of a structurally abnormal β^E-globin chain, which pairs with α chains to form hemoglobin E (HbE, $\alpha_2\beta^E_2$).[86,87]

Deletions involving the β-globin gene and sometimes extending to the δ-, γ-, and ε-globin genes may less frequently cause β-thalassemia (**Fig. 4**A). A 619 bp deletion that removes the 3' end of the β-globin gene is common in India and responsible for about 30% of thalassemia cases in this population.[82,88] Larger deletions involving part of the β-globin gene cluster sparing γ-globin genes may result in HPFH or δβ-thalassemia and are associated with increased production of γ-globin. γδβ-thalassemias occur when deletions include the γ-globin genes. Sporadically, deletion of the entire β-globin gene cluster or the upstream β-LCR produces εγδβ-thalassemia.[89–91] Deletions that abrogate embryonic (ε) and fetal (γ) β-like globin chains production have only been observed in the heterozygous state, likely because homozygous deletions are lethal in early gestation.[82] In heterozygosity, these conditions manifest clinically with self-limited neonatal anemia and hemolysis of variable severity, which sometimes requires blood transfusions and evolve in adults into the hematological phenotype of thalassemia trait with normal levels of HbA2 and HbF.[90]

In addition to deletions, unequal crossing over and recombination due to misalignment of homologous chromosomes during meiosis can produce rare forms of fusion globin genes, resulting in peculiar forms of thalassemia. Hb Lepore is the result of an in-frame fusion between the 5' end of the δ-globin gene and the 3' end of the β-globin gene. The fused δβ-globin seems to form stable and functional hemoglobin ($\alpha_2[\delta\beta]_2$) called Hb Lepore.[92] However, as the expression of the abnormal

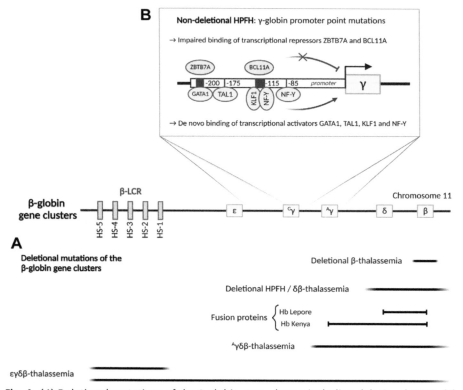

Fig. 4. (*A*) Deletional mutations of the β-globin gene cluster, including deletional HPFH. (*B*) Nondeletional HPFH caused by single point mutations at the level of promoters of γ-globin genes. (Created with BioRender.com.)

δβ-globin is under the control of the δ-globin promoter, which is only 2% to 3% as active as the β-globin promoter, there is severe underproduction of this globin chain manifesting as thalassemia of moderate-to-high severity in homozygotes. On the contrary, the fused βδ-globin chain, which pairs with α-globin to form Hb anti-Lepore, is under the control of the β-globin promoter and produced at much higher levels.[93]

Although β-thalassemia is normally inherited as a recessive disease, rarely it can be dominantly inherited. Some β-globin chain variants, although synthesized in normal amounts, display high instability and are unable to form stable and functional hemoglobin tetramers. These mutations display a dominant negative effect and result in the phenotype of β-thalassemia even when present as a single copy.[94] Dominant β-thalassemia mutations are mostly found in the third and second exons of the β-globin gene.[95]

In rare cases, β-thalassemia is caused by mutations which lie outside the β-globin gene cluster. Mutations in the general transcription factor gene *TFIIH* can result in β-thalassemia in association with xeroderma pigmentosum and trichothiodystrophy.[96] Moreover, mutations in the erythroid transcription factor genes *GATA1* and *KLF1* can dysregulate globin gene expression and give rise to a β-thalassemia phenotype.[97,98] More recently, variants in the gene *SUPT5H*, involved in the regulation of mRNA processing and transcription by RNA polymerase II, have also been associated with a β-thalassemia phenotype.[99] Somatic deletions of chromosome 11p15 involving the β-globin gene in a subpopulation of erythroid cells have been reported as a rare cause of β-thalassemia when co-occurring in individuals constitutionally heterozygous for a β-thalassemia mutation.[100,101] Moreover, uniparental isodisomy of a portion of chromosome 11p in β-thalassemia carriers has been described as a cause of β-thalassemia major.[102] Rarely, acquired somatic β-globin cluster deletions may be associated with myelodysplastic syndromes.[103]

Genotype-Phenotype Correlation of β-Thalassemia

In erythroid cells, the deficient production of β-globin chains leads to an imbalance between α-globin and β-globin chains. Unpaired α-globin chains accumulate, bind to heme, and form highly insoluble aggregates, called hemichromes, which precipitate, bind, or intercalate the plasma membrane, and promote the generation of cytotoxic reactive oxidant species.[104] These events hamper the maturation and viability of red blood cell precursors, causing ineffective erythropoiesis, and lead to premature hemolysis of circulating red cells, along with compensatory hematopoietic expansion.[105] Based on the clinical presentation, β-thalassemia is traditionally categorized as minor, intermedia, or major. Patients with β-thalassemia minor (also called β-thalassemia trait) have only one mutated allele and typically present with very mild microcytic hypochromic anemia. Patients with β-thalassemia major are homozygous or compound heterozygous for severe β-globin gene mutations (β^0/β^+ or β^0/β^0) and present with severe anemia in infancy, which requires lifelong transfusion therapy. Between these 2 extremes, β-thalassemia intermedia collects a group of genetically and phenotypically heterogeneous conditions that manifest later in life with mild-to-moderate anemia and variable transfusion requirement.[80] The decision to initiate transfusions in β-thalassemia intermedia may be influenced by clinical factors as well as patient and provider preferences and resource availability for regular access to a safe blood supply, iron chelation, and associated monitoring. Another classification scheme distinguishes transfusion-dependent thalassemia (TDT) from nontransfusion-dependent thalassemia (NTDT), which acknowledges that the regularity of transfusions might change over time.

The type of β-globin gene mutation is the primary determinant of β-thalassemia clinical severity. However, the remarkable clinical heterogeneity depends on several modifiers that modulate the degree of globin chain imbalance and thus the extent of ineffective erythropoiesis (**Fig. 5**).[106,107] Conditions that improve the α- to β-globin balance, either by decreasing the production of α-globin or by increasing that of β-like globins, namely γ-globin, ameliorate the clinical severity of β-thalassemia. Co-inheritance of α-thalassemia trait (-α/αα, −/αα, -α/-α) has been demonstrated to ameliorate the clinical manifestations of β-thalassemia and in some cases to abolish the need for lifelong transfusions in thalassemia major patients. On the contrary, an excess of α-globin genes (ααα/αα, ααα/ααα, αααα/αα) aggravates the phenotype.[108,109] Genetic modifiers that increase γ-globin chain production protect from the deleterious effect of excess α-globin and improve clinical manifestations. In a spectrum of disorders, which include HPFH and δβ-thalassemia, expression of γ-globin and HbF persist at high levels in adult erythroid cells. Although δβ-thalassemia is characterized by microcytosis and heterocellular HbF, HPFH is a benign condition that manifests with higher pancellular HbF and morphologically normal erythrocytes. Although the 2 conditions were originally differentiated based on hematological and clinical features, it is now evident that there is considerable overlap between the 2 conditions.[91] Both HPFH and δβ-thalassemia are usually caused by deletions of different sizes involving the β-globin gene cluster that dysregulate the repression of γ-globin expression.[89,91] Deletions are thought to cause incomplete suppression of fetal γ-globin gene activity postnatally by removing silencer elements, juxtaposing downstream enhancer elements to the γ-globin gene promoter, and relieving competition between the γ- and β-globin gene promoters for interaction with the β-LCR.[84] Less frequently, HPFH is due to single-base substitutions or small deletions in γ-globin gene promoters that impair binding of repressing factors, such as BCL11A and ZBTB7A, or introduce binding sites for activators, such as GATA1, TAL1, KLF1, and NF-Y (**Fig. 4**B).[34,39,110–115] Another condition associated with biochemical and clinical features of HPFH is Hb Kenya, which arises from unequal crossover and recombination between the 5' end of the Aγ-globin gene and the 3' end of the β-globin gene. The deletion of silencing elements located between the γ and δ genes and the closer apposition of a strong globin enhancer located at the 3' site of the β gene drive the high expression of Gγ- and the fusion Aγ-β-globin genes

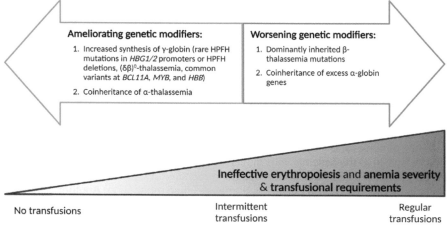

Fig. 5. Genetic modifiers of β-thalassemia. (Created with BioRender.com.)

and thus high level of HbF synthesis.[116,117] The observation that even modest elevations of HbF in adults can ameliorate the clinical course of inherited β-haemoglobinopathies has prompted effort in understanding the HbF to adult hemoglobin switch for the development of novel curative strategies. As previously described, common genetic variants at regulatory elements of *BCL11A* and *MYB* as well as variants at the β-globin gene cluster itself are associated with both HbF level and clinical severity of β-thalassemia.[40,47,51] Although the main modifiers of β-thalassemia phenotype are known, yet undescribed genetic modifiers might exist. Indeed, cases of asymptomatic homozygous β-thalassemia are documented.[118]

Other Genetic Modifiers that Influence Thalassemia Clinical Course

Factors involved in bilirubin metabolism, iron metabolism, bone diseases, and cardiac diseases, although not affecting the primary disease pathophysiology, can influence secondary manifestations of the disease and response to therapies. *UGT1A1* polymorphisms predispose to jaundice and the development of gallstones, common complications of thalassemia.[119] Moreover, some polymorphisms of genes involved in iron metabolism, such as the common *HFE* H63D variant, are known to predispose to iron overload.[120] Finally, genetic predisposition to osteoporosis and cardiac diseases can further affect the development of secondary complications.[107] Conversely, red blood cell traits themselves may act as disease modifiers. For instance, the β-thalassemia carrier state seems to confer cardiovascular protection through a favorable lipidic, blood pressure, and inflammatory profile and, in the future, might contribute to polygenic risk scores for common diseases.[121–123]

Co-inheritance of thalassemia with structural hemoglobin variants

Co-inheritance of thalassemia mutations with hemoglobin variants, characterized by structural and biochemical alterations that variably affect physiologic function, further complicates the molecular landscape of thalassemia syndromes and gives rise to complex clinical phenotypes. Hemoglobin S (HbS) is a common hemoglobin variant that results from a single point mutation of the β-globin gene (p. Glu6Val), which produces a hemoglobin tetramer ($\alpha_2\beta^S_2$) that is poorly soluble and tends to polymerize when deoxygenated, giving rise to sickle cell anemia when inherited in homozygosity.[124] Heterozygous sickle trait hemoglobin AS protects against severe malarial disease and is largely asymptomatic, although can be associated with clinical manifestations under extreme conditions. Coinheritance of the sickle cell β^S mutation and a β-thalassemia mutation results in sickle cell-β-thalassemia syndromes. Sickle cell-β thalassemia can be divided into sickle cell-β^0 thalassemia and sickle cell-β^+ thalassemia, according to the nature of the β-thalassemia mutation and thus the residual β-globin chain production, which in turn determines HbA levels and clinical severity. Patients with sickle cell-β^0 thalassemia do not produce HbA and are characterized by a clinical course as severe as homozygous sickle cell disease (HbSS). Higher HbA levels are generally associated with less severe clinical manifestations so individuals with HbS-β^+ thalassemia usually have a more benign clinical course than those with HbS-β^0 thalassemia or HbSS.[125]

Coinheritance of α-thalassemia is an important modulator of sickle cell disease. Individuals with sickle cell-α thalassemia are characterized by a lower degree of hemolysis and milder anemia, with fewer reticulocytes and sickle cells. Although some aspects of the clinical phenotype may be improved, it is yet not clear whether α-thalassemia increases survival in patients with sickle cell disease.[126–128] The higher hemoglobin may lead to hyperviscosity, which is associated with an increased risk of vaso-occlusive complications.

As described earlier, hemoglobin E (HbE) is a common structural hemoglobin variant, which results from the CD26 (GAG>AAG) β-globin mutation, which activates a cryptic splicing site, resulting in the synthesis of a structurally abnormal β^E-globin at low levels.[86] HbE occurs at high frequencies throughout many Asian countries. Coinheritance of HbE with β-thalassemia produces a wide variety of clinical disorders, which can range from mild NTDT to TDT, whose severity reflects the degree of globin chain imbalance and is modulated by HbF levels and coinheritance of α-thalassemia mutations. HbE β-thalassemia is the most common form of severe β-thalassemia in Asia.[87]

MOLECULAR TECHNIQUES FOR THE DIAGNOSIS OF THALASSEMIA SYNDROMES

Although protein-based methods, namely gel electrophoresis, high-performance liquid chromatography, capillary zone electrophoresis, and isoelectric focusing, remain the method of choice for initial qualitative and quantitative Hb analyses, DNA testing is necessary for the definitive diagnosis of thalassemia.[129,130] Numerous molecular genetics techniques for the detection of globin gene variants, each with specific strengths and limitations, have been developed. The choice of the most suitable diagnostic approach must consider the prevalence of specific thalassemia alleles in the population and the clinical phenotype. Different strategies are used to detect nondeletional variants, for which sequencing is generally sufficient, and large deletions and duplications, for which copy number variation (CNV) analysis is often necessary. Comprehensive analysis, including sequencing and CNV analysis, of both α- and β-globin gene loci is often necessary to accurately explain and predict the phenotype.

Direct DNA sequencing with Sanger sequencing is currently the most applicable method for detection of known and unknown nondeletional sequence variants. Allele-specific assays, such as allele-specific PCR or restriction fragment length polymorphism analysis, can be when a specific type of globin gene defect is suspected. Large deletions and duplications are usually detected with gap-polymerase chain reaction (gap-PCR) and multiplex ligation-dependent probe amplification (MLPA). Gap-PCR is applied for the detection of large deletions through the amplification of known breakpoints. MLPA exploits pairs of oligonucleotides that hybridize to adjacent target sequences, ligate, and get amplified by PCR to quantify copy numbers of the target sequences. Differently from gap-PCR, MLPA can be used for the identifications of both known and unknown deletions and duplications, although it cannot identify exact breakpoints. Next-generation sequencing (NGS), although not yet routinely used for hemoglobinopathy testing, is entering clinical practice and will allow the simultaneous sequencing of all the globin genes, along with genes known to affect hemoglobin expression, such as BCL11A, MYB, KLF1, and GATA1.[131] In August 2022, the first test based on NGS technology (combinatorial probe-anchor synthesis sequencing method) for the detection of thalassemia mutations was approved in Europe.[132,133] The introduction of such screening tools has important implications for reproductive practices.

Universal screening for the thalassemia carrier state in preconception or early prenatal period is recommended by the American College of Obstetricians and Gynecologists.[134,135] An appropriate screening includes a complete blood count, iron balance, and complete Hb separation (HbA2-HbF-Hb variant).[136] Low MCV or MCH is the most important screening test for thalassemia and/or iron deficiency. However, as red cell indices may fail to identify all carriers and distinguish iron deficiency from thalassemia, molecular-based screening is suggested in high-risk populations and to confirm the diagnosis. If the partners are at risk of offspring affected by thalassemia, they should be counseled about the cause, clinical manifestations, prognosis, and the full range of long-term outcomes of the expected disease. Prospective parents should be informed about the option of preimplantation genetic testing of embryos. Patients who are already pregnant should be offered early prenatal diagnosis, either through chorionic villus sampling or amniocentesis, to allow for informed decision-making about the pregnancy. Ultrasound markers can also be used to screen fetuses of couples at risk.[137,137] Finally, advancement in sequencing technologies has enabled the development of noninvasive prenatal diagnosis (NIPD) approaches based on NGS analysis of fetal DNA in maternal plasma for early diagnosis of monogenic diseases. The detection of low-level fetal variants in a high maternal background is still challenging, but methods are advancing and NIPD is becoming more widely available and will revolutionize prenatal diagnosis of thalassemia.[138] Different individual and cultural perspectives on screening before marriage, prenatal diagnosis, and pregnancy termination may influence the perinatal management of these diseases.[139]

CELL AND GENE THERAPY STRATEGIES FOR THE CURE OF THALASSEMIA

Allogeneic hematopoietic stem cell transplantation (HSCT) has represented for decades the only curative option for TDT.[140] However, the broad use of this therapeutic approach has been hindered by HLA-identical donor availability and transplant-related mortality and morbidity, in particular graft rejection, graft versus-host disease, infertility, and other treatment-related toxic effects.[141–143] Autologous HSCT after gene therapy, overcoming the major limitations of allogeneic HSCT, is theoretically a universal cure for TDT and, with the Food and Drug Administration approval of beti-beglogene autotemcel (Lenti BB305, BlubirdBio) in August 2022, now represents a real curative option for patients with TDT.[144–148] Several approaches are being investigated to genetically manipulate CD34+ hematopoietic stem and progenitor cells (HSPCs) ex vivo to correct the underlying genetic defects (**Fig. 6**).[149,150] Lentiviral vectors, derived from the HIV-1 virus, can be used to correct thalassemia by gene addition.[151] The new treatment betibeglogene autotemcel and other experimental lentiviral vector–based therapies exploit this transduction strategy to introduce fully functional β-like globin genes.[147,148,152,153] Interestingly, the same vectors can be used for the treatment of SCD when antisickling β-like globins, such as Hb^{T87Q} or γ-globin, are added.[150,154] Lentiviral vectors are also being explored to induce the constitutional expression of shRNA targeting and downregulating the expression of BCL11A to reactivate γ-globin expression or α-globin to ameliorate the α-to-β globin chain imbalance.[109,155,156] Numerous clinical trials evaluating different types of lentiviral vectors are currently underway around the world.[157]

Genome editing technologies, which have advanced tremendously over the last 2 decades, are also being explored to correct thalassemia-causing mutations or reactivate HbF.[158] Three generations of programmable nucleases, namely zinc finger nucleases, transcription activator-like effector nucleases, and CRISPR-associated nuclease Cas9 (CRISPR-Cas), have been developed to generate specific DNA double-strand breaks (DSBs).[159] In nondividing eukaryotic cells, DNA DSBs are normally repaired by the error-prone nonhomologous end joining (NHEJ) pathway, resulting in small indels that can disrupt specific DNA target sequences, such as the *BCL11A* erythroid-specific enhancer, or reproduce HPFH deletions or mimic *HBG1/2* promoter mutations, to reactivate HbF production.[160–164] When a homologous DNA donor template is provided, DSBs may be repaired by homologous recombination, allowing the insertion of specific DNA sequences and the possibility to correct disease-causing single nucleotide substitutions and small indels, although

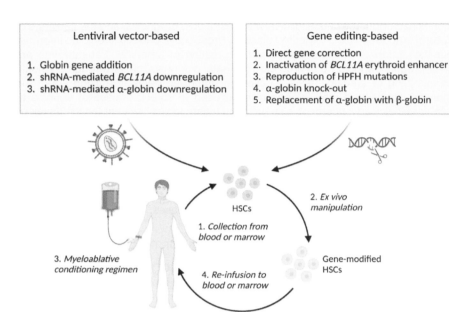

Lentiviral vector-based	Gene editing-based
1. Globin gene addition 2. shRNA-mediated *BCL11A* downregulation 3. shRNA-mediated α-globin downregulation	1. Direct gene correction 2. Inactivation of *BCL11A* erythroid enhancer 3. Reproduction of HPFH mutations 4. α-globin knock-out 5. Replacement of α-globin with β-globin

HSCs

2. Ex vivo manipulation

1. Collection from blood or marrow

3. Myeloablative conditioning regimen

Gene-modified HSCs

4. Re-infusion to blood or marrow

Fig. 6. Cell and gene therapy approaches for the cure of β-thalassemia. Numerous approaches could be used to add a globin gene, to activate a gene paralog (such as fetal globin), or to directly correct the mutation. Several examples are listed applicable to lentiviral transduction or gene editing. The process of ex vivo gene modification includes collection of hematopoietic stem and progenitor cells from mobilized peripheral blood or bone marrow harvest, ex vivo genetic manipulation, treatment of patient with myeloablative conditioning regimen, and reinfusion of modified cells to peripheral blood or bone marrow. (Created with BioRender.com.)

developing individual therapies to correct each of the hundreds of distinct mutations would be particularly challenging.[165–167] Gene therapies designed to reactivate HbF via ex vivo CRISPR/Cas9 gene editing at the erythroid enhancer region of *BCL11A* in autologous HSPCs are demonstrating promising results in clinical trials.[168–170] In addition to simple nucleases, CRISPR–Cas-derived genome editing agents, such as base editors and prime editors, are further expanding the genome editing toolbox.[159] Current base editors contain a catalytically impaired CRISPR–Cas nuclease fused to a cytosine or adenine deaminase enzyme and can efficiently correct all 4 possible transition mutations (C>T, A>G, T>C, G>A).[171,172] C•G-to-G•C base editors (CGBEs), able to correct C>G or G>C transversions, have been developed by linking editors with uracil DNA N-glycosylase or other DNA repair proteins.[173–176] About 58% of currently annotated β-thalassemia single nucleotide variants could be potentially corrected with this toolbox of base editors (**Fig. 7**). Prime editors are fusion proteins between a Cas nickase and an engineered reverse transcriptase that can potentially be used to introduce all types of point mutations, small insertions, and small deletions in a precise and targeted manner, although their efficiency in human HSCs remains uncertain.[177] Base editors and prime editors seem to be powerful and versatile tools, and base editors are currently moving into the clinic. The future development of orally bioavailable medicines that could potently and specifically upregulate HbF levels could be a boon for the treatment of β-thalassemia patients.

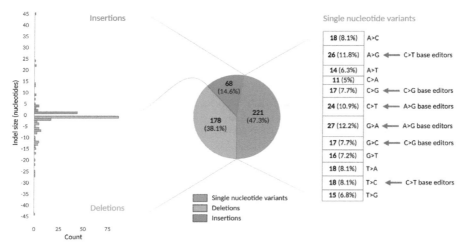

Fig. 7. Descriptive analysis of β-thalassemia mutations annotated on the IthaGenes database (https://www.ithanet.eu/db/ithagenes). Pie chart shows frequency of deletions, insertions, and single nucleotide variants among the listed β-thalassemia mutations. On the left is shown the distribution of insertions and deletions causing β-thalassemia according to indel size up to 50 nucleotides. Indels longer than 50 nucleotides, which comprise 32/246 (13%), are not shown in plot. On the right is shown the distribution of β-thalassemia variants according to nucleotide substitution. Number of unique mutations and deviation from expected 8.3% for each of the 12 substitution types are shown; 58% of currently annotated β-thalassemia single nucleotide variants could be potentially corrected with C>T, C>G, or A>G base editors. (Created with BioRender.com.)

In some instances, iatrogenic thalassemia could develop secondary to genetic manipulation of globin genes. The addition of an excessive number of globin genes could lead to the development of a secondary thalassemia syndrome, due to a secondary imbalance between α- and β-globin chains. For example, in the phase III trial of betibeglogene autotemcel in non-β⁰/β⁰ thalassemia, the vector copy number in peripheral-blood mononuclear cells ranged from 1.9 to 5.6 copies per diploid genome.[148] Anemia was observed in 2 patients carrying homozygous α⁺-thalassemia affected by SCD when treated with LentiGlobin due to apparent development of worsened α-thalassemia with excess of β to α-globin chains.[154] Moreover, it could be possible to convert sickle cell disease to β-thalassemia in cases where HDR is intended. Since NHEJ and HDR are competing DNA repair pathways, it is possible that some clones have both alleles repaired by NHEJ and could produce erythroid progeny with a β-thalassemia phenotype.[178] The overall clinical phenotype would likely reflect the cumulative erythroid output of all clones, including those that are unmodified and with various modifications.

SUMMARY

Thalassemia syndromes are among the commonest monogenic disorders and represent a substantial health burden worldwide. Here the authors have described globin genes, developmental production of hemoglobin, molecular lesions causing thalassemia syndromes, genotype-phenotype correlations, genetic modifiers, molecular diagnosis and prevention, and cell and gene therapy approaches. With the advent of improved diagnostic and genetic modification technologies, the clinical approach to thalassemias is on the precipice of revolution. Knowledge of the molecular basis of the thalassemias can be the foundation for the development and application of simple, safe, and effective therapies to be equitably delivered to patients in need.

CLINICS CARE POINTS

- Thorough knowledge of the molecular basis and genetic modifiers of thalassemias is important for accurate diagnosis and appropriate management of these conditions.
- Deletions of α-globin genes and point mutations of the β-globin gene are the predominant mutational mechanisms responsible for α-thalassemia and β-thalassemia, respectively.
- α-thalassemia trait carriers due to 2 deletions in cis are at risk of pregnancies affected by Bart's hydrops fetalis syndrome, whereas carriers due to 2 deletions in trans do not carry this risk.
- Although less frequent than deletions, nondeletional mutations can cause α-thalassemia. Nondeletional HbH disease tends to be more severe than deletional HbH disease.
- The clinical severity of β-thalassemia may be ameliorated by genetic factors that increase HbF production and by coinheritance of α-thalassemia.
- Although regular transfusions with iron chelation and allogeneic HSC transplantation still represent the standard of care options for severe thalassemia, numerous innovative and potentially curative molecular therapies are entering the clinic.

ACKNOWLEDGMENTS

All figures were created with BioRender.com. D.E. Bauer was supported by the National Heart, Lung, and Blood Institute (OT2HL154984, P01HL053749, R01HL150669), United States, Doris Duke Charitable Foundation, United States, and the St. Jude Children's Research Hospital Collaborative Research Consortium. N. Tesio expresses his gratitude to the Giovanni Armenise Harvard Foundation, United States, the Fondazione Ospedale Alba Bra, and the School of Medicine of the University of Torino, Italy for fellowship support and to Professor G. B. Ferrero for dedicated mentorship.

DISCLOSURE

The authors have nothing to disclose.

REFERENCES

1. Kattamis A, Kwiatkowski JL, Aydinok Y. Thalassaemia. Lancet 2022;399(10343): 2310–24.
2. Modell B, Darlison M. Global epidemiology of haemoglobin disorders and derived service indicators. Bull World Health Organ 2008;86(6):480–7.
3. Weatherall DJ. Genetic variation and susceptibility to infection: the red cell and malaria. Br J Haematol 2008;141(3):276–86.
4. Weatherall DJ. The evolving spectrum of the epidemiology of thalassemia. Hematol Oncol Clin North Am 2018;32(2):165–75.
5. Kattamis A, Forni GL, Aydinok Y, et al. Changing patterns in the epidemiology of β-thalassemia. Eur J Haematol 2020;105(6):692–703.

6. Rabbitts TH. Bacterial cloning of plasmids carrying copies of rabbit globin messenger RNA. Nature 1976;260(5548):221–5.

7. Muirhead H, Cox JM, Mazzarella L, et al. Structure and function of haemoglobin: III. A three-dimensional fourier synthesis of human deoxyhemoglobin at 5·5 Å resolution. J Mol Biol 1967;28(1):117–50.

8. Pauling L, Itano HA. Sickle cell anemia, a molecular disease. Science 1949; 109(2835):443.

9. Ingram VM. Gene mutations in human haemoglobin: the chemical difference between normal and sickle cell haemoglobin. Nature 1957;180(4581):326–8.

10. Myers RM, Tilly K, Maniatis T. Fine structure genetic analysis of a beta-globin promoter. Science 1986;232(4750):613–8.

11. Grosveld F, van Assendelft GB, Greaves DR, et al. Position-independent, high-level expression of the human beta-globin gene in transgenic mice. Cell 1987; 51(6):975–85.

12. Efstratiadis A, Posakony JW, Maniatis T, et al. The structure and evolution of the human beta-globin gene family. Cell 1980;21(3):653–68.

13. Higgs DR, Vickers MA, Wilkie AO, et al. A review of the molecular genetics of the human alpha-globin gene cluster. Blood 1989;73(5):1081–104.

14. Goh SH, Lee YT, Bhanu NV, et al. A newly discovered human alpha-globin gene. Blood 2005;106(4):1466–72.

15. Hughes JR, Cheng JF, Ventress N, et al. Annotation of cis-regulatory elements by identification, subclassification, and functional assessment of multispecies conserved sequences. Proc Natl Acad Sci U S A 2005;102(28):9830–5.

16. Mettananda S, Gibbons RJ, Higgs DR. Understanding α-globin gene regulation and implications for the treatment of β-thalassemia. Ann N Y Acad Sci 2016; 1368(1):16–24.

17. Tuan D, London IM. Mapping of DNase I-hypersensitive sites in the upstream DNA of human embryonic epsilon-globin gene in K562 leukemia cells. Proc Natl Acad Sci U S A 1984;81(9):2718–22.

18. Forrester WC, Takegawa S, Papayannopoulou T, et al. Evidence for a locus activation region: the formation of developmentally stable hypersensitive sites in globin-expressing hybrids. Nucleic Acids Res 1987;15(24):10159–77.

19. Wijgerde M, Grosveld F, Fraser P. Transcription complex stability and chromatin dynamics in vivo. Nature 1995;377(6546):209–13.

20. Bulger M, Groudine M. Looping versus linking: toward a model for long-distance gene activation. Genes Dev 1999;13(19):2465–77.

21. De Gobbi M, Anguita E, Hughes J, et al. Tissue-specific histone modification and transcription factor binding in alpha globin gene expression. Blood 2007; 110(13):4503–10.

22. Vernimmen D, Marques-Kranc F, Sharpe JA, et al. Chromosome looping at the human alpha-globin locus is mediated via the major upstream regulatory element (HS -40). Blood 2009;114(19):4253–60.

23. Vernimmen D, Lynch MD, De Gobbi M, et al. Polycomb eviction as a new distant enhancer function. Genes Dev 2011;25(15):1583–8.

24. Deng W, Rupon JW, Krivega I, et al. Reactivation of developmentally silenced globin genes by forced chromatin looping. Cell 2014;158(4):849–60.

25. Lee WS, McColl B, Maksimovic J, et al. Epigenetic interplay at the β-globin locus. Biochim Biophys Acta Gene Regul Mech 2017;1860(4):393–404.

26. Stamatoyannopoulos G. Control of globin gene expression during development and erythroid differentiation. Exp Hematol 2005;33(3):259–71.

27. Vinjamur DS, Bauer DE, Orkin SH. Recent progress in understanding and manipulating haemoglobin switching for the haemoglobinopathies. Br J Haematol 2018;180(5):630–43.

28. Menzel S, Garner C, Gut I, et al. A QTL influencing F cell production maps to a gene encoding a zinc-finger protein on chromosome 2p15. Nat Genet 2007; 39(10):1197–9.

29. Uda M, Galanello R, Sanna S, et al. Genome-wide association study shows BCL11A associated with persistent fetal hemoglobin and amelioration of the phenotype of beta-thalassemia. Proc Natl Acad Sci U S A 2008;105(5):1620–5.

30. Bauer DE, Kamran SC, Orkin SH. Reawakening fetal hemoglobin: prospects for new therapies for the β-globin disorders. Blood 2012;120(15):2945–53.

31. Xu J, Bauer DE, Kerenyi MA, et al. Corepressor-dependent silencing of fetal hemoglobin expression by BCL11A. Proc Natl Acad Sci U S A 2013;110(16): 6518–23.

32. Sankaran VG, Menne TF, Xu J, et al. Human fetal hemoglobin expression is regulated by the developmental stage-specific repressor BCL11A. Science 2008;322(5909):1839–42.

33. Liu N, Hargreaves VV, Zhu Q, et al. Direct promoter repression by BCL11A controls the fetal to adult hemoglobin switch. Cell 2018;173(2):430–42.e17.

34. Martyn GE, Wienert B, Yang L, et al. Natural regulatory mutations elevate the fetal globin gene via disruption of BCL11A or ZBTB7A binding. Nat Genet 2018;50(4):498–503.

35. Liu N, Xu S, Yao Q, et al. Transcription factor competition at the γ-globin promoters controls hemoglobin switching. Nat Genet 2021;53(4):511–20.

36. Bauer DE, Kamran SC, Lessard S, et al. An erythroid enhancer of BCL11A subject to genetic variation determines fetal hemoglobin level. Science 2013; 342(6155):253–7.

37. Basak A, Hancarova M, Ulirsch JC, et al. BCL11A deletions result in fetal hemoglobin persistence and neurodevelopmental alterations. J Clin Invest 2015; 125(6):2363–8.

38. Huang P, Peslak SA, Ren R, et al. HIC2 controls developmental hemoglobin switching by repressing BCL11A transcription. Nat Genet 2022;54(9):1417–26.

39. Doerfler PA, Feng R, Li Y, et al. Activation of γ-globin gene expression by GATA1 and NF-Y in hereditary persistence of fetal hemoglobin. Nat Genet 2021;53(8): 1177–86.

40. Masuda T, Wang X, Maeda M, et al. Transcription factors LRF and BCL11A independently repress expression of fetal hemoglobin. Science 2016;351(6270): 285–9.

41. Harju-Baker S, Costa FC, Fedosyuk H, et al. Silencing of Agamma-globin gene expression during adult definitive erythropoiesis mediated by GATA-1-FOG-1-Mi2 complex binding at the -566 GATA site. Mol Cell Biol 2008;28(10):3101–13.

42. Gnanapragasam MN, Scarsdale JN, Amaya ML, et al. p66Alpha-MBD2 coiled-coil interaction and recruitment of Mi-2 are critical for globin gene silencing by the MBD2-NuRD complex. Proc Natl Acad Sci U S A 2011;108(18):7487–92.

43. Sher F, Hossain M, Seruggia D, et al. Rational targeting of a NuRD subcomplex guided by comprehensive in situ mutagenesis. Nat Genet 2019;51(7):1149–59.

44. Vinjamur DS, Yao Q, Cole MA, et al. ZNF410 represses fetal globin by singular control of CHD4. Nat Genet 2021;53(5):719–28.

45. Lan X, Ren R, Feng R, et al. ZNF410 uniquely activates the NuRD component CHD4 to silence fetal hemoglobin expression. Mol Cell 2021;81(2):239–54.e8.

46. Zhou D, Liu K, Sun CW, et al. KLF1 regulates BCL11A expression and γ- to β-globin gene switching. Nat Genet 2010;42(9):742–4.

47. Borg J, Papadopoulos P, Georgitsi M, et al. Haploinsufficiency for the erythroid transcription factor KLF1 causes hereditary persistence of fetal hemoglobin. Nat Genet 2010;42(9):801–5.

48. Liu D, Zhang X, Yu L, et al. KLF1 mutations are relatively more common in a thalassemia endemic region and ameliorate the severity of β-thalassemia. Blood 2014;124(5):803–11.

49. Perkins A, Xu X, Higgs DR, et al. Krüppeling erythropoiesis: an unexpected broad spectrum of human red blood cell disorders due to KLF1 variants. Blood 2016;127(15):1856–62.

50. Menzel S, Jiang J, Silver N, et al. The HBS1L-MYB intergenic region on chromosome 6q23.3 influences erythrocyte, platelet, and monocyte counts in humans. Blood 2007;110(10):3624–6.

51. Thein SL, Menzel S, Peng X, et al. Intergenic variants of HBS1L-MYB are responsible for a major quantitative trait locus on chromosome 6q23 influencing fetal hemoglobin levels in adults. Proc Natl Acad Sci U S A 2007;104(27): 11346–51.

52. Sankaran VG, Menne TF, Śćepanović D, et al. MicroRNA-15a and -16-1 act via MYB to elevate fetal hemoglobin expression in human trisomy 13. Proc Natl Acad Sci U S A 2011;108(4):1519–24.

53. Qin K, Huang P, Feng R, et al. Dual function NFI factors control fetal hemoglobin silencing in adult erythroid cells. Nat Genet 2022;54(6):874–84.

54. Piel FB, Weatherall DJ. The α-thalassemias. N Engl J Med 2014;371(20): 1908–16.

55. Higgs DR. The molecular basis of α-thalassemia. Cold Spring Harb Perspect Med 2013;3(1):a011718.

56. Farashi S, Harteveld CL. Molecular basis of α-thalassemia. Blood Cells Mol Dis 2018;70:43–53.

57. Higgs DR, Wood WG. Long-range regulation of alpha globin gene expression during erythropoiesis. Curr Opin Hematol 2008;15(3):176–83.

58. Coelho A, Picanço I, Seuanes F, et al. Novel large deletions in the human α-globin gene cluster: clarifying the HS-40 long-range regulatory role in the native chromosome environment. Blood Cells Mol Dis 2010;45(2):147–53.

59. Sollaino MC, Paglietti ME, Loi D, et al. Homozygous deletion of the major alpha-globin regulatory element (MCS-R2) responsible for a severe case of hemoglobin H disease. Blood 2010;116(12):2193–4.

60. Wu MY, He Y, Yan JM, et al. A novel selective deletion of the major α-globin regulatory element (MCS-R2) causing α-thalassaemia. Br J Haematol 2017;176(6): 984–6.

61. Kalle Kwaifa I, Lai MI, Md Noor S. Non-deletional alpha thalassaemia: a review. Orphanet J Rare Dis 2020;15(1):166.

62. Wajcman H, Traeger-Synodinos J, Papassotiriou I, et al. Unstable and thalassemic alpha chain hemoglobin variants: a cause of Hb H disease and thalassemia intermedia. Hemoglobin 2008;32(4):327–49.

63. Clegg JB, Weatherall DJ. Hemoglobin constant spring, and unusual alpha-chain variant involved in the etiology of hemoglobin H disease. Ann N Y Acad Sci 1974;232(0):168–78.

64. Schrier SL, Bunyaratvej A, Khuhapinant A, et al. The unusual pathobiology of hemoglobin constant spring red blood cells. Blood 1997;89(5):1762–9.

65. Singer ST, Kim HY, Olivieri NF, et al. Hemoglobin H-constant spring in North America: an alpha thalassemia with frequent complications. Am J Hematol 2009;84(11):759–61.

66. Gibbons R. Alpha thalassaemia-mental retardation, X linked. Orphanet J Rare Dis 2006;1:15.

67. Clynes D, Higgs DR, Gibbons RJ. The chromatin remodeller ATRX: a repeat offender in human disease. Trends Biochem Sci 2013;38(9):461–6.

68. Truch J, Downes DJ, Scott C, et al. The chromatin remodeller ATRX facilitates diverse nuclear processes, in a stochastic manner, in both heterochromatin and euchromatin. Nat Commun 2022;13(1):3485.

69. Gibbons RJ, Higgs DR. The alpha-thalassemia/mental retardation syndromes. Medicine 1996;75(2):45–52.

70. Harteveld CL, Kriek M, Bijlsma EK, et al. Refinement of the genetic cause of ATR-16. Hum Genet 2007;122(3–4):283–92.

71. Lorey F, Charoenkwan P, Witkowska HE, et al. hydrops foetalis syndrome: a case report and review of literature. Br J Haematol 2001;115(1):72–8.

72. Lal A, Goldrich ML, Haines DA, et al. Heterogeneity of hemoglobin H disease in childhood. N Engl J Med 2011;364(8):710–8.

73. Songdej D, Babbs C, Higgs DR, BHFS International Consortium. An international registry of survivors with Hb Bart's hydrops fetalis syndrome. Blood 2017;129(10):1251–9.

74. MacKenzie TC, Amid A, Angastiniotis M, et al. Consensus statement for the perinatal management of patients with α thalassemia major. Blood Adv 2021; 5(24):5636–9.

75. King AJ, Higgs DR. Potential new approaches to the management of the Hb Bart's hydrops fetalis syndrome: the most severe form of α-thalassemia. Hematol Am Soc Hematol Educ Program 2018;2018(1):353–60.

76. Russell JE, Liebhaber SA. Reversal of lethal alpha- and beta-thalassemias in mice by expression of human embryonic globins. Blood 1998;92(9):3057–63.

77. King AJ, Songdej D, Downes DJ, et al. Reactivation of a developmentally silenced embryonic globin gene. Nat Commun 2021;12(1):4439.

78. Sancar GB, Tatsis B, Cedeno MM, et al. Proportion of hemoglobin G Philadelphia (alpha 268 Asn leads to Lys beta 2) in heterozygotes is determined by alpha-globin gene deletions. Proc Natl Acad Sci U S A 1980;77(11):6874–8.

79. Steensma DP, Gibbons RJ, Higgs DR. Acquired alpha-thalassemia in association with myelodysplastic syndrome and other hematologic malignancies. Blood 2005;105(2):443–52.

80. Taher AT, Musallam KM, Cappellini MD. β-thalassemias. N Engl J Med 2021; 384(8):727–43.

81. Thein SL. Molecular basis of β thalassemia and potential therapeutic targets. Blood Cells Mol Dis 2018;70:54–65.

82. Thein SL. The molecular basis of β-thalassemia. Cold Spring Harb Perspect Med 2013;3(5):a011700.

83. Huisman TH. Levels of Hb A2 in heterozygotes and homozygotes for beta-thalassemia mutations: influence of mutations in the CACCC and ATAAA motifs of the beta-globin gene promoter. Acta Haematol 1997;98(4):187–94.

84. Topfer SK, Feng R, Huang P, et al. Disrupting the adult globin promoter alleviates promoter competition and reactivates fetal globin gene expression. Blood 2022;139(14):2107–18.

85. Weatherall DJ. Phenotype-genotype relationships in monogenic disease: lessons from the thalassaemias. Nat Rev Genet 2001;2(4):245–55.

86. Orkin SH, Kazazian HH Jr, Antonarakis SE, et al. Abnormal RNA processing due to the exon mutation of beta E-globin gene. Nature 1982;300(5894):768–9.

87. Fucharoen S, Weatherall DJ. The hemoglobin E thalassemias. Cold Spring Harb Perspect Med 2012;2(8):a011734.

88. Thein SL, Old JM, Wainscoat JS, et al. Population and genetic studies suggest a single origin for the Indian deletion beta thalassaemia. Br J Haematol 1984; 57(2):271–8.

89. Orkin SH, Goff SC, Nathan DG. Heterogeneity of DNA deletion in gamma delta beta-thalassemia. J Clin Invest 1981;67(3):878–84.

90. Thein SL, Wood WG. The molecular basis of β thalassemia, δβ thalassemia, and hereditary persistence of fetal hemoglobin. In: Steinberg MH, Forget BG, Higgs DR, Weatherall DR, editors. Disorders of hemoglobin: genetics, pathophysiology, and clinical management. Cambridge, UK: Cambridge University Press; 2009. p. 323–56.

91. Forget BG. Molecular basis of hereditary persistence of fetal hemoglobin. Ann N Y Acad Sci 1998;850:38–44.

92. Baglioni C. The fusion of two peptide chains in hemoglobin Lepore and its interpretation as a genetic deletion. Proc Natl Acad Sci U S A 1962;48:1880–6.

93. Efremov GD. Hemoglobins Lepore and anti-Lepore. Hemoglobin 1978;2(3): 197–233.

94. Thein SL, Hesketh C, Taylor P, et al. Molecular basis for dominantly inherited inclusion body beta-thalassemia. Proc Natl Acad Sci U S A 1990;87(10):3924–8.

95. Thein SL. Is it dominantly inherited beta thalassaemia or just a beta-chain variant that is highly unstable? Br J Haematol 1999;107(1):12–21.

96. Viprakasit V, Gibbons RJ, Broughton BC, et al. Mutations in the general transcription factor TFIIH result in β-thalassaemia in individuals with trichothiodystrophy. Hum Mol Genet 2001;10(24):2797–802.

97. Yu C, Niakan KK, Matsushita M, et al. X-linked thrombocytopenia with thalassemia from a mutation in the amino finger of GATA-1 affecting DNA binding rather than FOG-1 interaction. Blood 2002;100(6):2040–5.

98. Perseu L, Satta S, Moi P, et al. KLF1 gene mutations cause borderline HbA(2). Blood 2011;118(16):4454–8.

99. Achour A, Koopmann T, Castel R, et al. A new gene associated with a β-thalassemia phenotype: the observation of variants in SUPT5H. Blood 2020;136(15): 1789–93.

100. Badens C, Mattei MG, Imbert AM, et al. A novel mechanism for thalassaemia intermedia. Lancet 2002;359(9301):132–3.

101. Galanello R, Perseu L, Perra C, et al. Somatic deletion of the normal beta-globin gene leading to thalassaemia intermedia in heterozygous beta-thalassaemic patients. Br J Haematol 2004;127(5):604–6.

102. Chang JG, Tsai WC, Chong IW, et al. {beta}-thalassemia major evolution from {beta}-thalassemia minor is associated with paternal uniparental isodisomy of chromosome 11p15. Haematologica 2008;93(6):913–6.

103. Brunner AM, Steensma DP. Myelodysplastic syndrome associated acquired beta thalassemia: "BTMDS". Am J Hematol 2016;91(8):E325–7.

104. Welbourn EM, Wilson MT, Yusof A, et al. The mechanism of formation, structure and physiological relevance of covalent hemoglobin attachment to the erythrocyte membrane. Free Radic Biol Med 2017;103:95–106.

105. Thein SL. Pathophysiology of beta thalassemia–a guide to molecular therapies. Hematol Am Soc Hematol Educ Program 2005;2005(1):31–7.

106. Danjou F, Anni F, Galanello R. Beta-thalassemia: from genotype to phenotype. Haematologica 2011;96(11):1573–5.
107. Thein SL. Genetic association studies in β-hemoglobinopathies. Hematol Am Soc Hematol Educ Program 2013;2013:354–61.
108. Voon HPJ, Vadolas J. Controlling alpha-globin: a review of alpha-globin expression and its impact on beta-thalassemia. Haematologica 2008;93(12):1868–76.
109. Mettananda S, Gibbons RJ, Higgs DR. α-Globin as a molecular target in the treatment of β-thalassemia. Blood 2015;125(24):3694–701.
110. Stoming TA, Stoming GS, Lanclos KD, et al. An A gamma type of nondeletional hereditary persistence of fetal hemoglobin with a T—C mutation at position -175 to the cap site of the A gamma globin gene. Blood 1989;73(1):329–33.
111. Fischer KD, Nowock J. The T—C substitution at -198 of the A gamma-globin gene associated with the British form of HPFH generates overlapping recognition sites for two DNA-binding proteins. Nucleic Acids Res 1990;18(19): 5685–93.
112. Wienert B, Funnell APW, Norton LJ, et al. Editing the genome to introduce a beneficial naturally occurring mutation associated with increased fetal globin. Nat Commun 2015;6:7085.
113. Wienert B, Martyn GE, Kurita R, et al. KLF1 drives the expression of fetal hemoglobin in British HPFH. Blood 2017;130(6):803–7.
114. Martyn GE, Wienert B, Kurita R, et al. A natural regulatory mutation in the proximal promoter elevates fetal globin expression by creating a de novo GATA1 site. Blood 2019;133(8):852–6.
115. Ravi NS, Wienert B, Wyman SK, et al. Identification of novel HPFH-like mutations by CRISPR base editing that elevate the expression of fetal hemoglobin. Elife 2022;11:e65421.
116. Huisman TH, Wrightstone RN, Wilson JB, et al. Hemoglobin Kenya, the product of fusion of amd polypeptide chains. Arch Biochem Biophys 1972;153(2):850–3.
117. Kendall AG, Ojwang PJ, Schroeder WA, et al. Hemoglobin Kenya, the product of a gamma-beta fusion gene: studies of the family. Am J Hum Genet 1973;25(5): 548–63.
118. Jiang Z, Luo HY, Huang S, et al. The genetic basis of asymptomatic codon 8 frame-shift (HBB:c25_26delAA) β(0) -thalassaemia homozygotes. Br J Haematol 2016;172(6):958–65.
119. Origa R, Galanello R, Perseu L, et al. Cholelithiasis in thalassemia major. Eur J Haematol 2009;82(1):22–5.
120. Melis MA, Cau M, Deidda F, et al. H63D mutation in the HFE gene increases iron overload in beta-thalassemia carriers. Haematologica 2002;87(3):242–5.
121. Sidore C, Busonero F, Maschio A, et al. Genome sequencing elucidates Sardinian genetic architecture and augments association analyses for lipid and blood inflammatory markers. Nat Genet 2015;47(11):1272–81.
122. Liu DJ, Peloso GM, Yu H, et al. Exome-wide association study of plasma lipids in >300,000 individuals. Nat Genet 2017;49(12):1758–66.
123. Triantafyllou AI, Farmakis DT, Lampropoulos KM, et al. Impact of β-thalassemia trait carrier state on inflammatory status in patients with newly diagnosed hypertension. J Cardiovasc Med 2019;20(5):284–9.
124. Kato GJ, Piel FB, Reid CD, et al. Sickle cell disease. Nat Rev Dis Primers 2018;4: 18010.
125. Vichinsky EP. Overview of compound sickle cell syndromes. 2021. Available at: https://www.uptodate.com/contents/overview-of-compound-sickle-cell-syndromes. Accessed October 3, 2022.

126. Embury SH, Dozy AM, Miller J, et al. Concurrent sickle-cell anemia and alpha-thalassemia: effect on severity of anemia. N Engl J Med 1982;306(5):270–4.
127. Billett HH, Nagel RL, Fabry ME. Paradoxical increase of painful crises in sickle cell patients with alpha-thalassemia. Blood 1995;86(11):4382.
128. Fertrin KY, Costa FF. Genomic polymorphisms in sickle cell disease: implications for clinical diversity and treatment. Expert Rev Hematol 2010;3(4):443–58.
129. Sabath DE. Molecular diagnosis of thalassemias and hemoglobinopathies: an ACLPS critical review. Am J Clin Pathol 2017;148(1):6–15.
130. Munkongdee T, Chen P, Winichagoon P, et al. Update in laboratory diagnosis of thalassemia. Front Mol Biosci 2020;7:74.
131. Achour A, Koopmann TT, Baas F, et al. The evolving role of next-generation sequencing in screening and diagnosis of hemoglobinopathies. Front Physiol 2021;12:686689.
132. He J, Song W, Yang J, et al. Next-generation sequencing improves thalassemia carrier screening among premarital adults in a high prevalence population: the Dai nationality. China Genet Med 2017;19(9):1022–31.
133. Zhang H, Li C, Li J, et al. Next-generation sequencing improves molecular epidemiological characterization of thalassemia in Chenzhou Region, P.R. China. J Clin Lab Anal 2019;33(4):e22845.
134. ACOG committee on obstetrics. ACOG practice bulletin No. 78: hemoglobinopathies in pregnancy. Obstet Gynecol 2007;109(1):229–37.
135. Committee opinion No. 691: carrier screening for genetic conditions. Obstet Gynecol 2017;129(3):e41–55.
136. Mandrile G, Barella S, Giambona A, et al. First and second level haemoglobinopathies diagnosis: best practices of the Italian Society of Thalassemia and Haemoglobinopathies (SITE). J Clin Med Res 2022;11(18):5426.
137. Yates AM. Prenatal screening and testing for hemoglobinopathy. 2021. Available at: https://www.uptodate.com/contents/prenatal-screening-and-testing-for-hemoglobinopathy. Accessed October 3, 2022.
138. Scotchman E, Shaw J, Paternoster B, et al. Non-invasive prenatal diagnosis and screening for monogenic disorders. Eur J Obstet Gynecol Reprod Biol 2020;253:320–7.
139. Committee opinion No. 690: carrier screening in the age of genomic medicine. Obstet Gynecol 2017;129(3):e35–40.
140. Copelan EA. Hematopoietic stem-cell transplantation. N Engl J Med 2006;354(17):1813–26.
141. Gragert L, Eapen M, Williams E, et al. HLA match likelihoods for hematopoietic stem-cell grafts in the U.S. registry. N Engl J Med 2014;371(4):339–48.
142. Baronciani D, Angelucci E, Potschger U, et al. Hemopoietic stem cell transplantation in thalassemia: a report from the European Society for Blood and Bone Marrow Transplantation Hemoglobinopathy Registry, 2000-2010. Bone Marrow Transplant 2016;51(4):536–41.
143. Li C, Mathews V, Kim S, et al. Related and unrelated donor transplantation for β-thalassemia major: results of an international survey. Blood Adv 2019;3(17):2562–70.
144. Cavazzana M, Bushman FD, Miccio A, et al. Gene therapy targeting haematopoietic stem cells for inherited diseases: progress and challenges. Nat Rev Drug Discov 2019;18(6):447–62.
145. Ferrari G, Thrasher AJ, Aiuti A. Gene therapy using haematopoietic stem and progenitor cells. Nat Rev Genet 2021;22(4):216–34.

146. Rosanwo TO, Bauer DE. Editing outside the body: Ex vivo gene-modification for β-hemoglobinopathy cellular therapy. Mol Ther 2021;29(11):3163–78.

147. Center for Biologics Evaluation. Research. ZYNTEGLO. U.S. Food and Drug Administration. Available at: https://www.fda.gov/vaccines-blood-biologics/zynteglo. Accessed September 21, 2022.

148. Locatelli F, Thompson AA, Kwiatkowski JL, et al. Betibeglogene Autotemcel gene therapy for Non-β0/β0 genotype β-thalassemia. N Engl J Med 2022; 386(5):415–27.

149. Cavazzana M, Antoniani C, Miccio A. Gene therapy for β-hemoglobinopathies. Mol Ther 2017;25(5):1142–54.

150. Leonard A, Tisdale JF, Bonner M. Gene therapy for hemoglobinopathies: beta-thalassemia, sickle cell disease. Hematol Oncol Clin North Am 2022;36(4): 769–95.

151. Naldini L, Blömer U, Gallay P, et al. In vivo gene delivery and stable transduction of nondividing cells by a lentiviral vector. Science 1996;272(5259):263–7.

152. Thompson AA, Walters MC, Kwiatkowski J, et al. Gene therapy in patients with transfusion-dependent β-thalassemia. N Engl J Med 2018;378(16):1479–93.

153. Marktel S, Scaramuzza S, Cicalese MP, et al. Intrabone hematopoietic stem cell gene therapy for adult and pediatric patients affected by transfusion-dependent ß-thalassemia. Nat Med 2019;25(2):234–41.

154. Kanter J, Walters MC, Krishnamurti L, et al. Biologic and clinical efficacy of LentiGlobin for sickle cell disease. N Engl J Med 2022;386(7):617–28.

155. Esrick EB, Lehmann LE, Biffi A, et al. Post-transcriptional genetic silencing of BCL11A to treat sickle cell disease. N Engl J Med 2021;384(3):205–15.

156. Liu B, Brendel C, Vinjamur DS, et al. Development of a double shmiR lentivirus effectively targeting both BCL11A and ZNF410 for enhanced induction of fetal hemoglobin to treat β-hemoglobinopathies. Mol Ther 2022;30(8):2693–708.

157. Musallam KM, Bou-Fakhredin R, Cappellini MD, et al. 2021 update on clinical trials in β-thalassemia. Am J Hematol 2021;96(11):1518–31.

158. Brusson M, Miccio A. Genome editing approaches to β-hemoglobinopathies. Prog Mol Biol Transl Sci 2021;182:153–83.

159. Anzalone AV, Koblan LW, Liu DR. Genome editing with CRISPR-Cas nucleases, base editors, transposases and prime editors. Nat Biotechnol 2020;38(7): 824–44.

160. Canver MC, Smith EC, Sher F, et al. BCL11A enhancer dissection by Cas9-mediated in situ saturating mutagenesis. Nature 2015;527(7577):192–7.

161. Chang KH, Smith SE, Sullivan T, et al. Long-term engraftment and fetal globin induction upon BCL11A gene editing in bone-marrow-derived CD34+ hematopoietic stem and progenitor cells. Mol Ther Methods Clin Dev 2017;4:137–48.

162. Antoniani C, Meneghini V, Lattanzi A, et al. Induction of fetal hemoglobin synthesis by CRISPR/Cas9-mediated editing of the human β-globin locus. Blood 2018; 131(17):1960–73.

163. Wu Y, Zeng J, Roscoe BP, et al. Highly efficient therapeutic gene editing of human hematopoietic stem cells. Nat Med 2019;25(5):776–83.

164. Métais JY, Doerfler PA, Mayuranathan T, et al. Genome editing of HBG1 and HBG2 to induce fetal hemoglobin. Blood Adv 2019;3(21):3379–92.

165. Wang J, Exline CM, DeClercq JJ, et al. Homology-driven genome editing in hematopoietic stem and progenitor cells using ZFN mRNA and AAV6 donors. Nat Biotechnol 2015;33(12):1256–63.

166. Cromer MK, Camarena J, Martin RM, et al. Gene replacement of α-globin with β-globin restores hemoglobin balance in β-thalassemia-derived hematopoietic stem and progenitor cells. Nat Med 2021;27(4):677–87.

167. Pavani G, Fabiano A, Laurent M, et al. Correction of β-thalassemia by CRISPR/Cas9 editing of the α-globin locus in human hematopoietic stem cells. Blood Adv 2021;5(5):1137–53.

168. Frangoul H, Altshuler D, Cappellini MD, et al. CRISPR-Cas9 Gene Editing for Sickle Cell Disease and β-Thalassemia. N Engl J Med 2021;384(3):252–60.

169. Locatelli F, Frangoul H, Corbacioglu S, et al. Efficacy and safety of a single dose of CTX011 for transfusion-dependent beta-thalassemia and severe sickle cell disease. In: European Hematology Association. 2022. Available at: https://library.ehaweb.org/eha/2022/eha2022-congress/366210/. Accessed September 21, 2022.

170. Fu B, Liao J, Chen S, et al. CRISPR-Cas9-mediated gene editing of the BCL11A enhancer for pediatric β0/β0 transfusion-dependent β-thalassemia. Nat Med 2022;28(8):1573–80.

171. Porto EM, Komor AC, Slaymaker IM, et al. Base editing: advances and therapeutic opportunities. Nat Rev Drug Discov 2020;19(12):839–59.

172. Zeng J, Wu Y, Ren C, et al. Therapeutic base editing of human hematopoietic stem cells. Nat Med 2020;26(4):535–41.

173. Chen L, Park JE, Paa P, et al. Programmable C: G to G: C genome editing with CRISPR-Cas9-directed base excision repair proteins. Nat Commun 2021;12(1):1384.

174. Kurt IC, Zhou R, Iyer S, et al. CRISPR C-to-G base editors for inducing targeted DNA transversions in human cells. Nat Biotechnol 2021;39(1):41–6.

175. Zhao D, Li J, Li S, et al. Glycosylase base editors enable C-to-A and C-to-G base changes. Nat Biotechnol 2021;39(1):35–40.

176. Koblan LW, Arbab M, Shen MW, et al. Efficient C•G-to-G•C base editors developed using CRISPRi screens, target-library analysis, and machine learning. Nat Biotechnol 2021;39(11):1414–25.

177. Zhang H, Sun R, Fei J, et al. Correction of beta-thalassemia IVS-II-654 mutation in a mouse model using prime editing. Int J Mol Sci 2022;23(11):5948.

178. Magis W, DeWitt MA, Wyman SK, et al. High-level correction of the sickle mutation is amplified in vivo during erythroid differentiation. iScience 2022;25(6):104374.

Fetal Hemoglobin Regulation in Beta-Thalassemia

Henry Y. Lu, PhD[a,b,c,d], Stuart H. Orkin, MD[a,b,d,e,f], Vijay G. Sankaran, MD, PhD[a,b,c,d,f],*

KEYWORDS

- Fetal hemoglobin • Beta-thalassemia • Anemia

KEY POINTS

- Therapeutic fetal hemoglobin (HbF) induction is a highly promising strategy for treating β-thalassemia.
- BCL11A is a potent HbF repressor that is being therapeutically targeted in multiple clinical trials in patients with β-thalassemia.
- Recent functional screens in cellular models have identified many new putative HbF modulators that may improve therapeutic HbF induction efforts.

INTRODUCTION

More than 50,000 infants are born annually with severe forms of one of the most common monogenic disorders in the world, β-thalassemia.[1] It is caused by mutations in the hemoglobin β subunit gene (*HBB*), which lead to reduced or absent β-globin production and anemia, as well as a range of associated complications.[2] This renders many patients transfusion and iron chelation dependent.[3,4] Although allogeneic bone marrow transplantation can be curative for some, it is limited by toxicity from conditioning and appropriate donor availability.[5] As such, more effective and definitive treatments are urgently needed.

a Division of Hematology/Oncology, Boston Children's Hospital, Harvard Medical School, Boston, MA, USA; b Department of Pediatric Oncology, Dana-Farber Cancer Institute, Harvard Medical School, Boston, MA, USA; c Broad Institute of Massachusetts Institute of Technology (MIT) and Harvard, Cambridge, MA, USA; d Karp Family Research Laboratories, Boston Children's Hospital, 1 Blackfan Street, Boston, MA 02115, USA; e Howard Hughes Medical Institute, Chevy Chase, MD, USA; f Harvard Stem Cell Institute, Cambridge, MA, USA
* Corresponding author. Karp Family Research Laboratories, Boston Children's Hospital, 1 Blackfan Street, Boston, MA 02115.
E-mail address: sankaran@broadinstitute.org
Twitter: @realhenrylu (H.Y.L.); @bloodgenes (V.G.S.)

Hematol Oncol Clin N Am 37 (2023) 301–312
https://doi.org/10.1016/j.hoc.2022.12.002
0889-8588/23/© 2022 Elsevier Inc. All rights reserved.

The last six decades are marked by enormous progress in the understanding of globin gene regulation and β-thalassemia that has placed us well on the way toward potentially curative therapies. Careful clinical and scientific observations have robustly shown a quantitative ameliorating effect of elevated fetal hemoglobin (HbF) levels on the severity, morbidity, and mortality of β-thalassemia.[5,6] Here, we briefly review original observations that spurred the study of HbF induction for β-thalassemia, the current understanding of HbF switching, and discuss recently identified regulators of HbF.

HEMOGLOBIN SWITCHING AND THE β-HEMOGLOBINOPATHIES

Hemoglobin is a tetrameric molecule consisting of two α-like and two β-like globin subunits each, which together with heme and iron mediate the oxygen-carrying function of erythrocytes.[6] In humans, multiple β-like globins with unique physiological properties are expressed and regulated across development. During the first weeks of embryonic development in humans, there is predominant expression of the embryonic ε-globin that is found in the transient primitive erythrocyte lineage, which is then replaced by γ-globin for the remainder of fetal development in definitive erythroid cells, forming a tetramer of $\alpha_2\gamma_2$ to produce HbF.[5] Soon after birth, the critical fetal-to-adult (γ-to β-globin) transcriptional switch occurs to form a tetramer of $\alpha_2\beta_2$ adult hemoglobin (HbA), which accounts for most hemoglobin in red cells throughout adulthood, with a small number of cells expressing HbF (~1%) or the minor adult hemoglobin $\alpha_2\delta_2$ (HbA$_2$).[5]

The β-globin genes are arranged in the order by which they are developmentally expressed ($\varepsilon > ^G\gamma > ^A\gamma > \delta > \beta$) downstream of a cluster of erythroid-specific enhancer elements termed the locus control region (LCR) (**Fig. 1**A).[5,7] The LCR, in concert with transcription factors (TFs), cofactors, and chromatin structural factors, forms physical loops that interact with the promoters of globin genes to activate their expression[5,7] (**Fig. 1**B, C). Notably, since its discovery in the late 1980s, this erythroid LCR mechanism now serves as a paradigm for regulatory enhancers, as well as enhancer clusters that act together known as "superenhancers," and the developmental regulation of other genes.

Genetic defects that affect *HBB* lead to the β-hemoglobinopathies, β-thalassemia and sickle cell disease (SCD).[2] SCD is caused by homozygous *HBB* mutations that create sickle hemoglobin, which can polymerize in hypoxic conditions, causing erythrocytes to sickle and be prone to hemolysis.[8] β-thalassemia is caused by diverse *HBB* mutations that result in reduced or absent β-globin, leading to unpaired α-globin and globin chain imbalance.[9,10] Accumulation of unstable excess α-globin chains leads to precipitation, the formation of inclusions, and the generation of reactive oxygen species in erythroid precursors, leading to hemolysis and ineffective erythropoiesis.[3,4]

THE CLINICAL BENEFIT OF FETAL HEMOGLOBIN

As β-thalassemia is caused by globin chain imbalance, strategies that can reduce this imbalance could be beneficial. Early clues toward accomplishing this arose from careful clinical observations of patients with β-hemoglobinopathies in the 1950 to 1970s. First, children with β-hemoglobinopathies are asymptomatic until after infancy when HbF expression wanes.[11] Second, rare patients with SCD or β-thalassemia who simultaneously harbor deletions leading to hereditary persistence of fetal hemoglobin (HPFH) are largely asymptomatic.[12] Decades later in the 1990s and early 2000s, the quantitative ameliorating effect of increased HbF was definitively established in large epidemiological studies of various β-thalassemia[13–17] and SCD[18–20] populations.

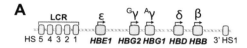

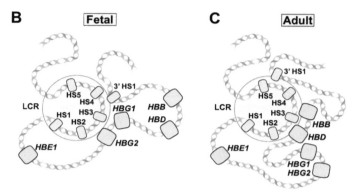

Fig. 1. LCR and β-globin gene cluster. (*A*) Schematic representation of the β-globin gene lo-cus. (*B, C*) Illustration of the physical looping of the LCR and its interaction with the pro-moter of the (*B*) *HBG1/2* genes for fetal hemoglobin and (*C*) *HBB* genes for adult hemoglobin at different stages of human development. *HBB*, hemoglobin subunit beta; *HBD*, hemoglobin subunit delta; *HBE1*, hemoglobin subunit epsilon 1; *HBG1/2*, hemoglobin subunit gamma 1/2; HS, DNAse 1-hypersensitive sites.

Indeed, enhanced HbF expression for β-thalassemia serves to reduce the globin chain imbalance as γ-globin can bind the excess α-chains to decrease inclusion body for-mation and hemolysis, thus improving erythropoiesis.[3,4] These findings spurred a longstanding and substantial interest in understanding regulation of the human fetal-to-adult hemoglobin switch for enabling therapeutic HbF induction.

A variety of findings during the 1980s provided further support for the therapeutic benefit of HbF induction and in the process highlighted the potential importance of DNA methylation and other epigenetic modifications in HbF switching. This started with the discovery that γ-globin genes are selectively silenced and methylated in adult, but not embryonic/fetal erythroid cells.[21] This motivated testing of various DNA hypo-methylating agents such as 5-azacytidine and decitabine in patients with β-thalas-semia[22] and SCD,[23,24] which reactivated HbF, at least in short-duration clinical studies. However, due to toxicity concerns, trials were halted and treatment courses remained limited. As 5-azacytidine is also a cell cycle S-phase inhibitor, it was reasoned that the observed HbF induction could be due to this effect.[24] This led to tri-als of hydroxyurea, which improved clinical parameters in SCD[25–27] and resulted in approval by the US Food and Drug Administration (FDA). However, hydroxyurea was not as effective for patients with β-thalassemia,[24] as the level of HbF induced is likely insufficient to counteract the globin imbalance present in this condition.

Around the same time, it was observed that infants born to diabetic mothers exhibit delayed HbF switching, which was attributed to elevated short-chain fatty acids.[28,29] Although small trials with hydroxybutyrate were encouraging,[30] larger trials showed inconsistent effectiveness.[31] As short-chain fatty acids behave as histone deacetylase (HDAC) inhibitors,[32] specific HDAC inhibitors are now under investigation for HbF in-duction.[33,34] More recently, mammalian target of rapamycin, phosphodiesterase 9, and 3,4-dihydroxyphenylalanine (DOPA) decarboxylase inhibitors were also in clinical trials for inducing HbF.[35] However, none of these nontargeted drugs offer lasting transfusion independence. In addition, the precise mechanistic links between the presumed mode of action of these agents and epigenetic changes that could modulate HbF expression remain unclear.

MOLECULAR REGULATION OF FETAL HEMOGLOBIN

For many years, direct molecular modulators of HbF remained elusive. Although master TFs, including GATA1, KLF1, and TAL1, influence HbF levels, they do not exhibit the requisite stage-specific expression or activity for regulating HbF switching and are known to have global roles in erythropoiesis and hematopoiesis.[5] As none of these factors appeared to be specific regulators of the HbF switch, the search continued.

The advent of genome-wide association studies (GWAS) in the mid-2000s empowered the effective study of naturally occurring human genetic variation and led to an important breakthrough. By applying this strategy to identify loci that regulate interindividual variation in HbF levels, a series of seminal studies identified common variation in three loci that account for a significant portion of the heritability of HbF, including the β-globin gene cluster, intergenic sequences between *HBS1L* and *MYB*, and a region within the gene *BCL11A*.[16,36–39]

BCL11A is a compelling hit as it is a TF that is not expressed in embryonic erythroid cells but is progressively turned on with the appearance of definitive adult erythroid cells.[40,41] Subsequently, a series of studies definitively established BCL11A as a repressor of HbF using a variety of genetic targeting strategies. Knockdown (KD) of *BCL11A* in primary human erythroid precursors[40] and knockout (KO) of *Bcl11a* in transgenic mice[42] leads to robust HbF induction without affecting erythropoiesis. Similarly, disruption of an erythroid-specific enhancer for *BCL11A* effectively increases HbF levels.[43,44] These findings were further strengthened with the discovery of patients with *BCL11A* haploinsufficiency, who present with a combination of neurodevelopmental abnormalities and significantly elevated HbF expression (**Fig. 2**).[45–47] Collectively, these studies strongly support *BCL11A* as a target for therapeutic HbF induction in β-hemoglobinopathies. As important proof of concept, erythroid-specific *Bcl11a* KO in SCD mice leads to normalization of red cell parameters.[48] This has paved the way for a variety of gene therapy and genome editing clinical trials that seek to suppress *BCL11A*, which have shown encouraging results.[35,49–51]

Although *BCL11A* targeting leads to effective HbF induction, it does not account for all *HBG1/2* silencing. Nearly a decade after the identification of *BCL11A*, a second TF and BCL11A-independent HbF repressor called ZBTB7A or LRF was identified.[52] Remarkably, single *BCL11A* or *ZBTB7A* KO in immortalized umbilical cord blood-derived erythroid progenitor (HUDEP) cell lines leads to ~40% to 50% HbF, whereas dual KO leads to ~90% to 100% HbF, at least in the context of this cell line model.[52] This suggests that BCL11A together with ZBTB7A and coregulators may mediate a significant extent of γ-globin transcriptional silencing in adult erythroid cells. Intriguingly, *BCL11A* and *ZBTB7A* genome editing in primary erythroid cells revealed that ZBTB7A may derepress *HBG1/2* beyond the typical degree observed in this setting, given the significant and disproportionate increase in *HBG1/2* relative to *HBB* silencing observed.[53] More clues about ZBTB7A-dependent HbF regulation can be gained from the study of human genetic variation. Recent work has resolved the DNA-binding domain of ZBTB7A complexed to DNA and showed that HPFH mutations might impair ZBTB7A-DNA interactions[54] to increase HbF levels.[55] Like *BCL11A*, rare patients with *de novo* heterozygous variants in *ZBTB7A* have also

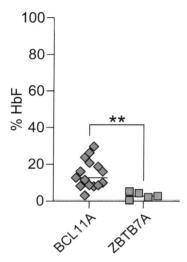

Fig. 2. HbF levels in individuals with heterozygous germline *BCL11A* and *ZBTB7A* mutations. Combined HbF levels from published patients with germline *BCL11A* and *ZBTB7A* variants as measured by high-performance liquid chromatography. Shaded region denotes the 0% to 1% reference range. One patient from[56] was excluded, as their HbF values were confounded by age (younger than 2 years of age). **P<.005.

recently been identified and they present with neurodevelopmental abnormalities and mildly elevated HbF levels.[56,57] Although germline *BCL11A* variants lead to markedly elevated HbF levels (median 13% HbF[45,46,58–60]), germline *ZBTB7A* variants appear to have a more modest effect on HbF levels (median 3% HbF[56,57]) (see **Fig. 2**). Collectively, these findings support *ZBTB7A* as a potential target for therapeutic HbF induction in the future, but also emphasize its more limited role in HbF silencing as compared with BCL11A *in vivo*, which appears to act as the primary physiologic regulator of hemoglobin switching.

Given the marked HbF induction conferred by *BCL11A* and *ZBTB7A* targeting, there is significant interest in uncovering the mechanism by which they repress the γ-globin gene to improve therapeutic efforts. Recent work has provided important insight into how this process is controlled. BCL11A and ZBTB7A directly bind unique regions in the γ-globin promoter,[55] with BCL11A selectively binding a distal TGACCA motif at approximately −115 bp[61] and ZBTB7A a GC-rich region at approximately −200 bp from the promoter (**Fig. 3**). BCL11A binding sterically hinders and displaces the binding of the *HBG1/2* NF-Y activator complex, which binds a −90 bp proximal region.[61] Both BCL11A and ZBTB7A independently associate with the nucleosome remodeling and deacetylase (NuRD) co-repressor complex to form BCL11A-NuRD and ZBTB7A-NuRD complexes and promote silencing.[40,43,52,62,63] BCL11A silencing additionally depends on interactions with other corepressors, including SIN3, SWI/SNF, NCoR/SMRT, LSD1/CoREST, and BCoR.[7,63] The altered chromatin organization that results from these interactions facilitates competitive LCR interactions with *HBB* over *HBG1/2* promoters[53] (see **Fig. 1**B, C). However, various aspects of this process remain to be identified, including factors that regulate BCL11A/ZBTB7A or NuRD/corepressor activity, as well as the precise mechanisms that are critical for *HBG1/2* silencing. Indeed, although these repressive cofactor interactions are likely to be important, long-range interactions might also have a critical role in enabling effective HbF silencing.[53]

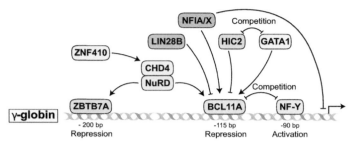

Fig. 3. Regulation of the γ-globin promoter. A simplified model of how the *HBG1/2* gene promoter is regulated. BCL11A and ZBTB7A independently associate with the NuRD/CHD4 complex and bind −115 bp and −200 bp of *HBG1/2*, respectively, to carry out repression. This process is modulated at various levels. The NuRD complex is negatively regulated by ZNF410. To bind *HBG1/2*, BCL11A must compete with the activator NF-Y, which binds −90 bp. BCL11A is additionally negatively regulated by LIN28B and HIC2, whereas NFIA/X promotes BCL11A expression. HIC2 itself is regulated by competition with GATA1 for BCL11A enhancers to regulate its expression. Not shown are other components of the NuRD complex, other corepressor and chromatin remodeling complexes that associate with BCL11A, and other positive and negative regulators of this process. Future studies are needed to clarify the relative quantitative importance of each of these pathways in HbF regulation *in vivo* in humans.

NEW REGULATORS OF FETAL HEMOGLOBIN

The combination of improved genome editing tools, the generation of the HUDEP1/2 transformed cell line in 2013,[64] and more effective tools to manipulate human CD34+ hematopoietic stem and progenitor cells (HSPCs) have empowered large-scale screening for and identification of additional potential HbF modulators in the past decade. These factors include RNA-binding proteins (RBPs), TFs, and epigenetic regulators. Here, we will review a few of these regulators that have been most effectively characterized.

RNA-Binding Factors: LIN28B

Posttranscriptional regulation of RNA stability, localization, splicing, modification, and translation is critical during ontogeny and is controlled by RBPs.[65] Indeed, a variety of RBPs belonging to the *let-7* miRNA pathway have been shown to act as posttranscriptional regulators of HbF, including LIN28B and IGF2BP1.[41,66,67] Overexpression of either RBP in adult erythroid cells leads to HbF induction. Recent work has clarified how LIN28B modulates HbF levels.[41] LIN28B exhibits developmental and stage-specific expression (fetal > newborn > adult) that is reciprocal to that of *BCL11A* (adult > newborn > fetal). It serves to directly bind *BCL11A* mRNA to impede its translation, independent of its effects on *let-7*, thus increasing HbF expression[41] (see **Fig. 3**). This represents one of the first demonstrations of posttranscriptional *BCL11A* regulation.

Transcription Factors: NFIA/X, HIC2

Trans-acting factors have long been appreciated for their role in regulating HbF.[6] Recent HUDEP-2 CRISPR (Clustered Regularly Interspaced Short Palindromic Repeats)/Cas9 screens have identified a variety of novel BCL11A regulators, including NFIA/X[68] and HIC2,[69] among others. Clues about their roles can be inferred from their pattern of expression, with NFIA/X following BCL11A (adult > newborn > fetal) and

HIC2 exhibiting reciprocal expression to BCL11A, analogous to LIN28B (fetal > newborn > adult). Accordingly, dual deletion of NFIA/X[68] and overexpression of HIC2[69] leads to reduced *BCL11A* expression and robust HbF induction in primary adult erythroblasts. These factors regulate *BCL11A* transcription through interaction with *BCL11A* enhancer elements,[43] with NFIA/X promoting expression by binding the +55, +58, +62 enhancers[68] and HIC2 repressing expression by competing with GATA1 for binding of the +55 enhancer by steric hindrance (see **Fig. 3**).[69] Regulation of these enhancer elements leads to changes in H3K27ac and chromatin accessibility, thus regulating *BCL11A* and HbF levels. Intriguingly, NFIA/X depletion may have therapeutic potential as this reactivates γ-globin in SCD patient-derived erythroblasts and reduces sickling.[68]

Epigenetic Regulators: ZNF410

As mentioned above, both BCL11A and ZBTB7A interact with the NuRD/CHD4 corepressor complex, and individual components of this complex are required for *HBG1/2* repression.[52,63,70] However, it is not known whether the NuRD complex is under direct regulation during HbF switching. Intriguingly, two recent CRISPR/Cas9 screens in HUDEP-2 have helped answer this question with the identification of a TF called ZNF410 that represses HbF.[71,72] Remarkably, ZNF410 only has a single transcriptional target, CHD4, and it selectively binds proximal and distal regulatory regions of *CHD4* to activate transcription (see **Fig. 3**). Deletion of *ZNF410* in HUDEP-2, primary adult erythroid cells, and mice leads to a significant increase in *HBG1/2* with a concurrent reduction in *HBB* and does not affect erythroid differentiation. As ZNF410 appears to be dispensable and only has a single target, it is a promising target for HbF reactivation in patients with β-hemoglobinopathies. Indeed, dual *BCL11A* and *ZNF410* KD in SCD and β-thalassemia patient-derived HSPCs lead to more HbF induction than with *BCL11A* KD alone and effectively reduces sickling and globin chain imbalance, respectively.[73]

Although the progress in identifying these and other new factors that might regulate switching has been exciting, there are often challenges extrapolating findings in cell lines or even in *in vitro* cultured primary cells to *in vivo* settings, emphasizing the need to continue to study *in vivo* diversity of HbF silencing in humans. With increased access to tools to study human biology and the increasing size of human genetic studies, there are tremendous opportunities to better understand the role these factors or others might play in HbF silencing. This is nicely illustrated by the case of ZBTB7A, which when haploinsufficient only mildly increases HbF expression *in vivo* in contrast to what is observed in cell models. In addition, the precise mechanisms of action for most of the HbF-associated genetic variation remains undefined and further studies are needed to connect variant-to-function at these loci.

CONCLUDING REMARKS

Since it was first observed that HbF could modify the clinical severity of β-thalassemia over 60 years ago, a massive amount of progress has been made toward identifying strategies that can therapeutically reactivate HbF. Although pharmacological strategies for HbF induction have historically seen limited efficacy for β-thalassemia patients, our improved understanding of how the β-globin gene cluster is regulated has now led to a variety of new HbF-inducing approaches actively being tested in clinical trials.[35]

Just 15 years ago, the study of natural human variation associated with HbF levels led to the discovery of BCL11A as a critical regulator of the fetal-to-adult hemoglobin switch.[40] Now, numerous gene therapy and genome editing clinical trials targeting *BCL11A* or γ-globin regulatory elements are already being tested in patients with β-thalassemia and SCD with very encouraging results. Rapidly advancing genomic and genome editing technologies and improved cellular and *in vivo* models will surely lead to an even finer dissection of HbF regulation. However, it is critical that these studies continue to examine the *in vivo* roles of specific nominated factors in humans when possible. In the coming decades, it is likely that patients with β-hemoglobinopathies will have a broad suite of therapeutic HbF induction options available to them, whether pharmacological or genetic, which will provide many with definitive cures.

CLINICS CARE POINTS

- Elevated fetal hemoglobin (HbF) levels can quantitatively ameliorate the severity of β-thalassemia
- BCL11A and ZBTB7A are two of the major repressors of HbF
- Gene therapies targeting BCL11A are currently undergoing clinical trials for patients with β-hemoglobinopathies and have led to effective and lasting HbF induction and transfusion independence
- Numerous novel HbF regulators are being identified and represent the next front as possible β-thalassemia treatment targets

DISCLOSURE

V.G. Sankaran serves as an advisor to and/or has equity in Branch Biosciences, Ensoma, Novartis, Forma, and Cellarity, all unrelated to the present work. The authors have no other competing interests to declare.

REFERENCES

1. Modell B, Darlison M. Global epidemiology of haemoglobin disorders and derived service indicators. Bull World Health Organ 2008;86(6):480–7.
2. Williams TN, Weatherall DJ. World distribution, population genetics, and health burden of the hemoglobinopathies. Cold Spring Harb Perspect Med 2012;2(9): a011692.
3. Sankaran VG, Nathan DG. Thalassemia: an overview of 50 years of clinical research. Hematol Oncol Clin North Am 2010;24(6):1005–20.
4. Taher AT, Musallam KM, Cappellini MD. beta-Thalassemias. N Engl J Med 2021; 384(8):727–43.
5. Orkin SH. MOLECULAR MEDICINE: Found in Translation. Med (N Y) 2021;2(2): 122–36.
6. Sankaran VG, Orkin SH. The switch from fetal to adult hemoglobin. Cold Spring Harb Perspect Med 2013;3(1):a011643.
7. Vinjamur DS, Bauer DE, Orkin SH. Recent progress in understanding and manipulating haemoglobin switching for the haemoglobinopathies. Br J Haematol 2018; 180(5):630–43.
8. Kato GJ, Piel FB, Reid CD, et al. Sickle cell disease. Nat Rev Dis Primers 2018;4: 18010.
9. Fessas P. Inclusions of hemoglobin erythroblasts and erythrocytes of thalassemia. Blood 1963;21:21–32.

10. Fessas P, Loukopoulos D, Thorell B. Absorption spectra of inclusion bodies in beta-thalassemia. Blood 1965;25:105–9.
11. Watson J. The significance of the paucity of sickle cells in newborn Negro infants. Am J Med Sci 1948;215(4):419–23.
12. Serjeant GR, Serjeant BE, Mason K. Heterocellular hereditary persistence of fetal haemoglobin and homozygous sickle-cell disease. Lancet 9 1977;1(8015):795–6.
13. Premawardhena A, Fisher CA, Olivieri NF, et al. Haemoglobin E beta thalassaemia in Sri Lanka. Lancet 2005;366(9495):1467–70.
14. Nuinoon M, Makarasara W, Mushiroda T, et al. A genome-wide association identified the common genetic variants influence disease severity in beta0-thalassemia/hemoglobin E. Hum Genet 2010;127(3):303–14.
15. Galanello R, Sanna S, Perseu L, et al. Amelioration of Sardinian beta0 thalassemia by genetic modifiers. Blood 2009;114(18):3935–7.
16. Uda M, Galanello R, Sanna S, et al. Genome-wide association study shows BCL11A associated with persistent fetal hemoglobin and amelioration of the phenotype of beta-thalassemia. Proc Natl Acad Sci U S A 2008;105(5):1620–5.
17. Musallam KM, Sankaran VG, Cappellini MD, et al. Fetal hemoglobin levels and morbidity in untransfused patients with beta-thalassemia intermedia. Blood 2012;119(2):364–7.
18. Platt OS, Thorington BD, Brambilla DJ, et al. Pain in sickle cell disease. Rates and risk factors. N Engl J Med 1991;325(1):11–6.
19. Platt OS, Brambilla DJ, Rosse WF, et al. Mortality in sickle cell disease. Life expectancy and risk factors for early death. N Engl J Med 1994;330(23):1639–44.
20. Castro O, Brambilla DJ, Thorington B, et al. The acute chest syndrome in sickle cell disease: incidence and risk factors. The Cooperative Study of Sickle Cell Disease. Blood 1994;84(2):643–9.
21. van der Ploeg LH, Flavell RA. DNA methylation in the human gamma delta beta-globin locus in erythroid and nonerythroid tissues. Cell 1980;19(4):947–58.
22. Ley TJ, DeSimone J, Anagnou NP, et al. 5-azacytidine selectively increases gamma-globin synthesis in a patient with beta+ thalassemia. N Engl J Med 1982;307(24):1469–75.
23. Ley TJ, DeSimone J, Noguchi CT, et al. 5-Azacytidine increases gamma-globin synthesis and reduces the proportion of dense cells in patients with sickle cell anemia. Blood 1983;62(2):370–80.
24. Musallam KM, Taher AT, Cappellini MD, et al. Clinical experience with fetal hemoglobin induction therapy in patients with beta-thalassemia. Blood 2013;121(12): 2199–212 [quiz: 2372].
25. Letvin NL, Linch DC, Beardsley GP, et al. Augmentation of fetal-hemoglobin production in anemic monkeys by hydroxyurea. N Engl J Med 1984;310(14):869–73.
26. Platt OS, Orkin SH, Dover G, et al. Hydroxyurea enhances fetal hemoglobin production in sickle cell anemia. J Clin Invest 1984;74(2):652–6.
27. Charache S, Terrin ML, Moore RD, et al. Effect of hydroxyurea on the frequency of painful crises in sickle cell anemia. Investigators of the Multicenter Study of Hydroxyurea in Sickle Cell Anemia. N Engl J Med 1995;332(20):1317–22.
28. Perrine SP, Greene MF, Faller DV. Delay in the fetal globin switch in infants of diabetic mothers. N Engl J Med 1985;312(6):334–8.
29. Bard H, Prosmanne J. Relative rates of fetal hemoglobin and adult hemoglobin synthesis in cord blood of infants of insulin-dependent diabetic mothers. Pediatrics 1985;75(6):1143–7.

30. Perrine SP, Ginder GD, Faller DV, et al. A short-term trial of butyrate to stimulate fetal-globin-gene expression in the beta-globin disorders. N Engl J Med 1993; 328(2):81–6.

31. Sher GD, Ginder GD, Little J, et al. Extended therapy with intravenous arginine butyrate in patients with beta-hemoglobinopathies. N Engl J Med 1995;332(24): 1606–10.

32. Fathallah H, Weinberg RS, Galperin Y, et al. Role of epigenetic modifications in normal globin gene regulation and butyrate-mediated induction of fetal hemoglobin. Blood 2007;110(9):3391–7.

33. Bradner JE, Mak R, Tanguturi SK, et al. Chemical genetic strategy identifies histone deacetylase 1 (HDAC1) and HDAC2 as therapeutic targets in sickle cell disease. Proc Natl Acad Sci U S A 2010;107(28):12617–22.

34. Mettananda S, Yasara N, Fisher CA, et al. Synergistic silencing of alpha-globin and induction of gamma-globin by histone deacetylase inhibitor, vorinostat as a potential therapy for beta-thalassaemia. Sci Rep 2019;9(1):11649.

35. Langer AL, Esrick EB. beta-Thalassemia: evolving treatment options beyond transfusion and iron chelation. Hematol Am Soc Hematol Educ Program 2021; 2021(1):600–6.

36. Menzel S, Garner C, Gut I, et al. A QTL influencing F cell production maps to a gene encoding a zinc-finger protein on chromosome 2p15. Nat Genet 2007; 39(10):1197–9.

37. Thein SL, Menzel S, Peng X, et al. Intergenic variants of HBS1L-MYB are responsible for a major quantitative trait locus on chromosome 6q23 influencing fetal hemoglobin levels in adults. Proc Natl Acad Sci U S A 2007;104(27):11346–51.

38. Lettre G, Sankaran VG, Bezerra MA, et al. DNA polymorphisms at the BCL11A, HBS1L-MYB, and beta-globin loci associate with fetal hemoglobin levels and pain crises in sickle cell disease. Proc Natl Acad Sci U S A 2008;105(33): 11869–74.

39. Galarneau G, Palmer CD, Sankaran VG, et al. Fine-mapping at three loci known to affect fetal hemoglobin levels explains additional genetic variation. Nat Genet 2010;42(12):1049–51.

40. Sankaran VG, Menne TF, Xu J, et al. Human fetal hemoglobin expression is regulated by the developmental stage-specific repressor BCL11A. Science 2008; 322(5909):1839–42.

41. Basak A, Munschauer M, Lareau CA, et al. Control of human hemoglobin switching by LIN28B-mediated regulation of BCL11A translation. Nat Genet 2020;52(2): 138–45.

42. Sankaran VG, Xu J, Ragoczy T, et al. Developmental and species-divergent globin switching are driven by BCL11A. Nature 2009;460(7259):1093–7.

43. Bauer DE, Kamran SC, Lessard S, et al. An erythroid enhancer of BCL11A subject to genetic variation determines fetal hemoglobin level. Science 2013; 342(6155):253–7.

44. Canver MC, Smith EC, Sher F, et al. BCL11A enhancer dissection by Cas9-mediated in situ saturating mutagenesis. Nature 2015;527(7577):192–7.

45. Basak A, Hancarova M, Ulirsch JC, et al. BCL11A deletions result in fetal hemoglobin persistence and neurodevelopmental alterations. J Clin Invest 2015; 125(6):2363–8.

46. Dias C, Estruch SB, Graham SA, et al. BCL11A Haploinsufficiency Causes an Intellectual Disability Syndrome and Dysregulates Transcription. Am J Hum Genet 2016;99(2):253–74.

47. Shen Y, Li R, Teichert K, et al. Pathogenic BCL11A variants provide insights into the mechanisms of human fetal hemoglobin silencing. Plos Genet 2021;17(10): e1009835.

48. Xu J, Peng C, Sankaran VG, et al. Correction of sickle cell disease in adult mice by interference with fetal hemoglobin silencing. Science 2011;334(6058):993–6.

49. Frangoul H, Altshuler D, Cappellini MD, et al. CRISPR-Cas9 Gene Editing for Sickle Cell Disease and beta-Thalassemia. N Engl J Med 21 2021;384(3):252–60.

50. Esrick EB, Lehmann LE, Biffi A, et al. Posttranscriptional Genetic Silencing of BCL11A to Treat Sickle Cell Disease. N Engl J Med 2021;384(3):205–15.

51. Fu B, Liao J, Chen S, et al. CRISPR-Cas9-mediated gene editing of the BCL11A enhancer for pediatric beta(0)/beta(0) transfusion-dependent beta-thalassemia. Nat Med 2022;28(8):1573–80.

52. Masuda T, Wang X, Maeda M, et al. Transcription factors LRF and BCL11A independently repress expression of fetal hemoglobin. Science 2016;351(6270): 285–9.

53. Shen Y, Verboon JM, Zhang Y, et al. A unified model of human hemoglobin switching through single-cell genome editing. Nat Commun 2021;12(1):4991.

54. Yang Y, Ren R, Ly LC, et al. Structural basis for human ZBTB7A action at the fetal globin promoter. Cell Rep 2021;36(13):109759.

55. Martyn GE, Wienert B, Yang L, et al. Natural regulatory mutations elevate the fetal globin gene via disruption of BCL11A or ZBTB7A binding. Nat Genet 2018;50(4): 498–503.

56. Ohishi A, Masunaga Y, Iijima S, et al. De novo ZBTB7A variant in a patient with macrocephaly, intellectual disability, and sleep apnea: implications for the phenotypic development in 19p13.3 microdeletions. J Hum Genet 2020;65(2):181–6.

57. von der Lippe C, Tveten K, Prescott TE, et al. Heterozygous variants in ZBTB7A cause a neurodevelopmental disorder associated with symptomatic overgrowth of pharyngeal lymphoid tissue, macrocephaly, and elevated fetal hemoglobin. Am J Med Genet A 2022;188(1):272–82.

58. Funnell AP, Prontera P, Ottaviani V, et al. 2p15-p16.1 microdeletions encompassing and proximal to BCL11A are associated with elevated HbF in addition to neurologic impairment. Blood 2015;126(1):89–93.

59. Yoshida M, Nakashima M, Okanishi T, et al. Identification of novel BCL11A variants in patients with epileptic encephalopathy: Expanding the phenotypic spectrum. Clin Genet 2018;93(2):368–73.

60. Wessels MW, Cnossen MH, van Dijk TB, et al. Molecular analysis of the erythroid phenotype of a patient with BCL11A haploinsufficiency. Blood Adv 2021;5(9): 2339–49.

61. Liu N, Hargreaves VV, Zhu Q, et al. Direct Promoter Repression by BCL11A Controls the Fetal to Adult Hemoglobin Switch. Cell 2018;173(2):430–442 e17.

62. Xu J, Sankaran VG, Ni M, et al. Transcriptional silencing of {gamma}-globin by BCL11A involves long-range interactions and cooperation with SOX6. Genes Dev 2010;24(8):783–98.

63. Xu J, Bauer DE, Kerenyi MA, et al. Corepressor-dependent silencing of fetal hemoglobin expression by BCL11A. Proc Natl Acad Sci U S A 2013;110(16): 6518–23.

64. Kurita R, Suda N, Sudo K, et al. Establishment of immortalized human erythroid progenitor cell lines able to produce enucleated red blood cells. PLoS One 2013;8(3):e59890.

65. Gebauer F, Schwarzl T, Valcarcel J, et al. RNA-binding proteins in human genetic disease. Nat Rev Genet 2021;22(3):185–98.

66. Lee YT, de Vasconcellos JF, Yuan J, et al. LIN28B-mediated expression of fetal hemoglobin and production of fetal-like erythrocytes from adult human erythroblasts ex vivo. Blood 2013;122(6):1034–41.
67. de Vasconcellos JF, Tumburu L, Byrnes C, et al. IGF2BP1 overexpression causes fetal-like hemoglobin expression patterns in cultured human adult erythroblasts. Proc Natl Acad Sci U S A 2017;114(28):E5664–72. https://doi.org/10.1073/pnas. 160955211.
68. Qin K, Huang P, Feng R, et al. Dual function NFI factors control fetal hemoglobin silencing in adult erythroid cells. Nat Genet 2022;54(6):874–84.
69. Huang P, Peslak SA, Ren R, et al. HIC2 controls developmental hemoglobin switching by repressing BCL11A transcription. Nat Genet 2022;54(9):1417–26.
70. Sher F, Hossain M, Seruggia D, et al. Rational targeting of a NuRD subcomplex guided by comprehensive in situ mutagenesis. Nat Genet 2019;51(7):1149–59.
71. Lan X, Ren R, Feng R, et al. ZNF410 Uniquely Activates the NuRD Component CHD4 to Silence Fetal Hemoglobin Expression. Mol Cell 2021;81(2):239–254 e8.
72. Vinjamur DS, Yao Q, Cole MA, et al. ZNF410 represses fetal globin by singular control of CHD4. Nat Genet 2021;53(5):719–28.
73. Liu B, Brendel C, Vinjamur DS, et al. Development of a double shmiR lentivirus effectively targeting both BCL11A and ZNF410 for enhanced induction of fetal hemoglobin to treat beta-hemoglobinopathies. Mol Ther 2022;30(8):2693–708.

Clinical Classification, Screening, and Diagnosis in Beta-Thalassemia and Hemoglobin E/Beta-Thalassemia

Morgan Pines, MD[a,b], Sujit Sheth, MD[a,*]

KEYWORDS

- Wide spectrum of disease • Major • Intermedia • Transfusion dependent
- Diagnostic algorithm • At-risk population screening

KEY POINTS

- The spectrum of disease in beta-thalassemia is wide as a result of the differences in genotype as well as other modifying factors.
- The previous classification of beta-thalassemia categorized individuals as having thalassemia major (severe genotype, usually transfusion dependent), thalassemia intermedia (less severe genotype, usually not transfusion dependent), and thalassemia minor (carriers).
- However, because the genotype/phenotype correlation was imperfect, and the clinical spectrum was variable, more recently individuals are being more broadly separated by transfusion status, as either transfusion dependent or non-transfusion-dependent.
- Evaluation for beta-thalassemia relies on red cell parameters on the complete blood count (CBC), and hemoglobin fractionation, with definitive genetic diagnostic testing recommended where possible for a clearer prediction of severity and course.
- Screening of individuals at risk is based on a composite picture including ethnicity or family history, CBC and hemoglobin fractionation, and genetic testing and counseling when indicated. Screening allows for earlier diagnosis and management in affected individuals while avoiding unnecessary and potentially harmful iron supplementation in both affected individuals and carriers.

INTRODUCTION

"Beta-thalassemia" is the general name given to a group of disorders which result from quantitative mutations in the beta-globin gene, including compound

The authors have no conflicts or commercial interests to disclose related to this work.

[a] Division of Pediatric Hematology/Oncology, Department of Pediatrics, Weill Cornell Medicine, P-695, 525 East 68th Street, New York, NY 10065, USA; [b] Department of Pediatrics, Memorial Sloan Kettering Cancer Center, 1275 York Avenue, H1117A, New York, NY 10065, USA
* Corresponding author.
E-mail address: shethsu@med.cornell.edu

Hematol Oncol Clin N Am 37 (2023) 313–325
https://doi.org/10.1016/j.hoc.2022.12.003
0889-8588/23/© 2022 Elsevier Inc. All rights reserved.

heterozygotes for hemoglobin E (HbE). The spectrum of disease is wide and clinical manifestations range from a complete lack of symptoms in individuals with beta-thalassemia trait to lifelong transfusion dependence in those with the most severe forms of the disease. Over the years, the terminology used to classify individuals has changed to be more descriptive and accommodate the nonstatic nature of the disease severity. The accurate diagnosis of these conditions has become easier in the developed world, with genetic testing providing a basis for classification and prognostication as well. Further, as the global burden of disease has changed over time, including as a result of increased immigration from parts of the world to areas where these conditions were infrequently found, the need for screening and early diagnosis has become more pressing. All of these topics are discussed in this article.

CLINICAL CLASSIFICATION

The epidemiology and molecular basis of beta-thalassemia have been described in detail in Soterios Soteriades and colleagues' article, "The Need for Translational Epidemiology in Beta Thalassaemia Syndromes: A Thalassaemia International Federation Perspective"; and Nicolò Tesio and Daniel Bauer's article, "Molecular Basis and Genetic Modifiers of Thalassemia," in this issue. Of the over 300 mutations described in the beta-globin gene, some are defined as β^+, and others as β^0 mutations, reflecting some or no production of beta-globin respectively.[1] Compound heterozygotes with one beta-thalassemia mutation and the other a HbE mutation are also included in the beta-thalassemias.

Clinical manifestations of the disease include anemia of variable severity, and complications related to the disease itself, bony changes, and osteopenia, extramedullary hematopoiesis, vascular disease, etc., and those related to the treatment, mainly iron overload and its sequelae.[2] These are described elsewhere in Rayan Bou-Fakhredin and colleagues' article, "Clinical Complications and Their Management," in this issue.

The most widely used classification defined individuals based on their genotype AND the degree of anemia and the need for transfusions (**Table 1**). It is important to keep in mind that the genotype-to-phenotype correlation is not perfect, and individuals with the same genotype, may have different severity of anemia, and thus if the disease as a whole.[3]

Table 1
Classification of beta-thalassemia

Syndrome	Genotype	Hematology	Disease Severity
Thalassemia major	β^0/β^0	• Complete absence of Hb A • Severe anemia requiring transfusions from infancy	• *TD* • Lifelong supportive care required
Thalassemia intermedia	β^+/β^+ or β^0/β^+ HbE/β^0 or HbE/β^+	• Diminished production of Hb A • Mild to moderate anemia	• *NTD* • May need occasional transfusions or may become *TD* • Significant variability in disease severity
Thalassemia minor	β^+/β or β^0/β	• Mild or no anemia	• *NTD* • May be asymptomatic

Abbreviations: NTD, non-transfusion dependent; TD, transfusion dependent.

At the mild end of the spectrum were individuals with thalassemia minor. These were individuals with one normal copy of the beta-globin gene who had lifelong mild anemia, with no need for transfusions, and no complications of the disease. Transfusion-dependent patients were classified as thalassemia major and included the most severe genotype with both mutations being β^0 mutations. These individuals typically began transfusions in the first year or two of life and required lifelong transfusion support.[4] However, there are many beta-globin mutations that are deemed "β^0-like," where the amount of beta-globin produced is very small, and these individuals would thus have more severe anemia and be more likely to need regular transfusions. As implied in the name, individuals with thalassemia major had the most clinical burden of the disease and its complications. Individuals were classified as thalassemia intermedia if they had less severe mutations, including a beta-plus or HbE mutations, and had moderate anemia, not requiring regular transfusions. These individuals may have required episodic or periodic transfusions, usually during periods of "stress," such is infections, perioperatively, or during pregnancy. There was also marked heterogeneity in clinical severity and manifestations of the disease itself as well as complications.[5,6]

However, the disease is not static, but often does progress over time (**Fig. 1**). With worsening anemia, potentially related to changes in the bone marrow iron content, or worsening splenomegaly and the development of hypersplenism, an individual who was initially transfusion independent, could become transfusion dependent, with all of the attendant complications. The classification would then become somewhat challenging because the genotype would still be intermediate but being clinically more severe, would have "major" disease.

Hence, it has become more common now to broaden the classification to only account for transfusion status and not define a genotype. Thus, individuals would be divided as having transfusion-dependent thalassemia (TDT) or non-transfusion-dependent thalassemia (NTDT). Similarly, the genotypic classification of beta-thalassemia and HbE/beta-thalassemia has been changed to two broad categories, β^0/β^0 thalassemia and non- β^0/β^0 thalassemia, with the latter category including compound heterozygotes for HbE and β^0 or β^+ mutations. Many of the more recent clinical trials have used the clinical classification to broadly divide subjects as TDT and NTDT, with subanalyses being performed based on the modified genotype status, that is, β^0/β^0 and non- β^0/β^0.

Screening for Beta-Thalassemia and Hemoglobin E Beta-Thalassemia

Screening for beta-thalassemia is complex and very relevant because of the changing prevalence of the disease in areas where this is not common and thus not recognized as it should be for appropriate intervention and management. Anemia is a very

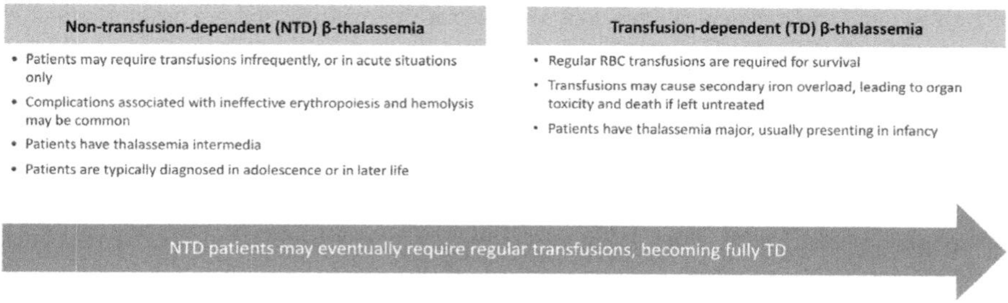

Non-transfusion-dependent (NTD) β-thalassemia	Transfusion-dependent (TD) β-thalassemia
• Patients may require transfusions infrequently, or in acute situations only	• Regular RBC transfusions are required for survival
• Complications associated with ineffective erythropoiesis and hemolysis may be common	• Transfusions may cause secondary iron overload, leading to organ toxicity and death if left untreated
• Patients have thalassemia intermedia	• Patients have thalassemia major, usually presenting in infancy
• Patients are typically diagnosed in adolescence or in later life	

NTD patients may eventually require regular transfusions, becoming fully TD

Fig. 1. Changing spectrum of disease in beta-thalassemia.

common diagnosis, and in the case of microcytic anemias, establishing the underlying pathology of the anemia is important to provide the correct treatment.

Why should we screen?

Screening for beta-thalassemia is important in three scenarios: (i) when the individual is anemic, to establish the correct diagnosis and therefore institute the correct management of anemia, (ii) for prenatal counseling for carrier parents at risk of having a child with the disease, and (iii) newborn screening for early diagnosis.[7]

Thalassemia carriers, and often those with mild thalassemia intermedia, are commonly misdiagnosed with iron deficiency anemia, and often receive prolonged courses of iron therapy, including occasional parenteral supplementation as well. Appropriate screening would prevent the unnecessary use of iron in carriers and prevent sequelae and chronic complications of iatrogenic iron overload in those with thalassemia intermedia.[8,9]

Prenatal screening can be used to identify adult carriers even before they have started families of their own. For known carriers, screening of partners leads to prenatal risk assessment and informs family planning counseling.[10] Pregnant women diagnosed with thalassemia trait should have partner screening to assess fetal risk, particularly for fetuses with the most severe form β^0/β^0 thalassemia, and receive education and counseling.[11]

Newborn screening programs allow early identification of affected infants, who can be monitored closely for the development of anemia, and start transfusions at the appropriate time, minimizing the risk for complications.[12]

Who should we screen?

1. Individuals should be screened based on demographics and personal and family history

   Adults and children of Asian, African, or Mediterranean ancestry, with a family history of thalassemia, family history of lifelong anemia, and those with a personal history of microcytic anemia unresponsive to iron supplementation, or microcytic anemia without iron deficiency, should all be screened for thalassemia.[7]

2. Prospective parents who should have Prenatal Screening

   The American College of Obstetrics and Gynecology (ACOG) recognizes that individuals with African, Mediterranean, and Southeast Asian ancestry are at increased risk for having mutations in alpha- and beta-globin genes predisposing to hemoglobinopathies including sickle cell and thalassemia.[11] With immigration patterns changing the prevalence of thalassemia in the United States, and with the more widespread mixing of populations, limiting screening to these ancestries may not be sufficient, and broader guidelines are necessary.[13]

   Prospective mothers who are identified as thalassemia carriers should have their partners screened, and if the pregnancy is at risk, the couple should receive prenatal genetic testing with counseling. Couples who are both thalassemia carriers can be offered in vitro fertilization and preimplantation genetic diagnosis.[11] For expectant parents, antepartum genetic testing can be offered before delivery along with counseling.[14]

3. Newborns

   At-risk newborns should be screened for thalassemia syndromes at birth.[15] This poses many technical challenges because the current methodology used for newborn hemoglobinopathy screening (mandated in all 50 states in the United States) is specifically designed to detect sickle hemoglobin.[16] The most severe form of beta-thalassemia, β^0/β^0 thalassemia could be diagnosed by the complete absence of HbA on the newborn screen. Less severe forms of beta-thalassemia, such as β^0/β^+ or β^+/β^+ could also be detected, but not usually the trait. Hb E/β^0 or HbE/β^+ thalassemia may be picked up as well, by the presence of HbE and low to absent HbA. In regions where thalassemia is more common, particularly in Asia, implementing newborn screening methodology to be able to detect thalassemia would be an important strategy for early diagnosis, counseling, and regular comprehensive care where appropriate. Technical and financial issues could be major impediments to the effective implementation of such programs.

4. Infants

The American Academy of Pediatrics (AAP) had a long-standing recommendation for screening all infants at 9 months of age with a hemoglobin/hematocrit (most often a finger-stick assessment), primarily with the intent of diagnosing iron deficiency early and instituting iron supplementation.[17] This remains important for breastfed infants. The iron-fortified formula is now the norm, and screening done at 12 months of age for formula-fed infants is not likely to show anemia. Severe, β^0/β^0 thalassemia, usually presents well before this age with progressive anemia and other clinical manifestations. However, more intermediate forms, including β^+/β^+ beta-thalassemia, HbE/β^0 or HbE/β^+ thalassemia may have few clinical manifestations besides mild to moderate anemia, and may be missed until the 9- to 12-month hemoglobin/hematocrit is done. Screening these infants would be important to establish a diagnosis, preclude unnecessary iron supplementation, and begin monitoring and comprehensive care to optimize outcomes and minimize morbidity.

How should we screen?

1. Newborn thalassemia screening

With the high prevalence and wide distribution of hemoglobinopathies, particularly sickle cell anemia, testing for these was incorporated into the newborn screen.[16] The normal newborn at term has ~80% to 90% HbF, and 10% to 20% HbA, with trace amounts of other hemoglobins such as HbA2, which are typically not reported.

Fetuses with β^0/β^0 mutations will produce no HbA and will have only HbF on newborn screen, only otherwise seen in extreme prematurity, where β-globin expression has not yet begun. Thus, gestational age is an important consideration and normal ranges should be established at various gestational ages for easier interpretation. Fetuses with one β^0-mutation and one β^+-mutation or two β^+-mutations (ie, non-β^0/β^0 thalassemia) will have some HbA on the newborn screen. If this is quantified, it is lower than the normal range–approximately 3% to 5% and may be flagged as possible beta-thalassemia.[7] Individuals with β^0/HbE may have no HbA, and only have HbF and HbE, whereas those with β^+/HbE will have some HbA in addition to the HbF and HbE. HbA2, which is elevated in carriers, is produced in very small quantities in the fetus (0.5%) and is not typically reported on the newborn screen.[5,18]

Newborn Screening in the United States.

There is currently no standard for thalassemia newborn screening across the United States, and recommendations for testing vary from state to state.[16] The AAP reviewed newborn hemoglobinopathy screening across 50 states in 2017. Thirty-one states had reporting and recommendations beyond sickle cell screening.[8] Five of the 31 states recommended hemoglobin electrophoresis and four recommended hematology referral. These could identify individuals with some forms of beta-thalassemia. Only one recommends initial genetic testing for a possible thalassemia screen. The other 19 states do not have beta-thalassemia screening recommendations. Twelve of these

19 states reported alpha thalassemia trait with no additional follow-up guideline and seven did not report alpha thalassemia or carrier status at all.

Another study from 2018 of the 53 newborn screening programs, including the 50 US states, the District of Columbia, Guam and Puerto Rico showed that all 46 of the programs that responded had at least one form of screening for beta-thalassemia.[12] Nine of these programs do one-step testing, whereas 37 did two-step testing. Additionally, many of these newborn screening programs also tested for HbE.

Initial newborn screening in most states is performed by high-performance liquid chromatography (HPLC) or Isoelectric focusing (IEF) on a spot of blood. These tests detect hemoglobin variants and may provide limited data to support the diagnosis of thalassemia syndrome. HPLC, either by cation exchange or reverse phase, quantifies hemoglobin variants such as Hemoglobin A, A2, F, S, H, and Barts.[19] However, different hemoglobin variants may co-elute on hemoglobin electrophoresis, making it difficult to distinguish one variant from another. Thus, HPLC is used for initial screening and is followed by a confirmatory test, either IEF or molecular testing.[12] IEF is more labor-intensive but identifies and quantifies hemoglobin variants more precisely than standard hemoglobin electrophoresis.[8] Molecular testing includes polymerase chain reaction (PCR)-based testing or DNA sequencing.[5] Allele-specific PCR-based methods are used to detect point mutations in alpha and beta-globin genes. Gap PCR is used to detect deletions, alpha duplications, deletional hemoglobin variants.[5] DNA sequencing is more expensive and more comprehensive and can be used to diagnose previously unidentified mutations.[5]

2. Thalassemia Screening in Children and adults

Prospectively screening all individuals with anemia for thalassemia is neither cost-effective nor indicated, since iron deficiency is relatively much more common and explains microcytic anemia. However, establishing the diagnosis of thalassemia trait is relevant, and avoidance of unnecessary iron supplementation is important from an individual and public health standpoint. It is also important to correctly diagnose individuals with an intermediate severity thalassemia syndrome, who have anemia, ineffective erythropoiesis, and complications that could be prevented if comprehensive care is provided early.[5]

Screening for thalassemia is recommended in the following situations:

a. Family history of thalassemia—trait or disease
b. Microcytic anemia with a negative history of iron deficiency-adequate dietary iron intake, absence of blood loss
c. Persistent microcytic anemia despite an adequate trial of supplemental iron

Definitive diagnostic testing of such individuals can be approached in a stepwise manner (**Fig. 2**).

3. Prenatal screening

The ACOG recommends that women with a low MCV should have a serum ferritin assessment. Those with normal levels and microcytic anemia should have hemoglobin fractionation testing (by HPLC or electrophoresis).[11] Women with increased Hemoglobin A2 (HbA2), with or without an increase in fetal hemoglobin (HbF), are diagnosed as having beta-thalassemia trait. Those with HbE and HbA would have the HbE trait, and those with HbE and no HbA would have HbE disease, and all of these women's partners should have tested, in case the partner carries a beta-thalassemia mutation. In each situation, partner testing is key to determining fetal risk and is based on

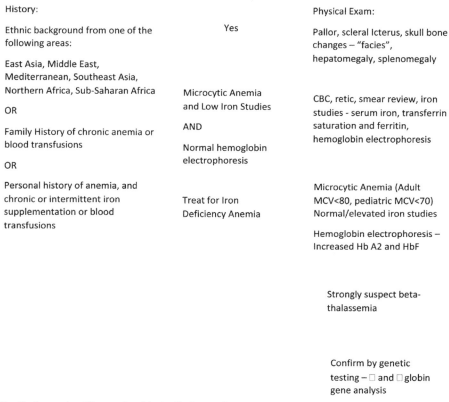

Fig. 2. Screening/diagnosis of beta-thalassemia.

hemoglobin fractionation or genetic testing as appropriate for beta- and alpha-thalassemia.[10] Couples who are both identified as carriers should receive genetic counseling to determine the risk of an affected fetus, and family decision support should be provided. Prenatal screening would identify the at-risk fetus and amniocentesis or chorionic villus sampling would confirm the diagnosis.[2,20] For women who are identified as having beta-thalassemia trait or sickle cell trait (based on finding sickle hemoglobin, HbS, and HbA on hemoglobin fractionation), partner hemoglobin characterization is imperative to assess fetal risk for beta-thalassemia or sickle cell disease (HbS-beta thal).[10]

Preimplantation genetic testing

The ACOG recommends preconception genetic testing and counseling for couples at high risk for thalassemia as noted.[11] In vitro fertilization and preimplantation genetic diagnosis can be offered to couples interested in avoiding elective termination.[11] For couples where both partners carry at-risk traits, and who were not identified as carriers before pregnancy, DNA testing via chronic villus sampling (CVS) or amniocentesis should be offered. Counseling should be offered in all such situations. This approach has resulted in a major reduction in the birth rate of infants with thalassemia throughout the Mediterranean region and the Middle East and in parts of the Indian subcontinent and Southeast Asia.[21] Novel approaches continue to be explored in an attempt to avoid the use of invasive procedures like CVS and amniocentesis, including harvesting fetal DNA from fetal cells in maternal blood or in maternal plasma.[21–24]

Suggested approach for screening of individuals at risk, all ages. As the demographics and epidemiology of thalassemia continue to change globally and in the United States, a comprehensive approach to early diagnosis will improve the health of patients and minimize risk. We would suggest the following, starting with preconceptions, and through adulthood:

1. Screening and identification of thalassemia carrier status and counseling early for all prospective mothers at risk based on ethnicity, family history, past medical history, and laboratory parameters. Confirmatory genetic testing of both partners and genetic counseling must be offered, and if available, preimplantation genetic diagnosis when appropriate.

2. If a pregnancy has already occurred in a mother at risk, the same screening tests should be performed, and if the thalassemia trait is confirmed as described previously, partner testing and genetic counseling are indicated. Testing of the fetus should be offered if both parents are carriers or if the father's status cannot be ascertained. More advanced techniques such as fetal DNA in maternal blood need to be tested more extensively to avoid more invasive testing procedures.[21] If the fetus is found to be affected, appropriate counseling should be provided.

3. Newborn screening should be standardized to include hemoglobin characterization and fractionation for all. Ideally, as genetic testing becomes more widely available, less expensive, and technically easier to perform, moving testing to a genome/exome or chip technology platform would be most effective in definitively identifying individuals with thalassemia. We recognize this may not be an approach with wide feasibility and application. Until such universal genetic testing can be performed, we recommend the optimal strategy of performing hemoglobin electrophoresis, HPLC, or IEF on all infants and reporting the hemoglobin variants, especially HbBarts and unstable hemoglobin variants, as well as quantifying HbA. Additions to the newborn screen are justified if a treatment introduced early would reduce morbidity and mortality. For thalassemia, this remains controversial and prospective data showing the benefits of this approach could provide a rationale.

4. We recommend screening all individuals (adults and children) with appropriate histories, certain physical exam findings, and microcytic anemia for thalassemia using the algorithm in **Fig. 2**.

Diagnosis of Beta-Thalassemia and Hemoglobin E Beta-Thalassemia

The early and complete diagnosis of beta-thalassemia is important for many reasons. It facilitates early intervention, preventing the development of complications, and avoids inappropriate treatments which could potentially be harmful. The diagnosis of the more severe forms of thalassemia, homozygous or compound heterozygous β-thalassemia is relatively straightforward. However, in milder phenotypes, it may be somewhat more nuanced. The essential elements of the diagnostic workup are shown in **Fig. 2**, and include the history, including family history and ethnicity, clinical features, and laboratory testing, including specific beta-globin gene analysis. With the easy availability of sophisticated DNA testing in the developed world, including whole exome or genome sequencing, it is now possible to characterize the disease more completely, including all of the possible genetic modifiers.[25] This forms the basis for a thorough characterization of all of the genotypes described in this section and offers some predictive insights into the clinical manifestation and future course. Although this is not routinely done for all patients, especially those with mild clinical manifestations, in more complex cases, it may be used to explain the clinical picture. The description below is tiered based on the severity of the syndrome, but the assessment of the history is the same. It is important to think about thalassemia in individuals whose ethnic origins are from the thalassemia belt, but with the increasing integration of ethnic communities, this is often not exclusive.

Homozygous β^0 thalassemia (β^0/β^0)

Individuals with the most severe forms of β thalassemia present in infancy with anemia. In the developed world, with better access to care, these infants may not progress to severe anemia or heart failure. In the developing world, infants are often profoundly anemic at diagnosis, with hemoglobin levels in the 2 to 4 g/dL range.[5] The clinical picture has elements of anemia, hepatosplenomegaly as a result of extramedullary hematopoiesis, and bone deformities to a variable extent from erythroid marrow expansion, depending on the age and severity of the genotype. The white cell and platelet counts, as well as the reticulocyte count, are all elevated, as a result of the marked marrow hyperplasia. Microcytosis and anisopoikilocytosis, hypochromia, target cells, nucleated red cells, and basophilic stippling are reported on peripheral smear examination. Red cell survival is markedly shortened, but there is some variability with cells containing more fetal hemoglobin, surviving longer. Characterization of the hemoglobin fractions by HPLC or hemoglobin electrophoresis shows no Hb A in β^0 homozygotes, with Hb F comprising the majority of the Hb, and a relative increase in Hb A_2 as a proportion of total hemoglobin. Serum iron and transferrin saturation are elevated, as is ferritin level, thus ruling out iron deficiency anemia as a cause for the microcytic, hypochromic anemia.

Although a bone marrow examination is not required for diagnosis, if performed, it shows marked erythroid hyperplasia with a maturation arrest, stippling, and inclusions in the red cell precursors, as well as increased iron content.

Homozygous or compound heterozygous β^+ thalassemia (β^+/β^0, β^+/β^+, HbE/β^0, or HbE/β^+)

At diagnosis, the hemoglobin levels are generally higher, but otherwise, the hematologic changes are similar to those with homozygous β^0 thalassemia. Clinical features include pallor, hepatosplenomegaly, and bone changes to varying degrees. In individuals with more severe anemia, the peripheral smear resembles that of β thalassemia major patient before starting transfusions, as noted above. HPLC shows a variable amount of Hb A depending on the mutations, and the rest is Hb F and A_2. If there is compound heterozygosity for Hb E, then this hemoglobin is also seen. In the absence of transfusions, iron studies will show a steady rise in serum iron, transferrin saturation, and ferritin, the rate of rise determined by the degree of ineffective erythropoiesis and thus increased intestinal absorption. Examination of the bone marrow, if performed, would confirm a variable degree of ineffective erythropoiesis, with hyperproliferation and some maturational arrest, as with more severe patients.

Heterozygous β thalassemia (β thalassemia trait, β/β^0 or β/β^+)

Individuals with one normal β globin gene do not have any clinical features. The classic picture of β-thalassemia minor is a mild microcytic anemia, with hemoglobin levels in the range from 9 to 11 g/dL, and mean corpuscular volume (MCV) values between 50 to 70 fL.[5] The red cell count is usually normal or elevated. The bone marrow in heterozygous β-thalassemia (not needed for diagnosis) shows slight erythroid hyperplasia with rare red cell inclusions. A mild degree of ineffective erythropoiesis is noted, but red cell survival is normal or nearly normal. On HPLC, the Hb A_2 level is increased to 3.5% to 7%. HbF is elevated in approximately 50% of cases, usually to 1% to 3%

and rarely to greater than 5%. Iron studies are normal, unless concomitant iron deficiency is also present, in which case the transferrin saturation and ferritin are low. In this situation, the hemoglobin is lower, as are the red cell indices, and the red cell count.

β-thalassemia with normal A₂ level

In some rare forms of β-thalassemia, heterozygotes have normal Hb A_2 levels. The hematologic picture may be completely normal or have a mild microcytic anemia with a normal hemoglobin pattern on electrophoresis or HPLC. These individuals may be misdiagnosed as having 2 gene deleted α-thalassemia and may cause difficulties in genetic counseling and prenatal diagnosis. Based on hematologic studies, two main classes of "normal Hb A_2 β-thalassemia" —sometimes called types 1 and 2—are seen.[26] Type 1 is the "silent" form of β-thalassemia. Type 2 is heterogeneous, with many cases representing the compound heterozygous state for β-thalassemia and δ-thalassemia.

"Silent" β-thalassemia is characterized by no hematologic changes in heterozygotes—a completely normal CBC.[27,28] Compound heterozygotes for this condition and $β^0$-thalassemia have a mild form of β-thalassemia intermedia. Normal Hb A_2 β-thalassemia type 2 in heterozygotes has a hematologic profile of mild microcytic anemia which is indistinguishable from typical β-thalassemia trait, except for the normal HbA2. The homozygous state has not been described. The compound heterozygous state for this gene and β-thalassemia with raised Hb A_2 levels is characterized by a clinical picture of severe transfusion-dependent β-thalassemia. Both of these can only be definitively diagnosed by DNA analysis.

Dominant β-thalassemia

The clinical features of the dominant β-thalassemias resemble the features of thalassemia intermedia.[29] Moderate anemia and splenomegaly are seen, with a blood picture showing thalassemic red cell changes. The marrow shows erythroid hyperplasia with well-marked inclusion bodies in the red cell precursors, which may be seen in the blood after splenectomy. Hemoglobin analysis shows Hb A and HbA₂ are present, Hb A_2 levels are always elevated and the Hb F level is usually elevated much higher than that seen in the β-thalassemia trait. This condition can only be definitively diagnosed by DNA analysis.[4]

Differential diagnosis. At all ages, the mild-to-moderate anemia of thalassemia minor or intermedia must be distinguished from iron deficiency anemia.[30] In the thalassemia trait, the red cell count is usually normal to high, and the mean corpuscular hemoglobin concentration is normal to low normal, both these values being low to very low in iron deficiency anemia. In thalassemia, the hemoglobin fractionation shows the typical pattern of elevated HbA2 and possibly HbF as well. In early childhood, it may occasionally be difficult to distinguish the most severe thalassemia syndromes from the congenital sideroblastic anemias, but the laboratory parameters and bone marrow appearances in the latter are quite characteristic. Fetal hemoglobin levels may be elevated in juvenile chronic myelogenous leukemia, and this disorder may superficially resemble β-thalassemia. However, the finding of primitive cells in the marrow, the absence of elevated Hb A_2 levels on hemoglobin electrophoresis, and the decrease in carbonic anhydrase in juvenile chronic myelogenous leukemia, readily differentiate this disorder from β-thalassemia.[2]

SUMMARY

With changing demographics and increasing migration from areas where thalassemia is more prevalent to those where it is less so, the population distribution of thalassemia is changing. It is now more prevalent in the developed world, and this has some public health implications. Thus, it is important to identify patients with thalassemia syndromes as well as thalassemia traits to be able to provide early comprehensive care, and also avoid unnecessary interventions, such as iron supplementation. Early diagnosis can prepare at-risk couples, and identify at-risk fetuses and newborns, allowing for the initiation of comprehensive care, and intervention before complications develop. Newborn screening for hemoglobin disorders pioneered with a sickle cell focus has advanced substantially, but there is still room for advances to achieve the goal of optimal screening for thalassemia. Early establishment of the diagnosis can facilitate appropriate management to reduce the morbidity of the disease in affected individuals.

CLINICS CARE POINTS

- Beta-thalassemia can lead to a microcytic anemia that can cause a range of clinical and laboratory manifestations.
- While previous classifications characterized patients based on their genotype that remained constant since birth, current classification divide patients based on their transfusion requirements, which can change over time.
- Beta-thalassemia should be considered in the differential diagnosis of anyone with microcytic anemia, especially in patients of Asian, African or Mediterranean ancestry or who have a family history of thalassemia or uncharacterized anemia.
- Screening should be considered in pregnant women and their partners if either individual is known to have beta-thalassemia or if thalassemia status is unknown and the individual is of high likelihood of having thalassemia based on ancestry or family history to promote earlier screening of the fetus or newborn.
- Preimplantation genetic testing can be offered for couples at high risk of conceiving a child with beta-thalassemia, while prenatal screening can be considered for a fetus at high risk for the diagnosis.
- Newborn screening as well as screening of children at risk for beta-thalassemia allows for earlier diagnosis and care, which may include transfusions in infancy/childhood if necessary.
- While both thalassemia and iron deficiency present with microcytic anemia, iron supplementation can lead to iron overload if given inappropriately to a patient with thalassemia.
- Persistent microcytic anemia despite iron supplementation should increase suspicion for beta-thalassemia and prompt evaluation for hemoglobin characterization with electrophoresis or other similar testing.
- A diagnosis of beta-thalassemia by hemoglobin analysis or genetic testing should prompt referral to hematology for comprehensive evaluation and care.

ACKNOWLEDGMENTS

M. Pines acknowledges support of the NCI Cancer Center Support Grant P30 CA008748. S. Sheth acknowledges support from HRSA (U1AMC28549-06) and CDC (NU58DD000001-01-00).

REFERENCES

1. Available at: https://globin.bx.psu.edu/hbvar/menu.html. Accessed September 19, 2022.

2. Origa R., Beta-thalassemia, In: Adam M.P., Everman D.B., Mirzaa G.M., et al., *GeneReviews®* [Internet], 2000, University of Washington, Seattle; Seattle (WA). p. 1993–2022. Available at: https://www.ncbi.nlm.nih.gov/books/NBK1426/.

3. Ho PJ, Hall GW, Luo LY, et al. Beta-thalassaemia intermedia: is it possible consistently to predict phenotype from genotype? Br J Haematol 1998;100(1):70–8.

4. Galanello R, Origa R. Beta-thalassemia. Orphanet J Rare Dis 2010;5:11.

5. Sheth S, Thein S. Thalassemia: A Disorder of Globin Synthesis. In: Kaushansky K, Prchal JT, Burns LJ, et al, editors. Williams Hematology. 10 edtion. McGraw Hill; 2021.

6. Weatherall DJ. Phenotype-genotype relationships in monogenic disease: lessons from the thalassaemias. Nat Rev Genet 2001;2(4):245–55.

7. Centers for Disease Control and Prevention, Association of Public Health Laboratories. Hemoglobinopathies: current practices for screening, confirmation and follow-up. 2015. Available at: https://www.cdc.gov/ncbddd/sicklecell/documents/nbs_hemoglobinopathy-testing_122015.pdf. Accessed November 1, 2022.

8. Fogel BN, Nguyen HLT, Smink G, et al. Variability in State-Based Recommendations for Management of Alpha Thalassemia Trait and Silent Carrier Detected on the Newborn Screen. J Pediatr 2018;195:283–7.

9. Mensah C, Sheth S. Optimal strategies for carrier screening and prenatal diagnosis of α- and β-thalassemia. Hematol Am Soc Hematol Educ Program 2021; 2021(1):607–13.

10. Rappaport VJ, Velazquez M, Williams K. Hemoglobinopathies in pregnancy. Obstet Gynecol Clin North Am 2004;31(2):287-vi.

11. ACOG Committee on Obstetrics. ACOG Practice Bulletin No. 78: hemoglobinopathies in pregnancy. Obstet Gynecol 2007;109(1):229–37.

12. Bender MA, Hulihan M, Dorley MC, et al. Newborn Screening Practices for Beta-Thalassemia in the United States. Int J Neonatal Screen 2021;7(4):83.

13. Shang X, Xu X. Update in the genetics of thalassemia: What clinicians need to know. Best Pract Res Clin Obstet Gynaecol 2017;39:3–15.

14. Leung TY, Lao TT. Thalassaemia in pregnancy. Best Pract Res Clin Obstet Gynaecol 2012;26(1):37–51.

15. Hoppe CC. Newborn screening for hemoglobin disorders. Hemoglobin 2011; 35(5–6):556–64.

16. Benson JM, Therrell BL Jr. History and current status of newborn screening for hemoglobinopathies. Semin Perinatol 2010;34(2):134–44.

17. Kohli-Kumar M. Screening for anemia in children: AAP recommendations–a critique. Pediatrics 2001;108(3):E56.

18. Taher AT, Weatherall DJ, Cappellini MD. Thalassaemia. *Lancet.* 2018;391(10116): 155–67.

19. Hoppe CC. Newborn screening for non-sickling hemoglobinopathies. Hematol Am Soc Hematol Educ Program 2009;19–25. https://doi.org/10.1182/asheducation-2009.1.19.

20. Cao A, Galanello R, Rosatelli MC. Prenatal diagnosis and screening of the haemoglobinopathies. Baillieres Clin Haematol 1998;11(1):215–38.

21. Cao A, Kan YW. The prevention of thalassemia. Cold Spring Harb Perspect Med 2013;3(2):a011775.

22. Cheung MC, Goldberg JD, Kan YW. Prenatal diagnosis of sickle cell anaemia and thalassaemia by analysis of fetal cells in maternal blood. Nat Genet 1996;14(3): 264–8.

23. Kuliev A, Rechitsky S, Verlinsky O, et al. Birth of healthy children after preimplantation diagnosis of thalassemias. J Assist Reprod Genet 1999;16(4):207–11.

24. Hung EC, Chiu RW, Lo YM. Detection of circulating fetal nucleic acids: a review of methods and applications. J Clin Pathol 2009;62(4):308–13.

25. Viprakasit V, Ekwattanakit S. Clinical Classification, Screening and Diagnosis for Thalassemia. Hematol Oncol Clin North Am 2018;32(2):193–211.

26. Kattamis C, Metaxotou-Mavromati A, Wood WG, et al. The heterogeneity of normal Hb A2-beta thalassaemia in Greece. Br J Haematol 1979;42(1):109–23.

27. Schwartz E. The silent carrier of beta thalassemia. N Engl J Med 1969;281(24): 1327–33.

28. Rund D, Filon D, Oppenheim A, et al. Silent carrier beta-thalassaemia due to a severe beta-globin mutation interacting with other genetic elements. Eur J Pediatr 1993;152(7):574–6.

29. Thein SL. Dominant beta thalassaemia: molecular basis and pathophysiology. Br J Haematol 1992;80(3):273–7.

30. Hoffmann JJ, Urrechaga E, Aguirre U. Discriminant indices for distinguishing thalassemia and iron deficiency in patients with microcytic anemia: a meta-analysis. Clin Chem Lab Med 2015;53(12):1883–94.

The Clinical Phenotypes of Alpha Thalassemia

Ashutosh Lal, MD*, Elliott Vichinsky, MD

KEYWORDS

- Alpha thalassemia trait • Hemoglobin H disease • Hydrops fetalis • Iron overload

KEY POINTS

- The clinical manifestations of α-thalassemia syndromes range from asymptomatic state to profound transfusion-dependent anemia with prenatal onset. Phenotype is correlated with the degree of α-globin chain deficit due to deletions or mutations affecting α-globin genes.
- Deletion of 1 or 2 α genes causes α-thalassemia trait, whereas deletion of all 4 α genes leads to α-thalassemia major (Hb Barts hydrops fetalis). All other genotypes of intermediate severity are grouped under HbH disease.
- HbH can develop from diverse combinations of α gene deletions and mutations. Deletional HbH disease is usually less severe than nondeletional HbH. Febrile illnesses can be associated with rapid worsening of anemia from increased hemolysis and need for urgent transfusion.
- The clinical spectrum of α-thalassemia is classified as mild, moderate, and severe based on symptoms and need for intervention. Certain forms of α-thalassemia manifest in the prenatal period as severe anemia and hydrops fetalis that can be fatal without intrauterine transfusion support.
- A judicious identification of patients with benign or severe disease allows appropriate counseling and planning of management. New therapies to modify severity of HbH disease or provide curative options for α-thalassemia major are under development.

INTRODUCTION

Alpha thalassemia is characterized by reduced output of α-globin genes leading to a relative excess of β-like globin chains (**Fig. 1**). The surplus chains during the fetal and early postnatal period are γ-globin that form γ_4 tetramers (Hb Barts), later replaced by β_4 tetramers (HbH) as β-globin synthesis increases after birth. The clinical spectrum of α-thalassemia is a continuum (**Fig. 2**) with clinical manifestations spanning the categories of thalassemia trait, intermedia, and major.[1] Molecular diagnosis is essential to predict the natural history of α-thalassemia[2–5] but this may be hindered by the

UCSF School of Medicine, UCSF Benioff Children's Hospital, 747 52nd Street, Oakland, CA 94609, USA
* Corresponding author.
E-mail address: Ashutosh.lal@ucsf.edu

Hematol Oncol Clin N Am 37 (2023) 327–339
https://doi.org/10.1016/j.hoc.2022.12.004
0889-8588/23/© 2022 Elsevier Inc. All rights reserved.

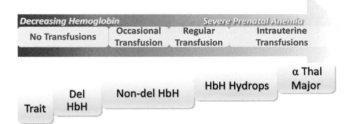

Fig. 1. Pathophysiology of α-thalassemia. Reduced synthesis of α-globin chains underlies the development of anemia. Excess γ-globin chains form tetramers detected as Hb Barts, which are replaced after birth by β tetramers (HbH). Both hemoglobins are unable to transport oxygen and contribute to tissue hypoxia when present in significant amounts. Precipitation of unstable hemoglobins (HbH, Hb Constant Spring) increases hemolysis.

limited availability of testing for mutations or deletions beyond the initial panel of common abnormalities.[6]

Normal individuals have 4 α-globin genes consisting of 2 linked α genes on each chromosome 16 (αα/αα). The most frequent cause of α-thalassemia is deletion of either one (–α or α⁺ thalassemia) or both (–DEL or α⁰ thalassemia) genes. Heterozygous α⁺ thalassemia (–α/αα) is a silent carrier state because it causes only mild changes in red cell indices that overlap with the normal reference range. When 2 out of 4 α-globin genes are missing (either –α/–α or –/αα), the microcytic and hypochromic anemia is readily appreciated but there are no clinical symptoms, splenomegaly, or laboratory evidence of hemolysis. The prevalence of α-thalassemia trait is high in sub-Saharan Africa, Mediterranean region, Middle East, Indian subcontinent, Southern China, and Southeast Asia, as well as in countries with immigrant populations from these regions.[7] Clinically significant forms of disease are observed where α⁰ thalassemia (–DEL)

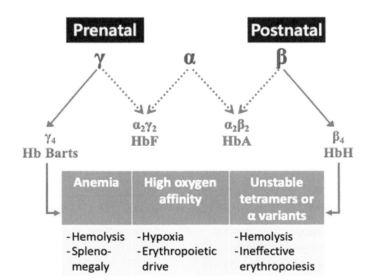

Fig. 2. Spectrum of clinical severity of α-thalassemia.

or α-globin gene mutations ($\alpha^T\alpha$) are prevalent (Middle East, Mediterranean, China, and Southeast Asia).[8] Distinguishing between homozygous α^+ thalassemia ($-\alpha/-\alpha$) and heterozygous α^0 thalassemia ($-^{DEL}/\alpha\alpha$) is vital for genetic counseling and estimating public health impact due to likelihood of severe disease and hydrops fetalis from the latter.

Patients who have anemia that is more severe than trait or exhibit evidence of hemolysis are grouped under HbH disease. The name refers to detection of HbH on electrophoresis or as RBC inclusions,[1,2,7,9] instead of a specific genotype. In fact, HbH disease comprises several different genotypes some of which do not have detectable HbH.[6,10] The clinical severity extends from mild anemia with no symptoms to severe anemia with transfusion-dependence, and some forms with prenatal onset are associated with hydrops fetalis (**Table 1** and **Fig. 2**).[1,11]

Individuals with deletional HbH disease (deletion of 3 α genes, $-\alpha/-$) usually have asymptomatic anemia that may not be diagnosed unless an incidental laboratory test prompts further investigation. Nondeletional HbH disease ($\alpha^T\alpha/-$, $\alpha^T\alpha/\alpha^T\alpha$, or $\alpha^T\alpha/-\alpha$) is generally more severe than deletional type, particularly when the mutation is located on the $\alpha2$ gene. In practice, heterogeneity in clinical manifestations is observed even among patients with identical genotype due to unexplained reasons. Environmental factors (recurrent infections, malaria, or nutrition) probably modify the phenotypic expression of HbH disease[2] and may explain variability in the use of transfusions in different regions.[2,9,12–15] Specific forms of HbH disease are associated with developmental delay (α-thalassemia mental retardation, ATR16, and ATRX) and myelodysplastic syndromes.[1]

The transfusion-dependent forms of α-thalassemia are α-thalassemia major (ATM), HbH disease with unstable α variants, and certain other nondeletional HbH genotypes. ATM is the deletion of all 4 α genes ($-/-$) and presents as Hb Barts hydrops fetalis, which requires prenatal and postnatal regular transfusions for survival.[11] Intrauterine anemia and hydrops also develop when unstable α variants are coinherited with α^0 thalassemia, and these patients continue to be transfusion-dependent (HbH hydrops fetalis).[16,17] Finally, some patients with HbH disease may initiate transfusions later in life to manage complications or symptoms from anemia.

DIAGNOSIS

Individuals with microcytic (MCV <80) and hypochromic (MCH <28) anemia should be investigated for thalassemia trait. This is recommended universally but is essential for persons of high-risk geographical ancestry (Southeast Asian, Chinese, South Asian, Pacific Islander, Middle Eastern, Mediterranean, Latin American, African American). Initial testing includes an iron panel to assess for iron deficiency and analysis of hemoglobin fractions with electrophoresis or high-performance liquid chromatography (HPLC). Hemoglobin electrophoresis is normal in α-thalassemia trait although occasional HbH inclusions in RBC can be demonstrated in peripheral blood smear.[18] Although an elevated HbA2 (>3.5%) is suggestive of β-thalassemia trait, it does not exclude coexisting α-thalassemia. Diagnosis is established on genetic testing, usually in the form of polymerase chain reaction to detect common deletions and mutations. Prenatal testing and genetic counseling are extremely important for individuals from ethnicities with high prevalence of α^0 thalassemia trait due to the reproductive risk of ATM and other severe genotypes.[19]

Laboratory testing for HbH disease shows lower hemoglobin with greater anisocytosis than observed with thalassemia trait. Reticulocyte count and indirect bilirubin are elevated to a variable extent. Hemoglobin electrophoresis shows HbA as the majority

Table 1
Phenotypic classification of α-thalassemia

Severity	Clinical Course	Genotype Examples*
HbH Disease		
Mild	Hemoglobin 9–11 g/dL in adults, no symptoms from anemia, transfusions are not needed	Del HbH disease ($-\alpha/-^{DEL}$) Hb CS homozygosity
Moderate	Hemoglobin 7–10 g/dL, mild symptoms, hemolytic episodes, occasional transfusions	HbH CS disease Other nondel HbH disease Some homozygous α mutations
Severe	Hemoglobin 6–9 g/dL, significant symptoms from anemia, marked splenomegaly, need for frequent or regular transfusions	HbH Constant Spring disease Other nondel HbH disease Some homozygous α mutations. Unstable variants
Hydrops fetalis		
With postnatal transfusion independence	Hydrops in second trimester, resolves spontaneously or with transfusions, regular transfusions not needed after birth	Homozygous CS or PA-1 mutations Nondel HbH disease
With continuing postnatal transfusion dependence	Hydrops in second trimester leads to fetal demise or premature birth with severe morbidity, patients remain transfusion-dependent for life	Alpha thalassemia major ($-^{DEL}/-^{DEL}$) HbH disease with hyperunstable variants ($-^{DEL}/\alpha^{T}\alpha$) Homozygous hyperunstable variants

* HbH genotypes are not exclusive to a category and overlap between adjacent groups.

fraction, normal to low HbA2, and 5% to 25% HbH. Coinheritance of β-thalassemia or HbE trait in HbH disease leads to either reduced or absent HbH with increase in Hb Barts (**Table 2**). Variant hemoglobin species such as Hb Constant Spring (CS) are observed in small quantities in patients with HbH CS disease and related disorders. Supravital staining with brilliant cresyl blue demonstrates HbH inclusions in red blood cells in a characteristic golf ball appearance. The diagnosis is confirmed with genetic testing for common deletions and mutations. If initial panel is negative, further testing is indicated with α-globin gene sequencing for rare mutations and multiplex ligation-dependent probe amplification for large deletions. Certain mutations such as CS (HBA2:c.427 T > C), polyadenylation site (HBA2:c.*92A > G), −5 nt (HBA2:c.95 + 2_95+6delTGAGG), and Adana (HBA1 or 2:c.179 G > A) achieve high prevalence in specific geographical regions and cause substantial morbidity.[8,11]

The presence of Hb Barts in newborn blood samples provides a unique opportunity to diagnose α-thalassemia.[20,21] HbH disease is highly likely when Hb Barts fraction is greater than 25% in blood sample collected within 48 hours after birth and analyzed by HPLC.[20] Lower levels of Hb Barts (10%–30%) are present in samples from newborns who have deletion of 2 α genes (trait).

Abnormal Hemoglobins in α-thalassemia

Anomalous and variant hemoglobin species play a significant role in the pathophysiology of α-thalassemia syndromes. A deficiency of α-globin relative to γ or β-globin chains leads to the formation of γ_4 (Hb Barts) and β_4 (HbH) tetramers. Unlike excess α-globin chains in β-thalassemia syndromes that precipitate in erythroblasts, γ_4 and β_4 tetramers are present in peripheral RBCs and contribute toward the total hemoglobin measured in routine complete blood count. Both these hemoglobins have extremely high oxygen affinity and do not participate in blood oxygen transport.[22] It is necessary to subtract the proportion of HbH and Hb Barts from the total hemoglobin to appreciate the true impact of anemia on tissue oxygenation in α-thalassemia syndromes.[11,23] The severity of α-globin chain deficiency roughly correlates with the proportion of HbH or Hb Barts.[20,24,25] In comparative studies, HbH forms 5% to 10% of the total hemoglobin in deletional HbH disease and 15% to 20% in nondeletional HbH disease.[24,25] α-globin synthesis is completely absent in ATM and Hb Barts constitutes 80% to 90% of the total hemoglobin in the fetus and the newborn.

Several α-globin gene mutations produce variant hemoglobins that modify the severity of HbH disease through posttranslational mechanisms.[1] For instance, CS mutation on $\alpha2$ terminal codon leads to elongated α-globin chain that is synthesized less efficiently[26] and is unstable.[27,28] Some α-globin structural variants such as Adana are hyperunstable and undergo rapid degradation in erythroblasts leading to ineffective erythropoiesis.[29–32]

HbH with Mild Clinical Course

Individuals in this group do not manifest symptoms of anemia and the diagnosis is usually made incidentally when a blood test reveals mild-to-moderate anemia. They can be misdiagnosed as iron deficiency anemia and prescribed supplemental iron, which increases the risk of iron overload. Newborn infants diagnosed at birth through screening programs have a normal perinatal period and infancy. Their hemoglobin trend follows the expected nadir around 3 months of age (usually staying above 8 g/dL), following which it slowly increases to reach 8.5–9.5 g/dL by 4 years. After puberty, hemoglobin in men increases from 10 to 12 g/dL, whereas in women, it is usually in the range of 9 to 10.5 g/dL.[1,2,5,7,9,12,13,25] Children demonstrate normal growth and development, and their physical activity is indistinguishable from peers. No skeletal changes are observed, and splenomegaly is absent or mild if present. Laboratory tests show hemolysis with slight increase in bilirubin and reticulocyte count. Gastrointestinal iron absorption is increased, which leads to a mild iron overload in the third decade or later.[12] Acute hemolytic episodes are not characteristic of this group and blood transfusion is almost never necessary.[2,12] Even during significant infections, hemoglobin

Table 2
Interaction of deletional HbH disease with β-thalassemia or variants

HbH Disease (−α/−)	Beta Genotype	Comment
AE Barts disease	$\beta^A\beta^E$	No H; ↑ Barts
EF Barts Disease	$\beta^E\beta^E$	No A or H; ↑ Barts
HbH with β-thal trait	$\beta^A\beta^0$ or $\beta^A\beta^+$	↑ A2; Barts, Low or absent H
HbH with HbE β-thal	$\beta^E\beta^0$ or $\beta^E\beta^+$	Severe anemia
HbH with Sickle trait	$\beta^A\beta^S$	S <20%, small amount of Barts, absent H

level is unlikely to reduce to less than 6 g/dL. In keeping with the benign disease physiology, cholelithiasis is uncommon and vascular complications are not reported. Women can go through pregnancy without an increase in adverse perinatal outcome or need for transfusion support. Some adults may develop fatigue, although quality of life has not been formally evaluated in HbH disease.

Common genotypes: The most frequent genotype in this group is deletional HbH disease from various combinations of α^+ ($-\alpha^{3.7}$, $-\alpha^{4.2}$, other) with α^0 ($-^{SEA}$, $-^{FIL}$, $-^{THAI}$, $-^{MED}$, other) thalassemia.[2,5,12,25,29,33,34] Coinheritance of β-thalassemia (particularly HbE) is not uncommon in regions where both conditions have high prevalence[10,35] but there is no significant impact on the disease severity. Homozygosity for Hb CS ($\alpha^{CS}\alpha/\alpha^{CS}\alpha$) also generally produces a hemolytic anemia with mild clinical course.[27] However, the severity of other homozygous nondeletional α^+ thalassemia varies according to the type of mutation.

HbH Disease of Moderate Severity

Hemoglobin level in this group is between 7 and 10 g/dL, which is 1 and 2 g/dL lower than the mild group, and these patients have symptoms from anemia. **Table 3** presents comparison of clinical manifestations in deletional and nondeletional HbH disease derived from a cumulative data from several studies[14] and recent data from California.[15] Although anemia is present in the neonatal period, severe hemolytic jaundice is not common.[12] Transfusions may be rarely necessary in early infancy due to low hemoglobin nadir. Subsequently, greater reticulocytosis and jaundice is observed compared with the mild group, and splenomegaly can sometimes be marked.[2,7,12,13] Some children manifest growth and pubertal delay but skeletal facial changes are infrequent and not typical of HbH disease. A distinguishing feature is the susceptibility to hemolytic episodes triggered by an infection where hemoglobin can rapidly reduce to less than 5 g/dL and blood transfusion may be needed.[2,9,12] There are several triggers that promote hemolytic crisis, such as infection, pyrexia, oxidative stress, marrow suppression, and hypersplenism.[2,9,14] Brisk hemolysis is accompanied by inadequate erythropoietic response during viral infections, therefore patients should be monitored closely for severe anemia. Young children may have multiple such episodes every year but the frequency decreases in older children and adults because the incidence of common viral infections wanes. Adults who have not undergone splenectomy can have significant anemia with decreased quality of life due to fatigue and reduced work performance. Patients can develop gall stones that may require cholecystectomy for management. Hemoglobin decreases from baseline during pregnancy, and there is an increase in adverse fetal outcome in the absence of regular transfusion support to the mother.[36] Iron overload due to intermittent transfusions and increased absorption is common[12,33] and usually exceeds the threshold for initiating iron chelation in adults. Liver fibrosis and cirrhosis can develop because of iron toxicity,[33] although cardiac and endocrine damage has not been reported.

Common genotypes: Genotypes that display clinical course of moderate severity are combinations of α^0 thalassemia with mutations affecting $\alpha2$ gene. Common mutations are CS, polyadenylation site (PA-1), IVSI splice site, initiation codon, and Quong Sze.[2,5,12,13,28,37-39] CS is one of a group of chain elongation α variants that includes Paksé, Icaria, Seal Rock, and Koya Dora, which may share similar pathophysiology and phenotype as HbH CS disease.[40-42] Homozygosity ($\alpha^T\alpha/\alpha^T\alpha$) for polyadenylation-site mutation (α^{PA-1}) and other $\alpha2$ mutations can cause HbH disease of moderate severity.[37,43]

Table 3
Manifestations of deletional and nondeletional HbH disease

Clinical Manifestation	Deletional HbH Disease	Nondeletional HbH Disease
Hemoglobin, g/dL (range)	8.5 (6.9–10.7)	7.2 (3.8–8.7)
MCV, fL (range)	54.0 (46.0–76.0)	65.2 (48.7–80.7)
MCH, pg (range)	16.6 (14.3–24.7)	18.6 (14.8–24.8)
Reticulocytosis	+	++
Bilirubin	+	++
Age at first transfusion[a] (years)	11 ± 5.5	1.5 ± 2.1
History of blood transfusion (%)	3–29	24–80
Type of transfusion[b] (%) • Never transfused • Intermittently transfused • Regularly transfused	92.4 7.6 0	46.2 44.9 9.0
Splenomegaly	+	+++
Gallstones	+	++
Growth retardation	Rare	Common
Decreased bone density	Rare	Common

[a] Cumulative data for published series.
[b] California data. See text for references.

HbH Disease with Severe Clinical Course

Patients who experience debilitating symptoms from anemia or have massive splenomegaly or growth failure are categorized as severe HbH disease. Intermittent transfusions are commonly used in the beginning but many patients will transition to regular transfusions. It is not well understood why individuals with identical genotype may have different disease severity.[44,45] Hemolytic episodes become less frequent in adults but baseline anemia can become symptomatic with age and need transfusions despite being tolerated during childhood.[45] There is a genuine concern about the long-term health of adults with moderate-to-severe anemia due to lack of information on natural history of even the common genotypes. Some patients undergo splenectomy as an alternative to frequent transfusions, which improves anemia and hemolytic episodes.[46] The mean hemoglobin following splenectomy is about 2 g/dL higher, although a few patients fail to respond.[14,46–48] The period immediately following splenectomy is high risk for thrombotic complications in splanchnic, portal and lower extremity veins, and pulmonary embolism.[48] There is also a long-term increased risk of thromboembolism and pulmonary hypertension, which is likely reduced with aspirin. Patients who initiate regular transfusions are susceptible to developing iron overload and red cell alloimmunization. Uncontrolled iron overload can lead to cardiac, hepatic, and endocrine complications as observed in transfusion-dependent β-thalassemia. Patients in moderate and severe groups would benefit from disease-modifying therapies currently under development. A recent preliminary study indicates that pyruvate kinase activators can increase hemoglobin level in HbH disease.[49] This phase 2 open label trial of mitapivat in non–transfusion-dependent thalassemia included 5 adults with HbH disease (4 with HbH CS disease), all of whom experienced sustained response with median improvement in hemoglobin of 1.2 g/dL.

Common genotypes: Along with the genotypes mentioned above (HbH CS, $-/\alpha^{PA-1}\alpha$, $\alpha^{PA-1}\alpha/\alpha^{PA-1}\alpha$), other rare nondeletional forms of HbH disease[42] are associated with severe clinical course that requires active intervention.

HbH Hydrops Fetalis

Because α-globin chains are essential for synthesis of HbF, fetal anemia in α-thalassemia starts during the switch from ζ to α-globin chains toward the end of first trimester of pregnancy.[7] In certain genotypes, anemia can be severe enough to induce fetal hydrops despite the preservation of 1 or 2 functional α genes.[44,50–53] Such anemia can be more severe during fetal life and hydrops can resolve spontaneously or with transfusions before or shortly after birth.[17,53] This phenomenon is reported with homozygosity for CS, PA-1, and Quong Sze mutations or their combination with α^0 thal.[44,52–54] Fetal anemia can be very severe with nadir hemoglobin 1.1 to 6.8 g/dL, and there is an increase in preterm birth and growth restriction. Response to intrauterine transfusion is observed with the resolution of hydrops occurring after 1 to 3 procedures.[31,53] Some newborns need transfusions after birth for a short period of time but eventually achieve transfusion independence. Careful prenatal evaluation and rapid confirmation of diagnosis is necessary to avoid misidentification as ATM or other nonimmune hydrops and to provide appropriate counseling for continuation of pregnancy.

At the severe end of the spectrum of HbH hydrops fetalis are genotypes where a hyperunstable $\alpha2$ variant (such as $\alpha2$ Hb Adana) is inherited as homozygous state or along with α^0 thalassemia trait.[16,17,32] The presentation and outcome of these cases is comparable to ATM but the diagnosis is difficult without a history of prior affected pregnancy to guide molecular testing. The presence of α^0 thalassemia in one parent should prompt α gene sequencing in the partner for detecting Adana and other severe mutations. As of now, survivors with HbH Adana disease are rare due to severe prenatal and perinatal complications, and its prevalence is likely to be underestimated despite high frequency of the mutation in certain regions.[55,56] As is the case for pregnancies affected by ATM, these patients require intensive multidisciplinary management with regular transfusions in the prenatal and postnatal periods.

Common genotypes: Hydrops fetalis followed by postnatal transfusion independence is likely with HbH CS disease, HbH with PA mutation, and homozygous CS or PA site mutation. Clinical similarity with ATM is observed with hyperunstable α variants, the most common being Hb Adana, although other rare codon 59 variants[57] are also observed.

Alpha Thalassemia Major

The deletion of all 4 α-globin genes due to homozygous α^0 thalassemia ($-^{DEL}/-^{DEL}$) is known as Hb Barts hydrops fetalis or ATM.[11,16] Because at least one preserved ζ chain is necessary for embryonic survival, most cases of ATM are due to homozygous Southeast Asian deletion ($-^{SEA}/-^{SEA}$) or $-^{SEA}$ in combination with another α^0 deletion. For this reason, ATM is prevalent in Southeast Asia and the Southern regions of China,[58,59] where it accounts for more than 50% of all pregnancies affected by nonimmune hydrops.[59] The fetus develops severe anemia with a midgestation hemoglobin around 6 g/dL, most of which is Hb Bart's that does not participate in transport of oxygen.[7,60] Severe fetal anemia and hypoxia in ATM lead to hydrops fetalis characterized by massive organomegaly, hypoalbuminemia, cardiomegaly, heart failure, ascites, pleural and pericardial effusions, edema, and growth failure.[11,60] In the absence of early diagnosis and intervention, fetal demise in the second trimester is expected in most cases. Prenatal diagnosis of ATM is suspected by the observation of hydrops on fetal ultrasound during the second trimester in conjunction with α^0 thalassemia trait in mother.[19] Diagnosis is confirmed with fetal tissue and termination of pregnancy is usually advised due to poor fetal outcome and concern over maternal complications (mirror syndrome).[19]

When parents choose to continue pregnancy, it is vital to initiate early intrauterine transfusions (IUT) starting at 18 to 20 weeks. Optimal management of fetal anemia is the strongest predictor of acceptable perinatal and postnatal outcome.[61–63] Preterm delivery or induction of labor is common due to concern for fetal health, although this is not necessary if regular IUTs are provided to achieve suppression of Hb Barts. Perinatal complications are exacerbated by preterm birth, low birth weight, and difficult resuscitation.[23] Intensive neonatal support may be needed to manage respiratory distress syndrome, persistent pulmonary hypertension, ascites, thrombocytopenia, and hyperbilirubinemia. Men have a high incidence of genitourinary anomalies such as hypospadias and undescended testes.

All infants with ATM remain transfusion-dependent from birth and develop iron overload much earlier than β-thalassemia major.[64] Transfusion support is complex as anemia promotes erythropoiesis and increases production of endogenous Hb Barts, later replaced by HbH, both of which do not contribute to oxygen transport.[65] Oxygen transport depends entirely on the transfused HbA, which should be quantified with HPLC to estimate corrected hemoglobin value for adequate transfusion support. Two international registries are tracking survivors of ATM to understand the impact of prenatal and postnatal management on long-term outcome.[62,66] In one registry, growth retardation was observed in 50% of the survivors of ATM and 20% had significant neurodevelopmental delays.[62] However, earlier initiation and higher number of IUT leads to improved outcomes, with most patients treated with at least 2 IUTs demonstrating normal neurodevelopmental scores.[66] Patients with suitable donors can be cured by bone marrow transplantation. A current phase 1 clinical trial (NCT02986698) is evaluating the utility of maternal haploidentical bone marrow transplant in the intrauterine period. Manipulation of ζ-globin genes is being explored to develop future therapies for ATM.[67,68]

Common genotypes: Homozygous Southeast Asian deletion ($-^{SEA}/-^{SEA}$), compound heterozygosity of $-^{SEA}$ with other α^0 thalassemia.

SUMMARY

HbH disease is a common condition that displays a full spectrum of severity determined by the underlying α-globin genotype, although significant heterogeneity exists even within the same diagnosis. HbH disease caused by deletion of 3 α-globin genes is typically a mild condition, whereas nondeletional HbH disease, which develops from diverse mutations and combinations with α-globin gene deletions, can have a more severe clinical course. The role of genetic factors outside of globin gene loci and environmental influences in determining severity has not been clarified. The nonfunctional Hb Barts and HbH, and several unstable α variants are important modifiers of phenotypic expression. There is a current need to improve access to molecular diagnosis of α-thalassemia and to investigate the natural history of HbH syndromes. All patients with α-thalassemia syndromes should receive specialized genetic counseling for assessing the risk of serious disorder in the offspring. Clinical management of HbH disease centers on monitoring of growth, bone health, spleen size, symptoms of cholecystitis, fatigue, and quality of life. Iron overload occurs in older patients but is observed much earlier in those who have been transfused. The severe forms of HbH disease and ATM begin in utero and the fetus is vulnerable in second trimester to developing anemia and hydrops. These complex disorders are managed by a multi-disciplinary team and require rapid diagnosis for appropriate counseling and fetal support to improve long-term outcome.

CLINICS CARE POINTS

- Diagnosing α0 thalassemia trait is important as there is potential for severe disease in the offspring if the partner is also a carrier. Individuals with microcytic and hypochromic anemia of high-risk geographical ancestry should undergo genetic testing if hemoglobin electrophoresis does not show elevated HbA2 suggestive of β thalassemia trait.

- Anomalous and variant hemoglobin species play a significant role in the pathophysiology of α thalassemia syndromes. Hb Barts (γ4) and HbH (β4) do not participate in oxygen transport, leading to underestimation of tissue hypoxia based on the total hemoglobin level alone.

- HbH disease is a heterogenous entity that requires genotypic diagnosis for counseling. Patients with deletional HbH disease have mild clinical course, but those with non-deletional HbH can have severe manifestations requiring transfusions.

- Some forms of α thalassemia are symptomatic in the prenatal period. Early risk assessment and fetal diagnosis is essential for effective management of anemia and hydrops to improve long-term outcomes.

FUNDING

(1) U.S. Department of Health and Human Services, Centers for Disease Control and Prevention, National Center on Birth Defects and Developmental Disabilities, Grant/Award Number: NU58DD000002 (2) This project was supported by the Health Resources and Services Administration (HRSA) of the US Department of Health and Human Services (HHS), grant number: U1AMC45369. This information or content and conclusions are those of the authors and should not be construed as the official position or policy of, nor should any endorsements be inferred by, HRSA, HHS, or the US Government.

REFERENCES

1. Harteveld CL, Higgs DR. α-thalassaemia. Orphanet J Rare Dis 2010;5(1):13.
2. Fucharoen S, Viprakasit V. Hb H disease: clinical course and disease modifiers. Hematology 2009;2009(1):26–34.
3. Kattamis C, Kanavakis E, Tzotzos S, et al. Correlation of clinical phenotype to genotype in haemoglobin H disease. The Lancet 1988;331(8583):442–4.
4. Kanavakis E, Papassotiriou I, Karagiorga M, et al. Phenotypic and molecular diversity of haemoglobin H disease: a Greek experience. Br J Haematol 2000; 111(3):915–23.
5. Origa R, Sollaino MC, Giagu N, et al. Clinical and molecular analysis of haemoglobin H disease in Sardinia: haematological, obstetric and cardiac aspects in patients with different genotypes. Br J Haematol 2007;136(2):326–32.
6. Farashi S, Harteveld CL. Molecular basis of α-thalassemia. Blood Cell Mol Dis 2017. https://doi.org/10.1016/j.bcmd.2017.09.004.
7. Vichinsky EP. Clinical manifestations of alpha-thalassemia. Cold Spring Harb Perspect Med 2013;3(5). https://doi.org/10.1101/cshperspect.a011742.
8. Piel FB, Weatherall DJ. The α-Thalassemias. N Engl J Med 2014;371(20): 1908–16.

9. Chui DHK, Fucharoen S, Chan V. Hemoglobin H disease: not necessarily a benign disorder. Blood 2003;101(3):791–800.

10. Chaibunruang A, Karnpean R, Fucharoen G, et al. Genetic heterogeneity of hemoglobin AEBart's disease: a large cohort data from a single referral center in northeast Thailand. Blood Cell Mol Dis 2014;52(4):176–80.

11. Vichinsky EP. Alpha thalassemia major—new mutations, intrauterine management, and outcomes. ASH Education Program Book 2009;2009(1):35–41.

12. Lal A, Goldrich ML, Haines DA, et al. Heterogeneity of hemoglobin H disease in childhood. N Engl J Med 2011;364(8):710–8.

13. Singer ST, Kim HY, Olivieri NF, et al. Hemoglobin H-constant spring in North America: An alpha thalassemia with frequent complications. Am J Hematol 2009; 84(11):759–61.

14. Vichinsky E. Advances in the treatment of alpha-thalassemia. Blood Rev 2012; 26(Suppl 1):S31–4.

15. Lal A, Wong TE, Andrews J, et al. Transfusion practices and complications in thalassemia. Transfusion 2018;58(12):2826–35.

16. Chan V, Chan VWY, Tang M, et al. Molecular defects in Hb H hydrops fetalis. Br J Haematol 1997;96(2):224–8.

17. Lorey F, Charoenkwan P, Witkowska HE, et al. Hb H hydrops foetalis syndrome: a case report and review of literature. Br J Haematol 2001;115(1):72–8.

18. Galanello R, Cao A. Alpha-thalassemia. Genet Med 2011;13(2):83–8.

19. MacKenzie TC, Amid A, Angastiniotis M, et al. Consensus statement for the perinatal management of patients with α thalassemia major. Blood Adv 2021;5(24): 5636–9.

20. Lorey F, Cunningham G, Vichinsky EP, et al. Universal Newborn Screening for Hb H Disease in California. Genet Test 2001;5(2):93–100.

21. Michlitsch J, Azimi M, Hoppe C, et al. Newborn screening for hemoglobinopathies in California. Pediatr Blood Cancer 2009;52(4):486–90.

22. Imai K, Tientadakul P, Opartkiattikul N, et al. Detection of haemoglobin variants and inference of their functional properties using complete oxygen dissociation curve measurements. Br J Haematol 2001;112(2):483–7.

23. Lal A, Lianoglou BR, Gonzalez Velez JM, et al. Alpha thalassemia major: Prenatal and postnatal management. 2022. Available at: https://www.uptodate.com/contents/alpha-thalassemia-major-prenatal-and-postnatal-management. Accessed October 31, 2022.

24. Wasi PAP. Levels of Haemoglobin H and Proportions of Red Cells with Inclusion Bodies in the Two Types of Haemoglobin H Disease. Br J Haematol 1980;46(3): 507–9.

25. Baysal E, Kleanthous M, Bozkurt G, et al. α-Thalassaemia in the population of Cyprus. Br J Haematol 1995;89(3):496–9.

26. Kan YW, Todd D, Dozy AM. Haemoglobin Constant spring synthesis in red cell precursors. Br J Haematol 1974;28(1):103–7.

27. Pootrakul P, Winichagoon P, Fucharoen S, et al. Homozygous haemoglobin constant spring: a need for revision of concept. Hum Genet 1981;59(3):250–5.

28. Schrier SL, Bunyaratvej A, Khuhapinant A, et al. The Unusual Pathobiology of Hemoglobin Constant Spring Red Blood Cells. Blood 1997;89(5):1762–9.

29. Higgs DR. The Molecular Basis of α-Thalassemia. Cold Spring Harb Perspect Med 2013;3(1):a011718.

30. Singh SA, Sarangi S, Appiah-Kubi A, et al. Hb Adana (HBA2 or HBA1: c.179G > A) and alpha thalassemia: Genotype–phenotype correlation. Pediatr Blood Cancer 2018;65(9):e27220.

31. Nainggolan IM, Harahap A, Ambarwati DD, et al. Interaction of Hb Adana (HBA2: c.179G>A) with Deletional and Nondeletional α+-Thalassemia Mutations: Diverse Hematological and Clinical Features. Hemoglobin 2013;37(3):297–305.

32. Henderson S, Pitman M, McCarthy J, et al. Molecular prenatal diagnosis of Hb H Hydrops Fetalis caused by haemoglobin Adana and the implications to antenatal screening for α-thalassaemia. Prenat Diagn 2008;28(9):859–61.

33. Chen FE, Ooi C, Ha SY, et al. Genetic and clinical features of hemoglobin H disease in chinese patients. N Engl J Med 2000;343(8):544–50.

34. Laosombat V, Viprakasit V, Chotsampancharoen T, et al. Clinical features and molecular analysis in Thai patients with HbH disease. Ann Hematol 2009;88(12): 1185–92.

35. Fucharoen S, Winichagoon P, Thonglairuam V, et al. EF Bart's disease: interaction of the abnormal α- and β-globin genes. Eur J Haematol 1988;40(1):75–8.

36. Ake-sittipaisarn S, Sirichotiyakul S, Srisupundit K, et al. Outcomes of pregnancies complicated by haemoglobin H-constant spring and deletional haemoglobin H disease: a retrospective cohort study. Br J Haematol 2022;199(1):122–9.

37. Fei YJ, Öner R, Bözkurt G, et al. Hb H Disease Caused by a Homozygosity for the AATAAA→ AATAAG Mutation in the Polyadenylation Site of the α2-Globin Gene: Hematological Observations. AHA 1992;88(2–3):82–5.

38. Hamamy HA, Al-Allawi NAS. Epidemiological profile of common haemoglobinopathies in Arab countries. J Community Genet 2013;4(2):147–67.

39. Sura T, Trachoo O, Viprakasit V, et al. Hemoglobin H disease induced by the common SEA deletion and the rare hemoglobin Quong Sze in a Thai female: longitudinal clinical course, molecular characterization, and development of a PCR/ RFLP-based detection method. Ann Hematol 2007;86(9):659–63.

40. Viprakasit V, Tanphaichitr VS, Pung-Amritt P, et al. Clinical phenotypes and molecular characterization of. Hb H-Paksé Dis 2002;87:9.

41. Kanavakis E, Traeger-Synodinos J, Papasotiriou I, et al. The interaction of α° thalassaemia with Hb Icaria: three unusual cases of haemoglobinopathy H. Br J Haematol 1996;92(2):332–5.

42. Wajcman H, Traeger-Synodinos J, Papassotiriou I, et al. Unstable and Thalassemic α Chain Hemoglobin Variants: A Cause of Hb H Disease and Thalassemia Intermedia. Hemoglobin 2008;32(4):327–49.

43. Al-Riyami AZ, Daar S, Kindi SA, et al. α-Globin genotypes associated with Hb H disease: a report from oman and a review of the literature from the eastern mediterranean region. Hemoglobin 2020;44(1):20–6.

44. Henderson S, Chapple M, Rugless M, et al. Haemoglobin H hydrops fetalis syndrome associated with homozygosity for the α2-globin gene polyadenylation signal mutation AATAAA→AATA. Br J Haematol 2006;135(5):743–5.

45. Haider M, Adekile A. Alpha-2-Globin Gene Polyadenylation (AATAAA→AATAAG) Mutation in Hemoglobin H Disease among Kuwaitis. MPP 2005;14(Suppl. 1):73–6.

46. Zhou YL, Zhang XH, Liu TN, et al. Splenectomy improves anaemia but does not reduce iron burden in patients with haemoglobin H Constant Spring disease. Blood Transfus 2014;12(4):471–8.

47. Yin XL, Zhang XH, Zhou TH, et al. Hemoglobin H disease in guangxi province, southern china: clinical review of 357 patients. AHA 2010;124(2):86–91.

48. Tso SC, Chan TK, Todd D. Venous thrombosis in haemoglobin H disease after splenectomy. Aust N Z J Med 1982;12(6):635–8.

49. Kuo KHM, Layton DM, Lal A, et al. Safety and efficacy of mitapivat, an oral pyruvate kinase activator, in adults with non-transfusion dependent α-thalassaemia or

β-thalassaemia: an open-label, multicentre, phase 2 study. The Lancet 2022; 400(10351):493–501.

50. Charoenkwan P, Sirichotiyakul S, Chanprapaph P, et al. Anemia and hydrops in a fetus with homozygous hemoglobin constant spring. J Pediatr Hematol Oncol 2006;28(12):827–30.

51. He Y, Zhao Y, Lou JW, et al. Fetal anemia and hydrops fetalis associated with homo-zygous Hb constant spring (HBA2: c.427T > C). Hemoglobin 2016;40(2):97–101.

52. Liao C, Li J, Li DZ. Fetal anemia and hydrops associated with homozygosity for hemoglobin Quong Sze. Prenatal Diagn 2008;28(9):862–4.

53. Sirilert S, Charoenkwan P, Sirichotiyakul S, et al. Prenatal diagnosis and management of homozygous hemoglobin constant spring disease. J Perinatol 2019;39(7):927–33.

54. Li J, Liao C, Zhou JY, et al. Phenotypic Variability in a Chinese Family with Non-deletional Hb H-Hb Quong Sze Disease. Hemoglobin 2011;35(4):430–3.

55. Akhtar MS, Qaw F, Borgio JF, et al. Spectrum of α-Thalassemia Mutations in Transfusion-Dependent β-Thalassemia Patients from the Eastern Province of Saudi Arabia. Hemoglobin 2013;37(1):65–73.

56. Lee TY, Lai MI, Ismail P, et al. Analysis of α1 and α2 globin genes among patients with hemoglobin Adana in Malaysia. Genet Mol Res 2016;15(2). https://doi.org/10.4238/gmr.15027400.

57. Yang X, Yan JM, Li J, et al. Hydrops Fetalis Associated with Compound Hetero-zygosity for Hb Zurich-Albisrieden (HBA2: C.178G > C) and the Southeast Asian (– –SEA/) Deletion. Hemoglobin 2016;40(5):353–5.

58. Fucharoen S, Winichagoon P. Hemoglobinopathies in Southeast Asia: Molecular Biology and Clinical Medicine. 2009. Available at: http://informahealthcare.com/doi/abs/10.3109/03630269709000664. Accessed December 3, 2012.

59. Liao C, Wei J, Li Q, et al. Nonimmune Hydrops Fetalis Diagnosed during the Sec-ond Half of Pregnancy in Southern China. FDT 2007;22(4):302–5.

60. Srisupundit K, Piyamongkol W, Tongsong T. Identification of fetuses with hemo-globin Bart's disease using middle cerebral artery peak systolic velocity. Ultra-sound Obstet Gynecol 2009;33(6):694–7.

61. Kreger EM, Singer ST, Witt RG, et al. Favorable outcomes after in utero transfu-sion in fetuses with alpha thalassemia major: a case series and review of the liter-ature. Prenat Diagn 2016;36(13):1242–9.

62. Songdej D, Babbs C, Higgs DR. An international registry of survivors with Hb Bart's hydrops fetalis syndrome. Blood 2017;129(10):1251–9.

63. Zhang HJ, Amid A, Janzen LA, et al. Outcomes of haemoglobin Bart's hydrops fetalis following intrauterine transfusion in Ontario, Canada. Arch Dis Child - Fetal Neonatal Edition 2021;106(1):51–6.

64. Amid A, Chen S, Athale U, et al. Iron overload in transfusion-dependent survivors of hemoglobin Bart's hydrops fetalis. Haematologica 2018;103(5):e184–7.

65. Amid A, Chen S, Brien W, et al. Optimizing chronic transfusion therapy for survi-vors of hemoglobin Barts hydrops fetalis. Blood J Am Soc Hematol 2016;127(9):1208–11.

66. Schwab ME, Lianoglou BR, Gano D, et al. The impact of in utero transfusions on perinatal outcomes in patients with alpha thalassemia major: the UCSF registry. Blood Adv 2022. https://doi.org/10.1182/bloodadvances.2022007823.

67. Gregory GL, Wienert B, Schwab M, et al. Investigating zeta globin gene expres-sion to develop a potential therapy for alpha thalassemia major. Blood 2020; 136:3–4.

68. King AJ, Songdej D, Downes DJ, et al. Reactivation of a developmentally silenced embryonic globin gene. Nat Commun 2021;12(1):4439.

Pathogenic Mechanisms in Thalassemia I

Ineffective Erythropoiesis and Hypercoagulability

Rayan Bou-Fakhredin, MSc[a], Stefano Rivella, PhD[b],
Maria Domenica Cappellini, MD, PhD[a,c], Ali T. Taher, MD, PhD[d],*

KEYWORDS

- β-Thalassemia • Ineffective erythropoiesis • Coagulopathy • Hypercoagulability
- Thrombosis • Vascular disease • Silent cerebral infarcts

KEY POINTS

- Ineffective erythropoiesis is the driving cause of many of the morbidities associated with β-thalassemia, including hypercoagulability and vascular disease.
- Several factors attribute to the pathophysiology of hypercoagulability in β-thalassemia.
- Splenectomy, anemia, iron overload, transfusion naivety, and high nucleatedred blood cells and platelet counts have all been identified as risk factors for thrombosis development in patients with β-thalassemia, especially in patients with non–transfusion-dependent thalassemia.

INTRODUCTION

Ineffective erythropoiesis in β-thalassemia occurs because of a complex interplay between different molecular mechanisms resulting in the production of pathological red blood cells (RBCs) in the bone marrow and its bidirectional cross talk between the erythron and other organs in the body such as the liver, spleen, and gut.[1] In β-thalassemia, the altered differentiation of erythroid progenitors combined with increased proliferation and apoptosis seem to exacerbate the process of ineffective erythropoiesis, ultimately leading to hemolysis, and anemia. This leads to a cascade of events responsible for the morbidities associated with β-thalassemia, among which is

[a] Department of Clinical Sciences and Community Health, University of Milan, Milan, Italy; [b] Division of Hematology, Department of Pediatrics, Children's Hospital of Philadelphia, Philadelphia, PA, USA; [c] UOC General Medicine, Fondazione IRCCS Ca' Granda Ospedale Maggiore Policlinico, Milan, Italy; [d] Division of Hematology-Oncology, Department of Internal Medicine, American University of Beirut Medical Center, Beirut, Lebanon
* Corresponding author.
E-mail address: ataher@aub.edu.lb

Hematol Oncol Clin N Am 37 (2023) 341–351
https://doi.org/10.1016/j.hoc.2022.12.005
0889-8588/23/© 2022 Elsevier Inc. All rights reserved.

thrombosis. We herein describe the main features of erythropoiesis and its regulation in addition to the mechanisms behind ineffective erythropoiesis development in β-thalassemia. Finally, we review the pathophysiology of hypercoagulability and vascular disease development in β-thalassemia and the currently available prevention and treatment modalities.

THE PROCESS OF ERYTHROPOIESIS AND ITS REGULATION

Erythropoiesis is a tightly regulated process that results in the production of RBCs.[2,3] Erythropoiesis involves the proliferation and differentiation of RBC progenitor cells and precursor cells to form mature RBCs. This process occurs in specialized niches within both the bone marrow and the spleen.[4] The formation of mature RBC represents a highly regulated process that begins with the differentiation of multipotent hematopoietic progenitor cells in a single lineage.[5] After this step, erythroid precursors undergo an extensive phase of proliferation. Finally, a progressive stage of maturation takes place, which is characterized by modifications in gene expression toward the formation of mature erythrocytes.[6–8] These events are aided by macrophages, forming a functional structure known as an erythroblastic island that controls the crucial regulation of this balance.[9–11] This whole and complex process is facilitated by a set of transcription factors, cytokines, and signaling molecules. GATA Binding Protein 1 (GATA1), a primary transcription factor, regulates the expression of numerous genes involved in process of erythropoiesis, including those for heme and globin production, antiapoptotic factors, and the receptor for erythropoietin (EPO).[12] EPO, which is produced in response to hypoxic conditions by the activation of hypoxia-inducible factor 2 alpha (HIF-2α) in the kidney, also regulates erythropoiesis in the early and late stages of erythroid progenitor differentiation.[13,14] EPO binds to the erythropoietin receptor (EPO-R), which causes receptor homodimerization. One of the main signaling pathways mediated by the EPO/EPO-R interaction is JAK2 activation, which subsequently phosphorylates and activates STAT5.[15] The JAK2/STAT5 pathway has been shown to activate genes fundamental for erythroid progenitor survival, proliferation, and differentiation.[16] Furthermore, STAT5 phosphorylation is essential for the acceleration of erythropoiesis during times of hypoxic stress. The JAK2/STAT5 pathway is chronically activated in β-thalassemia due to the chronic hypoxia state leading to increased levels of EPO synthesis.[17] Other downstream activation pathways include mitogen-activated protein kinase and phosphoinositide 3-kinase (PI3K). Similarly, these pathways are involved in the differentiation and proliferation of erythroid progenitors.[18]

In the later stages of erythroid precursor maturation, the involvement of other molecules such as transforming growth factor beta (TGF-β) superfamily ligands and other pathways such as the SMAD signaling pathway regulates the progression of erythropoiesis.[19] Paracrine and endocrine mediators involved in oxidative stress, inflammation, and apoptosis also have influence on the maturation stage of the erythropoiesis process.[20,21] Moreover, and in order to allow the synthesis of hemoglobin (Hb), iron metabolism is tightly regulated throughout the whole process.[22]

Under conditions of low oxygen delivery, the rate of erythropoiesis may be expanded significantly to increase oxygen delivery to the tissues.[23] This physiological adaptation is defined as stress erythropoiesis and is characterized by an imbalance of erythroid proliferation and the differentiation axis, resulting in an expansion of the erythroid progenitor pool to meet the demands of increased RBC generation and oxygenation.[23] In conditions of pathologically altered erythropoiesis or ineffective erythropoiesis, such as β-thalassemia, the reduced ability of erythrocytes to differentiate, survive, and deliver oxygen stimulates a state of stress erythropoiesis that leads to the ineffective production of RBCs[24] (**Fig. 1**).

INEFFECTIVE ERYTHROPOIESIS IN β-THALASSEMIA

In a state of decreased β-globin chain production such as β-thalassemia, excess α-globin chains aggregate resulting in hemolysis and, as a consequence, a reduction in RBC life span in circulation.[25] The excess α-globin chains accumulate on erythroid membranes, leading to the formation of methemoglobin and hemichromes conducive to an oxidative stress environment, contributing to reduced differentiation and apoptosis.[26] As a result of this, a continuous state of chronic stress erythropoiesis arises, and the expanded pool of erythroid precursors is unable to generate enough RBCs, thereby resulting in anemia. The severity of this anemia depends on the degree of α/β-globin chain imbalance.[25,26] Moreover, the resulting anemia is accompanied by a decrease in the expression of hepcidin (HAMP), the hormone that limits how much iron is taken up from the duodenum, thereby leading to increased iron absorption and iron overload.[4] Another factor responsible for iron overload is that the intestinal HIF2α, which is activated under condition of hypoxia in β-thalassemia and leads to upregulation of genes responsible for duodenal iron absorption.[27,28]

Macrophages have also been described to play a role in the pathophysiology of ineffective erythropoiesis. In fact, studies conducted on thalassemic mice have shown that the depletion of macrophages substantially ameliorated anemia and splenomegaly.[29,30] Other factors that have also been implicated in anemia associated with ineffective erythropoiesis such as that seen in β-thalassemia, include those that are primarily associated with the α/β globin chain imbalance. The formation of α-globin aggregates has cytotoxic effects that lead to sequestration of heat shock protein 70, leaving GATA1 accessible for caspase-3 cleavage.[31] This results in apoptosis at the polychromatophilic stage of erythroid maturation, and generation of ROS.[22,30,32] However, it has been shown that the pathway of heme-regulated inhibitor kinase and eukaryotic translational initiation factors 2 (eIF2alpha) seem to play a role in preventing denatured α-globin aggregates from accumulating, indirectly favoring GATA1-mediated maturation.[33,34]

Certain members of the TGF-β family are thought to have a prominent role in ineffective erythropoiesis through the inhibition of RBC maturation, mediated by the activation of class II activin receptors A (ActRIIA) and B (ActRIIB).[35] Growth differentiation

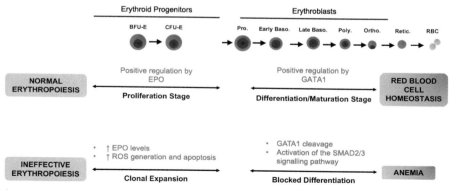

Fig. 1. Comparison between normal erythropoiesis and ineffective erythropoiesis.

factor 11 (GDF11) has been shown to be elevated in diseases exhibiting hallmarks of ineffective erythropoiesis such as β-thalassemia. The activation of the inhibitory SMAD2/3 pathway by GDF11 may lead to reduced erythroid differentiation and a lack of mature erythrocytes. However, the role of GDF11 in this mechanism has been questioned because lack of GDF11 does not improve mice with anemia affected by β-thalassemia.[36]

Furthermore, the resulting anemia and hypoxia cause an increase in EPO production, which in turn exacerbates the increased proliferation and accumulation of immature erythroid precursors.[26] These increased production of abnormal nucleated erythroid cells leads to 2 major endpoints: (1) elevated levels of the erythroid-secreted hormone erythroferrone, which contributes to the suppression of HAMP and iron overload in β-thalassemia; (2) synthesis of other factors such as growth differentiation factor 15, which correlate positively with markers of ineffective erythropoiesis, such as EPO, soluble TfR1, and nucleated RBC levels, and with the clinical severity of the pathologic condition itself.[37–39]

HYPERCOAGULABILITY AND VASCULAR DISEASE IN BETA-THALASSEMIA
Pathophysiology

Several factors that lead to the hypercoagulable state in patients with β-thalassemia have been identified and described[40] (**Fig. 2**). One of these factors is chronic activation of platelets and enhancement of platelet aggregation.[41] Compared with healthy individuals, patients with β-thalassemia have been shown to have elevated markers of hemostatic activity, as evident by studies that have measured the levels of thromboxane A2 and prostacyclins.[42] Splenectomized patients with β-thalassemia in particular tend to have an increased platelet count and platelet adhesion compared with their nonsplenectomized counterpart.[43]

In β-thalassemia, the oxidation of globin subunits in erythroid cells leads to the formation of hemichromes, which precipitate and prompt the subsequent release of toxic radicals leading to the formation of ROS.[44] This then causes oxidation of membrane proteins and exposure of phosphatidylserine through a flip-flop mechanism, which in turn increases the rigidity, deformability, and aggregation of RBCs, resulting in premature cell removal.[45,46] Thalassemic RBCs containing a high content of such negatively charged phospholipids often lead to an increase in thrombin generation.[47,48]

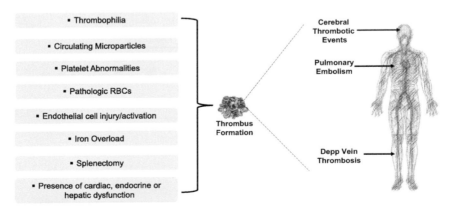

- Thrombophilia
- Circulating Microparticles
- Platelet Abnormalities
- Pathologic RBCs
- Endothelial cell injury/activation
- Iron Overload
- Splenectomy
- Presence of cardiac, endocrine or hepatic dysfunction

Thrombus Formation

Cerebral Thrombotic Events

Pulmonary Embolism

Depp Vein Thrombosis

Fig. 2. Factors that lead to the pathophysiology of hypercoagulability in patients with β-thalassemia and the subsequent thromboembolic events.

Again, splenectomized patients have a considerably higher number of these negatively charged pathologic RBCs and thus higher levels of thrombin generation are often seen in these patients.[49] Free iron also induces lipid oxidation and elevates the level of membrane-bounded hemichromes and immunoglobulins causing alteration of the structures of spectrin and band 3 protein of RBC membrane and consequently resulting in aggregation and adhesion of abnormal RBCs to endothelial cells.[50]

Other peripheral blood elements that can contribute to the procoagulant state in β-thalassemia include elevated levels of endothelial adhesion proteins (including E-selectin, intercellular adhesion molecule-1 and von Willebrand factor), and vascular cell adhesion molecule 1.[51] In addition, circulating endothelial cells expressing adhesion molecules and tissue factor have been documented in patients with β-thalassemia.[52]

Inherited thrombophilia does not play a role in the hypercoagulable state of β-thalassemia.[53] However, deficiencies of protein C and protein S, and antithrombin III have been reported in patients with β-thalassemia.[54-56] In addition, an increased incidence of antiphospholipid antibodies, such as lupus anticoagulant, anticardiolipin, and anti-beta 2-glycoprotein 1, is commonly found in patients with β-thalassemia disease. Those antibodies are considered as strong thrombophilic risk factors causing thromboembolism.[57,58]

Decreased nitric oxide, secondary to hemolysis caused by the decreased level of arginine, leads to pulmonary vasoconstriction and subsequently results in chronic pulmonary thromboembolism.[57,59] Iron overload per se can lead to an increase in NTBI formation and subsequent vessel injury and formation of atherosclerotic plaques.[60,61]

Incidence and Prevalence

Based on the results of a study conducted on 8860 patients with β-thalassemia in the Mediterranean area and in Iran, it was found that the incidence of thrombosis is about 4-fold higher in patients with non–transfusion-dependent thalassemia (NTDT) compared with patients with transfusion-dependent thalassemia (TDT) is mostly venous and is a leading cause of mortality.[62,63] The frequency of thrombosis in NTDT is significantly higher in patients aged older than 35 years (28.2%) compared with patients aged 18 to 35 years (14.9%), or younger than 18 years (4.1%).[64] Patients with NTDT who were at higher risk of developing thrombosis were those aged older than 20 years, those who were splenectomized, or those who have a personal or family history of thrombosis.[62] A cross-sectional study from the OPTICAL CARE on 584 patients with NTDT with from 6 comprehensive care centers in the Middle East and Italy further showed that thrombotic disease, mostly venous, was the fifth most common complication, affecting about 14% of the subject population.[64] Splenectomy, anemia (Hb level <9 g/dL), transfusion naivety and iron overload (serum ferritin >800 mg/L or liver iron concentration >5 mg Fe/g dry weight) have all been identified as risk factors.[49,62,64] Additionally, high nucleated RBCs ($\geq$300 $\times$ 10^6/L) and platelet counts ($\geq$500 $\times$ 10^9/L) were shown to further substantiate the risk in splenectomized patients with NTDT.[63,64]

Cerebral thrombotic events, overt and silent, resulting from a chronic hypercoagulable state, have been reported in β-thalassemia. Although the incidence of overt strokes is relatively low (about 5%), silent strokes have been described in up to 60% of splenectomized adults (mean age, 32 years) with NTDT, with a clear correlation with advancing age.[62,63,65,66] A cross-sectional study from Lebanon using brain MRI was conducted on 30 splenectomized patients with NTDT (mean age 32 years). None of the patients included in the study was receiving antiplatelet or anticoagulant therapy. Eighteen patients (60%) showed evidence of 1 or more ischemic lesions, all involving the subcortical white matter. Most of the patients showed evidence of multiple lesions. The frontal subcortical white matter was usually involved, followed by the occipital and parietal subcortical white matter. Increasing age and no transfusion history were both noted as independently associated with a higher occurrence and multiplicity of lesions.[66] Using the same cohort of patients in this study, a magnetic resonance angiography (MRA) scan was also done. Of 29 evaluable patients, 8 (27.6%) had evidence of arterial stenosis on MRA.[67] The majority of lesions had mild narrowing and mostly involved the internal carotid artery. Five patients (17.2%) had evidence of aneurysms. Among the 18 patients with silent brain infarction on MRI, 3 had evidence of stenosis on MRA with only 1 patient having lesions that could explain the silent infarcts.[67] Another cross-sectional study from Iran was conducted on 30 patients with NTDT who were splenectomized, and who had a platelet count $500 \times 10^9/L$ or greater and a Hb level greater than 7 g/dL. The investigators noted 8 patients (26.7%) with silent ischemic lesions.[68]

Patients with TDT were also shown to be at risk of developing silent cerebral ischemia (SCI). One study from Iran reported that the frequency of SCI in patients with TDT was determined to be 37.5% and concluded that frequent transfusions and low platelet counts may not always be associated with a low frequency of SCI.[69] Another study conducted on 28 patients with TDT aged older than 18 years demonstrated a high rate of SCI as evident by the MRI studies that showed focal bright foci, single or multiple (up to 73 lesions) in the cerebral white matter in 17 (60.7%) patients.[70] Most lesions were observed in frontal lobes of the brain, bilateral, with maximal diameter of 7 mm. Although not causing identifiable symptoms, SCI still causes damage to the brain and places the patient at increased risk for both transient ischemic attack and major stroke in the future.

Prevention and Management

All patients with β-thalassemia who develop thrombotic or cerebrovascular disease should be treated as per standard local or international guidelines.[71] It is also strongly recommended that these patients are regarded as high-risk individuals in medical or surgical settings.

The use of blood transfusion therapy has been established for the primary or secondary prevention of thrombotic or cerebrovascular disease. These blood transfusions may control the hypercoagulability in patients with NTDT by improving ineffective erythropoiesis and decreasing the levels of pathological RBCs with thrombogenic potential. Data from observational studies conducted on patients with NTDT showed that transfusion therapy was associated with lower rates of silent strokes and thromboembolic events.[64,66] Transfusion therapy in fact may also explain the lower rates of thrombotic events that are seen in patients with TDT compared with patients with NTDT.

Hematopoietic stem cell transplantation has been reported as a modality that could normalize the abnormal hemostatic derangement seen in pediatric patients with β-thalassemia by increasing natural anticoagulant proteins and decreasing microparticles and RBC-expressing phosphatidyl serine and activating platelets in the circulation.[72,73]

There are currently no available results from clinical trials on the role of antiplatelet or anticoagulant therapy for the prevention of thrombotic or cerebrovascular disease in patients with β-thalassemia. However, some studies have also elucidated to the role of aspirin in lowering the recurrence rate of thrombotic events in splenectomized patients with NTDT.[63] Unlike sickle cell disease, the evidences of using direct oral anticoagulants in patients with β-thalassemia who develop thromboembolism are limited.[74] However, the recent study showed that using rivaroxaban in patients with hemoglobinopathies including thalassemia was effective and did not increase the risk of bleeding or thrombosis.[75]

The role of iron chelation therapy has not yet been evaluated in this setting. As for the use of hydroxyurea, some studies have shown that this agent could reduce hemostatic activation and phospholipid expression on the surface of RBCs.[76,77] Further studies are necessary, however, to elucidate the role of hydroxyurea and iron chelation therapy in the prevention of thrombotic disease.

Assessment with brain or cerebrovascular imaging for high-risk patients may be considered. In fact, one study further highlighted the role of transcranial Doppler as a screening tool for the evaluation of brain ischemia risk in patients with β-thalassemia, and its association with makers such as NSE (biomarker of neuronal loss) and S100 B (biomarker of glial destruction).[78] Simple and practical tools to better understand the related risk for thrombosis in patients with thalassemia have also been developed. A β-thalassemia-related thrombosis risk scoring system (TRT-RSS) now exists to better understand and aid practitioners in categorizing patients for thrombosis risk based on their underlying disease characteristics, and hence support all management decisions.[79] The TRT-RSS is aimed at predicting first thrombotic events in patients without prior incidents and provides long-term risk (>10 years) assessment considering the chronic, lifelong nature of the disease.[79]

SUMMARY

Ineffective erythropoiesis is the driving cause of many of the morbidities associated with β-thalassemia. One of the most notable of these morbidities is hypercoagulability and vascular disease. Several factors that contribute to the hypercoagulable state in patients with β-thalassemia have been identified. In most cases, a combination of these factors leads to clinical thromboembolic events. An individualized approach is recommended to establish an optimal strategy for preventing the occurrence of this complication in patients with β-thalassemia. Establishment of disease-specific thromboprophylaxis guidelines should be the target of future efforts in this patient population.

CLINICS CARE POINTS

- All patients with β-thalassemia who develop thrombotic or cerebrovascular disease should be treated as per standard local or international guidelines
- When it comes to management, an individualized approach is recommended
- Future efforts should include establishing disease-specific thromboprophylaxis guidelines for this patient population

DISCLOSURE

The authors have nothing to disclose.

REFERENCES

1. Longo F, Piolatto A, Ferrero GB, et al. Ineffective erythropoiesis in beta-thalassaemia: key steps and therapeutic options by drugs. Int J Mol Sci 2021;22(13): 7229.

2. Eggold JT, Rankin EB. Erythropoiesis, EPO, macrophages, and bone. Bone 2019; 119:36–41.

3. Zivot A, Lipton JM, Narla A, et al. insights into pathophysiology and treatments in 2017. Mol Med 2018;24(1):1–15.

4. Gupta R, Musallam KM, Taher AT, et al. Ineffective erythropoiesis: anemia and iron overload. Hematol Oncol Clin North Am 2018;32(2):213–21.

5. Tusi BK, Wolock SL, Weinreb C, et al. Population snapshots predict early haematopoietic and erythroid hierarchies. Nature 2018;555(7694):54–60.

6. Chen K, Liu J, Heck S, et al. Resolving the distinct stages in erythroid differentiation based on dynamic changes in membrane protein expression during erythropoiesis. Proc Natl Acad Sci U S A 2009;106(41):17413–8.

7. Dulmovits BM, Hom J, Narla A, et al. Characterization, regulation, and targeting of erythroid progenitors in normal and disordered human erythropoiesis. Curr Opin Hematol 2017;24(3):159–66.

8. An X, Schulz VP, Li J, et al. Global transcriptome analyses of human and murine terminal erythroid differentiation. Blood 2014;123(22):3466–77.

9. Chasis JA, Mohandas N. Erythroblastic islands: niches for erythropoiesis. Blood 2008;112(3):470–8.

10. Chasis JA. Erythroblastic islands: specialized microenvironmental niches for erythropoiesis. Curr Opin Hematol 2006;13(3):137–41.

11. Mohandas N, Chasis JA. The erythroid niche: molecular processes occurring within erythroblastic islands. Transfus Clin Biol 2010;17(3):110–1.

12. Valent P, Busche G, Theurl I, et al. Normal and pathological erythropoiesis in adults: from gene regulation to targeted treatment concepts. Haematologica 2018;103(10):1593–603.

13. Bhoopalan SV, Huang LJ, Weiss MJ. Erythropoietin regulation of red blood cell production: from bench to bedside and back, *F1000Res*, 9, 2020, F1000 Faculty Rev-1153.

14. Kapitsinou PP, Liu Q, Unger TL, et al. Hepatic HIF-2 regulates erythropoietic responses to hypoxia in renal anemia. Blood 2010;116(16):3039–48.

15. Witthuhn BA, Quelle FW, Silvennoinen O, et al. JAK2 associates with the erythropoietin receptor and is tyrosine phosphorylated and activated following stimulation with erythropoietin. Cell 1993;74(2):227–36.

16. Grebien F, Kerenyi MA, Kovacic B, et al. Stat5 activation enables erythropoiesis in the absence of EpoR and Jak2. Blood 2008;111(9):4511–22.

17. Libani IV, Guy EC, Melchiori L, et al. Decreased differentiation of erythroid cells exacerbates ineffective erythropoiesis in beta-thalassemia. Blood 2008;112(3): 875–85.

18. Zhang Y, Wang L, Dey S, et al. Erythropoietin action in stress response, tissue maintenance and metabolism. Int J Mol Sci 2014;15(6):10296–333.

19. Blank U, Karlsson S. TGF-beta signaling in the control of hematopoietic stem cells. Blood 2015;125(23):3542–50.

20. Koulnis M, Liu Y, Hallstrom K, et al. Negative autoregulation by Fas stabilizes adult erythropoiesis and accelerates its stress response. PLoS One 2011;6(7): e21192.

21. Parisi S, Finelli C, Fazio A, et al. Clinical and molecular insights in erythropoiesis regulation of signal transduction pathways in myelodysplastic syndromes and beta-thalassemia. Int J Mol Sci 2021;22(2):827.

22. Kim A, Nemeth E. New insights into iron regulation and erythropoiesis. Curr Opin Hematol 2015;22(3):199.

23. Paulson RF, Shi L, Wu DC. Stress erythropoiesis: new signals and new stress progenitor cells. Curr Opin Hematol 2011;18(3):139–45.

24. Crielaard BJ, Rivella S. beta-Thalassemia and Polycythemia vera: targeting chronic stress erythropoiesis. Int J Biochem Cell Biol 2014;51:89–92.

25. Nandakumar SK, Ulirsch JC, Sankaran VG. Advances in understanding erythropoiesis: evolving perspectives. Br J Haematol 2016;173(2):206–18.

26. Camaschella C, Nai A. Ineffective erythropoiesis and regulation of iron status in iron loading anaemias. Br J Haematol 2016;172(4):512–23.

27. Anderson ER, Taylor M, Xue X, et al. Intestinal HIF2alpha promotes tissue-iron accumulation in disorders of iron overload with anemia. Proc Natl Acad Sci U S A 2013;110(50):E4922–30.

28. Gardenghi S, Marongiu MF, Ramos P, et al. Ineffective erythropoiesis in beta-thalassemia is characterized by increased iron absorption mediated by down-regulation of hepcidin and up-regulation of ferroportin. Blood 2007;109(11): 5027–35.

29. Ramos P, Casu C, Gardenghi S, et al. Macrophages support pathological erythropoiesis in polycythemia vera and beta-thalassemia. Nat Med 2013;19(4): 437–45.

30. Arlet J-B, Ribeil J-A, Guillem F, et al. HSP70 sequestration by free α-globin promotes ineffective erythropoiesis in β-thalassaemia. Nature 2014;514(7521): 242–6.

31. De Maria R, Zeuner A, Eramo A, et al. Negative regulation of erythropoiesis by caspase-mediated cleavage of GATA-1. Nature 1999;401(6752):489–93.

32. Arlet JB, Dussiot M, Moura IC, et al. Novel players in beta-thalassemia dyserythropoiesis and new therapeutic strategies. Curr Opin Hematol 2016;23(3):181–8.

33. Chen JJ. Regulation of protein synthesis by the heme-regulated eIF2alpha kinase: relevance to anemias. Blood 2007;109(7):2693–9.

34. Chen J-J, Zhang S. Heme-regulated eIF2α kinase in erythropoiesis and hemoglobinopathies. Blood 2019;134(20):1697–707.

35. Rivella S. Iron metabolism under conditions of ineffective erythropoiesis in beta-thalassemia. Blood 2019;133(1):51–8.

36. Guerra A, Oikonomidou PR, Sinha S, et al. Lack of Gdf11 does not improve anemia or prevent the activity of RAP-536 in a mouse model of beta-thalassemia. Blood 2019;134(6):568–72.

37. Tanno T, Noel P, Miller JL. Growth differentiation factor 15 in erythroid health and disease. Curr Opin Hematol 2010;17(3):184–90.

38. Musallam KM, Taher AT, Duca L, et al. Levels of growth differentiation factor-15 are high and correlate with clinical severity in transfusion-independent patients with beta thalassemia intermedia. Blood Cells Mol Dis 2011;47(4):232–4.

39. Salussoglia I, Volpe G, Fracchia S, et al. Growth differentiation factor 15 (GDF15) and erythropoietin (EPO) levels in beta talassemia major patients. Blood 2008; 112(11):1881.

40. Taher AT, Cappellini MD, Bou-Fakhredin R, et al. Hypercoagulability and vascular disease. Hematol Oncol Clin North Am 2018;32(2):237–45.

41. Winichagoon P, Fucharoen S, Wasi P. Increased circulating platelet aggregates in thalassaemia. Southeast Asian J Trop Med Public Health 1981;12(4):556–60.

42. Eldor A, Lellouche F, Goldfarb A, et al. In vivo platelet activation in β-thalassemia major reflected by increased platelet-thromboxane urinary metabolites. Blood 1991;77(8):1749–53.

43. Goldschmidt N, Spectre G, Brill A, et al. Increased platelet adhesion under flow conditions is induced by both thalassemic platelets and red blood cells. Thromb Haemost 2008;100(05):864–70.

44. Hershko C, Graham G, Bates GW, et al. Non-specific serum iron in thalassaemia: an abnormal serum iron fraction of potential toxicity. Br J Haematol 1978;40(2): 255–63.

45. Kuypers FA, de Jong K. The role of phosphatidylserine in recognition and removal of erythrocytes. Cell Mol Biol (Noisy-le-grand) 2004;50(2):147–58.

46. Tavazzi D, Duca L, Graziadei G, et al. Membrane-bound iron contributes to oxidative damage of beta-thalassaemia intermedia erythrocytes. Br J Haematol 2001; 112(1):48–50.

47. Borenstain-Ben Yashar V, Barenholz Y, Hy-Am E, et al. Phosphatidylserine in the outer leaflet of red blood cells from beta-thalassemia patients may explain the chronic hypercoagulable state and thrombotic episodes. Am J Hematol 1993; 44(1):63–5.

48. Helley D, Eldor A, Girot R, et al. Increased procoagulant activity of red blood cells from patients with homozygous sickle cell disease and beta-thalassemia. Thromb Haemost 1996;76(3):322–7.

49. Cappellini MD, Robbiolo L, Bottasso BM, et al. Venous thromboembolism and hypercoagulability in splenectomized patients with thalassaemia intermedia. Br J Haematol 2000;111(2):467–73.

50. Eldor A, Rachmilewitz EA. The hypercoagulable state in thalassemia. Blood 2002; 99(1):36–43.

51. Butthep P, Bunyaratvej A, Funahara Y, et al. Alterations in vascular endothelial cell-related plasma proteins in thalassaemic patients and their correlation with clinical symptoms. Thromb Haemost 1995;74(4):1045–9.

52. Butthep P, Rummavas S, Wisedpanichkij R, et al. Increased circulating activated endothelial cells, vascular endothelial growth factor, and tumor necrosis factor in thalassemia. Am J Hematol 2002;70(2):100–6.

53. Iolascon A, Giordano P, Storelli S, et al. Thrombophilia in thalassemia major patients: analysis of genetic predisposing factors. Haematologica 2001;86(10): 1112–3.

54. Taher AT, Otrock ZK, Uthman I, et al. Thalassemia and hypercoagulability. Blood Rev 2008;22(5):283–92.

55. Huang Y, Long Y, Deng D, et al. Alterations of anticoagulant proteins and soluble endothelial protein C receptor in thalassemia patients of Chinese origin. Thromb Res 2018;172:61–6.

56. Angchaisuksiri P, Atichartakarn V, Aryurachai K, et al. Hemostatic and thrombotic markers in patients with hemoglobin E/beta-thalassemia disease. Am J Hematol 2007;82(11):1001–4.

57. Sirachainan N. Thalassemia and the hypercoagulable state. Thromb Res 2013; 132(6):637–41.

58. Sharma S, Raina V, Chandra J, et al. Lupus anticoagulant and anticardiolipin antibodies in polytransfused beta thalassemia major. Hematology 2006;11(4): 287–90.

59. Tantawy AA, Adly AA, Ismail EA, et al. Endothelial nitric oxide synthase gene intron 4 variable number tandem repeat polymorphism in beta-thalassemia major: relation to cardiovascular complications. Blood Coagul Fibrinolysis 2015;26(4): 419–25.

60. Auer JW, Berent R, Weber T, et al. Iron metabolism and development of atherosclerosis. Circulation 2002;106(2):e7 [author reply: e7].

61. Aessopos A, Tsironi M, Andreopoulos A, et al. Heart disease in thalassemia inter-media. Hemoglobin 2009;33(Suppl 1):S170–6.
62. Taher A, Isma'eel H, Mehio G, et al. Prevalence of thromboembolic events among 8,860 patients with thalassaemia major and intermedia in the Mediterranean area and Iran. Thromb Haemost 2006;96(10):488–91.
63. Taher AT, Musallam KM, Karimi M, et al. Splenectomy and thrombosis: the case of thalassemia intermedia. J Thromb Haemost 2010;8(10):2152–8.
64. Taher AT, Musallam KM, Karimi M, et al. Overview on practices in thalassemia in-termedia management aiming for lowering complication rates across a region of endemicity: the OPTIMAL CARE study. Blood 2010;115(10):1886–92.
65. Musallam KM, Taher AT, Karimi M, et al. Cerebral infarction in beta-thalassemia intermedia: breaking the silence. Thromb Res 2012;130(5):695–702.
66. Taher AT, Musallam KM, Nasreddine W, et al. Asymptomatic brain magnetic reso-nance imaging abnormalities in splenectomized adults with thalassemia interme-dia. J Thromb Haemost 2010;8(1):54–9.
67. Musallam KM, Beydoun A, Hourani R, et al. Brain magnetic resonance angiog-raphy in splenectomized adults with beta-thalassemia intermedia. Eur J Haema-tol 2011;87(6):539–46.
68. Karimi M, Bagheri H, Rastgu F, et al. Magnetic resonance imaging to determine the incidence of brain ischaemia in patients with beta-thalassaemia intermedia. Thromb Haemost 2010;103(5):989–93.
69. Karimi M, Toosi F, Haghpanah S, et al. The frequency of silent cerebral ischemia in patients with transfusion-dependent beta-thalassemia major. Ann Hematol 2016;95(1):135–9.
70. Pazgal I, Inbar E, Cohen M, et al. High incidence of silent cerebral infarcts in adult patients with beta thalassemia major. Thromb Res 2016;144:119–22.
71. Taher A, Vichinsky E, Musallam K, et al. Guidelines for the Management of Non Transfusion Dependent Thalassaemia (NTDT). Nicosia (Cyprus). Thalassaemia International Federation 2013.
72. Sirachainan N, Thongsad J, Pakakasama S, et al. Normalized coagulation markers and anticoagulation proteins in children with severe β-thalassemia dis-ease after stem cell transplantation. Thromb Res 2012;129(6):765–70.
73. Klaihmon P, Vimonpatranon S, Noulsri E, et al. Normalized levels of red blood cells expressing phosphatidylserine, their microparticles, and activated platelets in young patients with β-thalassemia following bone marrow transplantation. Ann Hematol 2017;96(10):1741–7.
74. Shet AS, Wun T. How I diagnose and treat venous thromboembolism in sickle cell disease. Blood J Am Soc Hematol 2018;132(17):1761–9.
75. Apostolou C, Klonizakis P, Mainou M, et al. Rivaroxaban use in patients with he-moglobinopathies. Hemoglobin 2017;41(3):223–4.
76. Singer ST, Vichinsky EP, Larkin S, et al. Hydroxycarbamide-induced changes in E/beta thalassemia red blood cells. Am J Hematol 2008;83(11):842–5.
77. Ataga KI, Cappellini MD, Rachmilewitz EA. Beta-thalassaemia and sickle cell anaemia as paradigms of hypercoagulability. Br J Haematol 2007;139(1):3–13.
78. Kanavaki A, Spengos K, Moraki M, et al. Serum levels of S100b and NSE proteins in patients with non-transfusion-dependent thalassemia as biomarkers of brain ischemia and cerebral vasculopathy. Int J Mol Sci 2017;18(12):2724.
79. Taher AT, Cappellini MD, Musallam KM. Development of a thalassemia-related thrombosis risk scoring system. Am J Hematol 2019;94(8):E207–9.

Pathogenic Mechanisms in Thalassemia II: Iron Overload

Tomas Ganz, PhD, MD*, Elizabeta Nemeth, PhD

KEYWORDS

- Ineffective erythropoiesis • Hepcidin • Erythroferrone • Nontransferrin-bound iron

KEY POINTS

- Iron overload in thalassemia is caused by erythrocyte transfusions and hyperabsorption of dietary iron.
- Hepcidin is inappropriately low in thalassemia with ineffective erythropoiesis, allowing dietary iron to be excessively absorbed.
- Erythroferrone secreted by thalassemic erythroblasts is an important erythroid suppressor of hepcidin in thalassemia with ineffective erythropoiesis.

INTRODUCTION/HISTORY/DEFINITION/BACKGROUND

Organismal iron physiology. Organismal trafficking of iron is dominated by the recycling of the iron content of senescent erythrocytes. Macrophages of the spleen and the liver process daily approximately 20 mg of iron from erythrocytes. This iron is loaded onto plasma transferrin for distribution to all tissues but is predominantly destined for erythropoiesis. Erythrocytes contain 2 to 3 g of iron in adults and have a lifespan of 120 days so erythrocyte replacement requires 17 to 25 mg/d of iron. The plasma transferrin compartment normally contains about 3 mg of iron, implying that transferrin-bound iron turns over approximately every 3 h. Intestinal iron absorption normally accounts for 1 to 2 mg iron/day and balances obligatory losses of similar size, mostly from the desquamation of intestinal cells and minor blood losses. Iron losses are not regulated, and do not appreciably increase in iron overload states, so total body iron content of 3 to 4 g in adults is entirely regulated by intestinal iron absorption. Iron storage in hepatocytes and macrophages accounts for approximately 0.2 to 1g of iron in adults, with the lower range seen in menstruating women. The stored iron is available for mobilization during periods of increased iron requirements, for example, after hemorrhage or during pregnancy or somatic growth.

Department of Medicine, David Geffen School of Medicine at UCLA, Los Angeles, CA 90095-1690, USA
* Corresponding author.
E-mail address: tganz@mednet.ucla.edu

Hematol Oncol Clin N Am 37 (2023) 353–363
https://doi.org/10.1016/j.hoc.2022.12.006
0889-8588/23/© 2022 Elsevier Inc. All rights reserved.

Iron overload in thalassemia. Iron overload, a major life-threatening complication of thalassemias, is a consequence of (i) increased iron delivery through erythrocyte transfusions that bypasses physiologic control mechanisms, and (ii) increased intestinal iron absorption, both in the face of physiologic inability to excrete excess iron. In transfusion-dependent thalassemia (thalassemia major), the current recommendations are for transfusions every 2 to 4 weeks, maintaining pretransfusion hemoglobin above 90 to 105 g/L or up to 110 to 120 g/L for patients with cardiac complications.[1] Each transfused unit of red blood cells (RBC) delivers between 200 and 250 mg of iron, so a patient receiving 1 to 2 unit RBC every 2 weeks accumulates additional iron at the rate of 14 to 33 mg/d. The iron load generated by these regimens may reach clinically toxic levels in a timespan of a few years (**Fig. 1**). Patients on such transfusion schedules require chelation therapy to remove excess iron from the body and prevent iron-mediated organ damage. By contrast, iron overload in nontransfusion-dependent thalassemias (thalassemia intermedia) develops over decades and is caused by increased dietary iron absorption estimated to cause a net iron gain of 3 to 9 mg/d.[2] Although the iron overload generated by repeated transfusions is readily understood, the molecular pathogenesis of hyperabsorption of iron in thalassemias and other anemias with ineffective erythropoiesis remained a mystery until quite recently.

Iron toxicity. Iron normally circulates in plasma bound to the carrier protein transferrin whose two iron binding sites are on the average 20% to 45% occupied by iron. Cells take up transferrin-bound iron, release the iron for intracellular uses and recycle the empty transferrin molecules back to plasma. During iron overload states, iron may accumulate in plasma and its concentration may exceed the binding capacity of transferrin. The surplus iron binds to lower affinity alternative binders that include organic acid anions (eg, citrate) and albumin, forms of iron collectively referred to as nontransferrin-bound iron (NTBI).[3] NTBI is transported into cells by cell-type specific alternative iron transporters that include ZIP14[4–6] in hepatocytes and pancreatic islet cells. How cardiomyocytes take up NTBI is still an unresolved question, but L-type and T-type calcium channels (L-type calcium channel [LTCCs] and T-type calcium channel [TTCCs]) seem to contribute.[4] The liver functions as the primary clearance organ for NTBI.[7] Hepatic toxicity manifesting as fibrosis correlates with an iron concentration in the liver and duration of exposure to excess iron.[8] The development of cardiac toxicity in thalassemia strongly correlates with NTBI concentrations,[9] perhaps because the liver takes up most NTBI unless the rate of NTBI generation exceeds the capacity of the liver to remove NTBI from circulation. Cardiac toxicity is uncommon in conditions where iron accumulation is slow and NTBI concentrations are relatively low (eg, HFE hemochromatosis and nontransfusion-dependent thalassemia[10]) compared with those conditions where iron accumulation is rapid and NTBI concentrations are high (eg, juvenile hemochromatosis and transfusion-dependent β-thalassemia). Excessive concentration of iron that is unchaperoned by carrier proteins can cause intracellular damage by catalyzing chemical modifications of proteins, lipids, and nucleic acids,[11] causing initially reversible functional deficits (eg, early cardiomyopathy) but eventually progressive fibrosis, organ failure, and carcinogenesis. Extracellularly, NTBI is highly bioavailable to gram-negative bacteria[12,13] and other pathogenic microbes that cause frequent infections in iron-overloaded patients with thalassemias.[14,15]

Molecular basis of organismal iron homeostasis. The hepatic peptide hormone hepcidin[16] is the endocrine regulator of intestinal iron absorption, and therefore of total body iron content. In this role, hepcidin controls the transfer of iron from duodenal enterocytes to blood plasma. In addition, on a much shorter time scale, hepcidin also regulates the plasma concentration of iron by controlling the transfer to blood

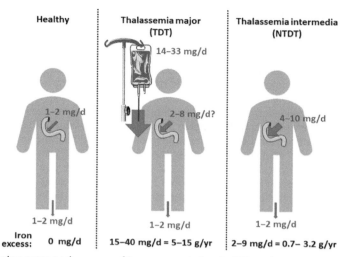

Fig. 1. Differing rates and sources of iron accumulation in TDT and NTDT. Iron overload develops rapidly in TDT compared with NTDT because of the large amount of iron in transfused blood and physiologic inability to increase iron excretion above baseline. Hyperabsorption of iron is the main cause of iron overload in NTDT but may contribute to TDT also when hemoglobin concentrations are inadequate to suppress ineffective erythropoiesis.

plasma of recycled, stored, and absorbed iron from macrophages, hepatocytes, and duodenal enterocytes, respectively. In both capacities, hepcidin acts by binding to the cellular iron exporter ferroportin, occluding the transporter and inducing its endocytosis and proteolysis.[17,18] As ferroportin is the sole known exporter of elemental iron from macrophages, hepatocytes, and duodenal enterocytes, the delivery of iron to blood plasma is proportional to the ferroportin concentration on the membranes of iron-exporting cells in contact with blood plasma. Effectively, hepcidin is a negative regulator of iron delivery from all its cellular sources to plasma. When hepcidin concentrations become pathologically inadequate, ferroportin activity on macrophages and duodenal enterocytes increases, driving greater iron delivery to blood plasma from both dietary sources and from iron stores in macrophages and hepatocytes.

Regulation of hepcidin. The major biological inputs that regulate hepcidin are iron status (plasma iron concentration and hepatic iron stores), inflammation, and erythropoietic activity. Although multiple other signals also affect hepcidin synthesis, two principal pathways have been identified to date. Iron and erythropoietic regulation center on a bone morphogenetic receptor complex consisting of BMP6 or BMP2 ligands, the BMP co-receptor hemojuvelin (HJV), bone morphogenetic protein (BMP) type I receptors activin receptor like kinase 2 or 3 (ALK2 or ALK3), and BMP type II receptors ACVRIIA or BMPR-II.[19] This complex interacts in an as yet incompletely characterized manner with iron-transferrin sensing molecules transferrin receptor 1 (TFR1) and TFR2 and additional ancillary molecules including homeostatic protein regulator (HFE) and neogenin.[19] The signaling by the BMP receptor complex is carried out by the suppressor of mothers against decaplegic (SMAD) signaling pathway[20] involving SMADs 1, 5, and 8, which bind to the common co-factor SMAD4 to enter the nucleus. There they attach to BMP response elements in the hepcidin gene promoter to regulate the transcription of the hepcidin gene. The second set of pathways controlling hepcidin production mediates the effects of inflammation and innate immunity on hepcidin. Its predominant effector is interleukin-6[21] acting through the JAK-STAT3 pathway,[22–24] again regulating the transcription of the hepcidin gene.

In thalassemia, multiple signals could regulate hepcidin in an opposing manner: increased erythroid activity would suppress hepcidin; iron loading would increase hepcidin, and any presence of inflammation would also increase hepcidin. The level of hepcidin expression ultimately depends on the relative strength of the stimuli.

Erythropoietic activity and iron homeostasis. Measurements of intestinal iron absorption and ferrokinetics in the 1950s documented that humans and laboratory mice respond to blood loss by increasing iron absorption several-fold and also mobilizing iron from stores, and that this response required functional marrow. A similar response was seen after injections of erythropoietin (EPO). It was noted then that iron absorption was very high in thalassemia, and much higher than in compensated hemolytic anemias such as hereditary spherocytosis, despite similar rates of peripheral erythrocyte destruction.[25] These observations gave rise to the idea that ineffective erythropoiesis led to a greatly enlarged mass of erythroblasts that exerted a dominant effect on iron homeostasis, leading to iron overload even in the absence of erythrocyte transfusions.

Ineffective erythropoiesis generates a suppressor of hepcidin. Following the discovery of hepcidin and its role as the iron-regulatory hormone, studies in humans and in mice showed that erythropoietic stimulation exerted its effect on iron regulation by suppressing hepcidin,[26–28] and that this response required functioning marrow.[27,28] Hepcidin mRNA or serum hepcidin was found to be low in human β-thalassemia[29–33] and in its mouse Th3/+ model,[34–36] especially when considered relative to the severity of iron overload. Hepcidin levels were also low in other iron-loading anemias with ineffective erythropoiesis, including congenital dyserythropoietic anemias.[37–39]

Candidate hepcidin suppressors GDF15 and TWSG1. The first strategy in the search for specific marrow-derived molecules that functioned as hepcidin suppressors in β-thalassemia focused on members of the TGFβ superfamily expressed in erythroblasts.[40] The rationale for this approach was based on the involvement of BMPs, members of the TGFβ superfamily, in hepcidin regulation. The two genes that stood out because of very high relative expression in human primary erythroblasts were GDF15 and TWSG1. GDF15 concentrations were increased 20- to 70-fold in the blood of patients with β-thalassemia compared with patients with sickle cell anemia or MDS, and 90-fold compared with patients with hemochromatosis. Moreover, GDF15 suppressed the expression of hepcidin mRNA in human primary hepatocytes and the hepatocyte cell line HuH7. Sera from patients with β-thalassemia also suppressed hepcidin expression in primary hepatocytes and the suppression could be partially reversed with neutralizing antibodies to GDF15. Compared with GDF15, TWSG1 is highly expressed earlier during erythroblast development and shows hepcidin-suppressive activity when assayed in murine primary hepatocytes. With human primary hepatocytes, TWSG1 antagonizes the hepcidin-stimulating effect or BMP2 or BMP4. However, GDF15 gene ablation or knockout (KO) mice have similar erythroid and iron parameters to WT mice and suppress hepcidin mRNA similarly after major blood loss. TWSG1 is not altered by blood loss in this model. Moreover, marrows of Th3/+ mice do not express high levels of GDF15. Although it is still possible that GDF15 or TWSG1 contribute to hepcidin suppression in human β-thalassemia and other iron-loading anemias with ineffective erythropoiesis, mouse models may not be an appropriate way to test this hypothesis.

Erythroferrone. The second strategy in the search for erythroid hepcidin suppressors focused on the early physiologic marrow response to blood loss or EPO administration in mice, preceding the nadir of hepcidin suppression at 12 to 15 h.[41]

Time-dependent expression profiling of the marrow after blood loss identified a transcript that was induced already at 4h and encoded a secreted protein with the systematic name Fam132b, later renamed erythroferrone (ERFE) based on its activity as an erythroid regulator of systemic iron homeostasis. ERFE was highly expressed in erythroblasts and its expression was stimulated by EPO through a pathway that could be inhibited by signal transducer and activator of transcription 5 (STAT5) inhibitors pimozide and N'-((4-oxo-4H-chromen-3-yl)methylene) nicotinohydrazide. Importantly, ERFE KO mice nearly completely failed to suppress hepcidin acutely in response to hemorrhage or EPO, demonstrating that ERFE was essential for early suppression of hepcidin in response to erythropoietic stimulation. Recombinant ERFE suppressed hepcidin mRNA expression and serum hepcidin in mice and hepcidin mRNA in primary hepatocytes, confirming its role as the physiologic erythroid hepcidin suppressor. In the aggregate, these findings are strong evidence for the essential role of ERFE as an erythroid regulator of hepcidin. However, chronic EPO treatment suppresses hepcidin even in ERFE KO mice indicating that other mechanisms must exist to compensate for the absence of ERFE, albeit with a time delay.[42]

Mechanism of action of ERFE. ERFE belongs to the C1q-TNFα family of proteins, many of which have as yet undefined receptors and signaling pathways. Unexpectedly, the search for ERFE receptors has so far been unsuccessful. Instead, ERFE seems to lower hepcidin by interfering with the signaling pathways that regulate hepcidin transcription. Hepcidin transcription is regulated by the interaction of two cell types, hepatic sinusoidal endothelial cells that secrete BMP2 and BMP6, and hepatocytes that synthesize and secrete hepcidin, under the control of the BMP receptor and its SMAD signaling pathway.[19] Erythroferrone prevents the normal interaction of BMPs with the BMP receptor,[43] most likely by trapping BMPs before they can bind to their receptors[43,44] (**Fig. 2**).

Erythroferrone in β-thalassemia. High levels of ERFE were detected by enzyme immunoassay[45] in patients with nontransfusion-dependent β-thalassemia or in patients with transfusion-dependent thalassemia before RBC transfusions but were much lower within days after transfusion. Moreover, hepcidin suppression anticorrelated with serum ERFE concentrations. Th3/+ thalassemic mice have elevated ERFE and characteristically decreased hepcidin, and deleting ERFE in Th3/+ mice reversed the suppression of hepcidin. However, this only partially prevented the development of iron overload[46] so that hepcidin was still lower than appropriate for the

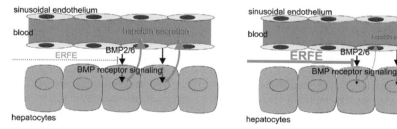

Fig. 2. Molecular basis of erythroferrone-mediated hepcidin suppression. Normal erythropoiesis (*left panel*) is shown for comparison with ineffective erythropoiesis (*right panel*). In ineffective erythropoiesis, high concentrations of ERFE, generated in the hyperexpanded and stimulated marrow, bind BMP2/6 to decrease signaling from sinusoidal endothelium (*cyan*) to hepatocytes (*orange-brown*). As a result, BMP receptor signaling in hepatocytes decreases, the transcription of the hepcidin gene slows, and the secretion of hepcidin declines.

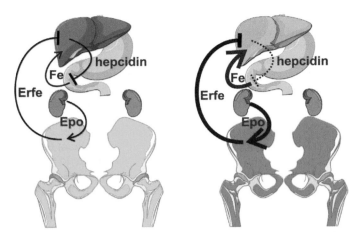

Fig. 3. Pathophysiology of iron overload in ineffective erythropoiesis. Normal erythropoiesis (*left panel*) is shown for comparison with ineffective erythropoiesis (*right panel*). In ineffective erythropoiesis, anemia drives increased production of EPO by the kidneys to stimulate erythropoiesis in the marrow. However, the resulting erythroblast expansion does not produce enough mature erythrocytes because most erythroblasts apoptose before completing the differentiation sequence. Hyperexpanded erythroid marrow (*red*) stimulated by EPO secretes a large amount of ERFE which inhibits hepcidin production in the liver. Inadequate hepcidin concentrations (*dotted line*) fail to inhibit dietary iron absorption in the duodenum. Over years, the hyperabsorbed iron (*blue*) accumulates predominantly in the liver.

degree of iron loading. Although this implies the existence of additional pathologic suppressors of hepcidin and possibly also hepcidin-independent contributors to iron overload in β-thalassemia and other iron-loading anemias, it also makes a strong case for the contribution of ERFE to the pathogenesis of iron overload in β-thalassemia and other anemias with ineffective erythropoiesis. Increased secretion of ERFE by the expanded and stimulated population of thalassemic erythroblasts blocks BMP signaling in the liver and suppresses hepcidin synthesis and secretion (see **Fig. 2**; **Fig. 3**). Low hepcidin would in turn allow greater iron absorption, saturation of circulating transferrin, generation of NTBI, and eventually iron loading of the liver and other parenchyma (see **Fig. 3**).

Transferrin receptor 1 (TFR1). Like ERFE mRNA, TFR1 mRNA is rapidly induced in erythroblasts within 5 h of EPO administration in mice.[47] Unlike for ERFE, the peak of TFR1 mRNA at 5 h is followed by a gradual decrease over 24 h. The initial induction of TFR1 causes a transient small decrease in serum iron and transferrin saturation but a more profound decrease, lasting several hours, in the concentration of diferric transferrin, the preferred ligand of TFR1. Because diferric transferrin is a well-established regulator of hepcidin[48,49] via the BMP-SMAD pathway, this mechanism may account for the transient small decrease in hepcidin concentrations seen in ERFE KO mice at 12 h after hemorrhage. It is not clear whether this mechanism contributes to iron overload in β-thalassemia or other iron-loading anemias. In addition, the TFR1 receptor is shed from erythroblasts,[50] generating the soluble form found in serum (sTFR1). Levels of sTFR1 are greatly elevated in β-thalassemia and other iron-loading anemias, reflective of both the increased mass of erythroblasts and the stimulation of TFR1 expression by EPO leading to the hypothesis that sTFR1 may have a role in the pathogenesis of iron overload. However, in mice, raising the concentrations of sTFR1 by its transient overexpression in the liver did not affect hepcidin concentrations or iron absorption.[51]

Local regulation of iron absorption in the duodenum. Nontransfusional iron overload in β-thalassemia and other iron-loading anemias is ultimately caused by hyperabsorption of dietary iron. An important direction of inquiry is whether dysregulated local duodenal factors in iron-loading anemias could increase iron absorption along with the altered systemic regulation by decreased hepcidin. The key transporters of iron in the duodenum include the apical divalent metal transporter DMT1 that imports Fe^{2+} from the diet into the enterocyte, its accessory ferric reductase duodenal cytochrome B (DCYTB) which converts the much more abundant dietary Fe^{3+} into Fe^{2+}, and the basolateral Fe^{2+} exporter ferroportin that uses ferroxygenases hephaestin and ceruloplasmin to convert Fe^{2+} into Fe^{3+}, the form of iron-loaded onto transferrin. The apical membrane of duodenal enterocytes can also efficiently take up dietary heme in humans (not in mice[52]), but the specific transporter mechanism involved is not yet known. The available evidence suggests that heme iron is extracted within the enterocyte and joins the stream of Fe^{2+} exported by ferroportin. The hypoxia-inducible factor (predominantly HIF-2α) enhances the transcription of DCYTB, DMT1, ferroportin, and hepatic ceruloplasmin and therefore promotes iron transport in response to hypoxia and iron deficiency. The cellular levels of HIF are posttranslationally controlled by HIF prolyl hydroxylases that direct the degradation of HIF when oxygen and iron are abundant and are inactive during hypoxia and iron deficiency, permitting HIF levels to rise. The duodenal enterocytes are hypoxic at baseline and their iron content is regulated by the iron exporter ferroportin under the control of its ligand hepcidin, effectively allowing hepcidin to control HIF-2α levels and the levels of HIF-2α-regulated iron transporters.[53] In view of these recent studies, it is unclear whether hepcidin-independent but still HIF-dependent duodenal mechanisms contribute to hyperabsorption of iron and systemic iron overload[54] in hemolytic anemias including β-thalassemia, and if so what the pathogenic non-hepcidin modulators of iron absorption are.

Tissue distribution of iron in NTDT compared with TDT. The nature of the predominant mechanism of iron accumulation (dietary in non transfusion-dependent thalassemia [NTDT] and transfusional in transfusion-dependent thalassemia [TDT]) has important consequences not only for the rate of iron accumulation that is much greater in TDT but also for organismal iron distribution. Hemolysis of transfused erythrocytes causes iron-loading of macrophage compartments in the spleen and the liver, as well as of hepatocytes. Macrophages seem to be the predominant secretors of serum ferritin[55,56] so this marker of iron overload rises more relative to body iron stores in TDT than in NTDT.[30] The more rapid accumulation of iron in hepatocytes in TDT reinforces this trend by stimulating hepcidin synthesis and increasing plasma hepcidin that binds to ferroportin on macrophages and inhibits their export of iron,[30] further stimulating ferritin secretion. Moreover, erythrocyte transfusions decrease plasma EPO levels and suppress exuberant erythropoiesis, thereby decreasing plasma ERFE concentrations and allowing hepcidin levels to rise,[45] particularly early during the transfusion cycle. In comparison, NTDT is characterized by much lower macrophage iron storage, as well as lower serum hepcidin and ferritin concentrations relative to iron stores documented by biopsy or MRI. Relying solely on serum ferritin concentrations in NTDT to estimate their iron burden while using criteria developed in patients with TDT may therefore underestimate the risk of iron toxicity in NTDT, with potentially adverse consequences for the long-term prognosis of these patients.[57]

SUMMARY

Iron overload in thalassemia remains an important clinical problem whose pathogenesis has two major components: (1) transfusional iron overload and (2) hyperabsorption of dietary iron caused by systemic effects of ineffective erythropoiesis. Typically, transfusional iron overload can reach toxic levels rapidly, within a few years, whereas hyperabsorption of dietary iron loads iron into tissues more slowly. Rapid iron loading generates high concentrations of NTBI, overwhelming the capacity for NTBI clearance by the liver and causing toxicity to the heart and endocrine system. Slow accumulation of iron generates lower concentrations of NTBI, which can be cleared by the liver, making that organ a primary target of iron overload in NTDT. The secretion of erythroferrone by a greatly expanded and stimulated population of erythroblasts, and the resulting suppression of hepcidin transcription in the liver is a major contributor to the pathogenesis of iron overload in NTDT but other mediators may contribute. Pharmacologic approaches to increase hepcidin activity or decrease erythroferrone may help ameliorate iron loading in thalassemias and other anemias with ineffective erythropoiesis.

CLINICS CARE POINTS

- Iron overload is a major cause of morbidity and mortality in beta-thalassemia, with or without regular transfusions.
- Iron overload is preventable or reversible by timely administration of iron chelators.

FUNDING

Research relevant to this review was funded by NIH NIDDK grant 1R01DK126680 (PI: Ganz).

DISCLOSURE

T. Ganz and E. Nemeth are shareholders in Intrinsic LifeSciences and Silarus Pharma, and have received consulting fees from Disc Medicine, FibrogenAstraZeneca, Ionis Pharmaceuticals, and Rallybio. T. Ganz has also received consulting fees from Alnylam Pharmaceuticals, Akebia Therapeutics, Global Blood Therapeutics, Gossamer Bio, Pharmacosmos, Sierra Oncology and Silence Therapeutics, Elizabeta Nemeth from GSK, Novo Nordisk, Protagonist, and Shield Therapeutics.

REFERENCES

1. Farmakis D, Porter J, Taher A, et al. 2021 Thalassaemia International Federation Guidelines for the Management of Transfusion-dependent Thalassemia. HemaSphere 2022;6(8):e732.
2. Pippard MJ, Callender ST, Warner GT, et al. Iron absorption and loading in beta-thalassaemia intermedia. Lancet 1979;2(8147):819–21.
3. Breuer W, Ronson A, Slotki IN, et al. The assessment of serum nontransferrin-bound iron in chelation therapy and iron supplementation. Blood 2000;95(9): 2975–82.
4. Knutson MD. Non-transferrin-bound iron transporters. Free Radic Biol Med 2019; 133:101–11.
5. Jenkitkasemwong S, Wang CY, Coffey R, et al. SLC39A14 Is Required for the Development of Hepatocellular Iron Overload in Murine Models of Hereditary Hemochromatosis. Cell Metab 2015;22(1):138–50.

6. Coffey R, Knutson MD. The plasma membrane metal-ion transporter ZIP14 contributes to non-transferrin-bound iron uptake by human beta cells. Am J Physiol Cell Physiol 2016;312(2):C169–75.

7. Craven CM, Alexander J, Eldridge M, et al. Tissue Distribution and Clearance Kinetics of Non-Transferrin-Bound Iron in the Hypotransferrinemic Mouse: A Rodent Model for Hemochromatosis. Proc Natl Acad Sci 1987;84(10):3457–61.

8. Chin J, Powell LW, Ramm LE, et al. Utility of hepatic or total body iron burden in the assessment of advanced hepatic fibrosis in HFE hemochromatosis. Sci Rep 2019;9(1):20234.

9. Piga A, Longo F, Duca L, et al. High nontransferrin bound iron levels and heart disease in thalassemia major. Am J Hematol 2009;84(1):29–33.

10. Origa R, Barella S, Argiolas GM, et al. No evidence of cardiac iron in 20 never- or minimally-transfused patients with thalassemia intermedia. Haematol-hematol J 2008;93(7):1095–6.

11. Ramm GrantA, Ruddell R. Hepatotoxicity of Iron Overload: Mechanisms of Iron-Induced Hepatic Fibrogenesis. Semin Liver Dis 2005;25(04):433–49.

12. Stefanova D, Raychev A, Arezes J, et al. Endogenous hepcidin and its agonist mediate resistance to selected infections by clearing non-transferrin-bound iron. Blood 2017;130(3):245–57.

13. Stefanova D, Raychev A, Deville J, et al. Hepcidin Protects against Lethal Escherichia coli Sepsis in Mice Inoculated with Isolates from Septic Patients. Infect Immun 2018;86(7):e00253–318.

14. Wang SC, Lin KH, Chern JP, et al. Severe bacterial infection in transfusion-dependent patients with thalassemia major. Clin Infectdis 2003;37(7):984–8.

15. Vento S, Cainelli F, Cesario F. Infections and thalassaemia. Lancet Infect Dis 2006;6(4):226–33.

16. Coffey R, Ganz T. Iron homeostasis: An anthropocentric perspective. J Biol Chem 2017;292(31):12727–34.

17. Aschemeyer S, Qiao B, Stefanova D, et al. Structure-function analysis of ferroportin defines the binding site and an alternative mechanism of action of hepcidin. Blood 2018;131(8):899–910.

18. Nemeth E, Tuttle MS, Powelson J, et al. Hepcidin regulates cellular iron efflux by binding to ferroportin and inducing its internalization. Science 2004;306(5704): 2090–3.

19. Fisher AL, Babitt JL. Coordination of iron homeostasis by bone morphogenetic proteins: Current understanding and unanswered questions. Dev Dyn 2022; 251(1):26–46.

20. Wang CY, Xiao X, Bayer A, et al. Ablation of Hepatocyte Smad1, Smad5, and Smad8 Causes Severe Tissue Iron Loading and Liver Fibrosis in Mice. Hepatology 2019;70(6):1986–2002.

21. Nemeth E, Rivera S, Gabayan V, et al. IL-6 mediates hypoferremia of inflammation by inducing the synthesis of the iron regulatory hormone hepcidin. J Clininvest 2004;113(9):1271–6.

22. Pietrangelo A, Dierssen U, Valli L, et al. STAT3 is required for IL-6-gp130-dependent activation of hepcidin in vivo. Gastroenterology 2007;132(1):294–300.

23. Verga Falzacappa MV, Vujic SM, Kessler R, et al. STAT3 mediates hepatic hepcidin expression and its inflammatory stimulation. Blood 2007;109(1):353–8.

24. Wrighting DM, Andrews NC. Interleukin-6 induces hepcidin expression through STAT3. Blood 2006;108(9):3204–9.

25. Finch C. Regulators of iron balance in humans. Blood 1994;84(6):1697–702.

26. Ashby DR, Gale DP, Busbridge M, et al. Erythropoietin administration in humans causes a marked and prolonged reduction in circulating hepcidin. Haematologica 2010;95(3):505–8.
27. Pak M, Lopez MA, Gabayan V, et al. Suppression of hepcidin during anemia requires erythropoietic activity. Blood 2006;108(12):3730–5.
28. Vokurka M, Krijt J, Sulc K, et al. Hepcidin mRNA levels in mouse liver respond to inhibition of erythropoiesis. Physiol Res 2006;55(6):667–74.
29. Kearney SL, Nemeth E, Neufeld EJ, et al. Urinary hepcidin in congenital chronic anemias. PediatrBlood Cancer 2007;48(1):57–63.
30. Origa R, Galanello R, Ganz T, et al. Liver iron concentrations and urinary hepcidin in beta-thalassemia. Haematologica 2007;92(5):583–8.
31. Kattamis A, Papassotiriou I, Palaiologou D, et al. The effects of erythropoetic activity and iron burden on hepcidin expression in patients with thalassemia major. Haematologica 2006;91(6):809–12.
32. Nemeth E, Ganz T. Hepcidin and iron-loading anemias. Haematologica 2006; 91(6):727–32.
33. Papanikolaou G, Tzilianos M, Christakis JI, et al. Hepcidin in iron overload disorders. Blood 2005;105(10):4103–5.
34. Gardenghi S, Marongiu MF, Ramos P, et al. Ineffective erythropoiesis in beta-thalassemia is characterized by increased iron absorption mediated by down-regulation of hepcidin and up-regulation of ferroportin. Blood 2007;109(11): 5027–35.
35. Breda L, Gardenghi S, Guy E, et al. Exploring the Role of Hepcidin, an Antimicrobial and Iron Regulatory Peptide, in Increased Iron Absorption in {beta}-Thalassemia. Ann New York Acad Sci 2005;1054:417–22.
36. Adamsky K, Weizer O, Amariglio N, et al. Decreased hepcidin mRNA expression in thalassemic mice. Br J Haematol 2004;124(1):123–4.
37. Kawabata H, Doisaki S, Okamoto A, et al. A case of congenital dyserythropoietic anemia type 1 in a Japanese adult with a CDAN1 gene mutation and an inappropriately low serum hepcidin-25 level. Intern Med 2012;51(8):917–20.
38. Casanovas G, Swinkels DW, Altamura S, et al. Growth differentiation factor 15 in patients with congenital dyserythropoietic anaemia (CDA) type II. J Molmed(berl) 2011;89(8):811–6.
39. Tamary H, Shalev H, Perez-Avraham G, et al. Elevated growth differentiation factor 15 expression in patients with congenital dyserythropoietic anemia type I. Blood 2008;112(13):5241–4.
40. Tanno T, Bhanu NV, Oneal PA, et al. High levels of GDF15 in thalassemia suppress expression of the iron regulatory protein hepcidin. Nat Med 2007;13(9): 1096–101.
41. Kautz L, Jung G, Valore EV, et al. Identification of erythroferrone as an erythroid regulator of iron metabolism. Nat Genet 2014;46(7):678–84.
42. Coffey R, Sardo U, Kautz L, et al. Erythroferrone is not required for the glucoregulatory and hematologic effects of chronic erythropoietin treatment in mice. Physiol Rep 2018;6(19):e13890.
43. Arezes J, Foy N, McHugh K, et al. Erythroferrone inhibits the induction of hepcidin by BMP6. Blood 2018;132(14):1473–7.
44. Wang CY, Xu Y, Traeger L, et al. Erythroferrone lowers hepcidin by sequestering BMP2/6 heterodimer from binding to the BMP type I receptor ALK3. Blood 2020; 135(6):453–6.
45. Ganz T, Jung G, Naeim A, et al. Immunoassay for human serum erythroferrone. Blood 2017;130(10):1243–6.

46. Kautz L, Jung G, Du X, et al. Erythroferrone contributes to hepcidin suppression and iron overload in a mouse model of beta-thalassemia. Blood 2015;126(17): 2031–7.
47. Mirciov CSG, Wilkins SJ, Hung GCC, et al. Circulating iron levels influence the regulation of hepcidin following stimulated erythropoiesis. Haematologica 2018; 103(10):1616–26.
48. Ramos E, Kautz L, Rodriguez R, et al. Evidence for distinct pathways of hepcidin regulation by acute and chronic iron loading in mice. Hepatology 2011;53(4): 1333–41.
49. Corradini E, Meynard D, Wu Q, et al. Serum and liver iron differently regulate the bone morphogenetic protein 6 (BMP6)-SMAD signaling pathway in mice. Hepatology 2011;54(1):273–84.
50. Guillemot J, Canuel M, Essalmani R, et al. Implication of the proprotein convertases in iron homeostasis: proprotein convertase 7 sheds human transferrin receptor 1 and furin activates hepcidin. Hepatology 2013;57(6):2514–24.
51. Flanagan JM, Peng H, Wang L, et al. Soluble Transferrin Receptor-1 Levels in Mice Do Not Affect Iron Absorption. Acta Haematol 2006;116(4):249–54.
52. Fillebeen C, Gkouvatsos K, Fragoso G, et al. Mice are poor heme absorbers and do not require intestinal Hmox1 for dietary heme iron assimilation. Haematologica 2015;100(9):e334–7.
53. Schwartz AJ, Das NK, Ramakrishnan SK, et al. Hepatic hepcidin/intestinal HIF-2alpha axis maintains iron absorption during iron deficiency and overload. J Clin Invest 2019;129(1):336–48.
54. Anderson ER, Taylor M, Xue X, et al. Intestinal HIF2alpha promotes tissue-iron accumulation in disorders of iron overload with anemia. Proc Natl Acad Sci U S A 2013;110(50):E4922–30.
55. Truman-Rosentsvit M, Berenbaum D, Spektor L, et al. Ferritin is secreted via 2 distinct nonclassical vesicular pathways. Blood 2018;131(3):342–52.
56. Cohen LA, Gutierrez L, Weiss A, et al. Serum ferritin is derived primarily from macrophages through a nonclassical secretory pathway. Blood 2010;116(9): 1574–84.
57. Musallam KM, Cappellini MD, Taher AT. Iron overload in beta-thalassemia intermedia: an emerging concern. Curr Opin Hematol 2013;20(3):187–92.

Clinical Complications and Their Management

Rayan Bou-Fakhredin, MSc[a], Irene Motta, MD[a,b],
Maria Domenica Cappellini, MD, PhD[a,b], Ali T. Taher, MD, PhD[c],*

KEYWORDS

- β-Thalassemia • Complications • Management • Heart • Liver • Endocrine
- Iron overload • Ineffective erythropoiesis

KEY POINTS

- Ineffective erythropoiesis and peripheral hemolysis can lead to a state of chronic anemia that can result in several of the complications seen in β-thalassemia.
- Iron overload is very prominent in both patients with transfusion-dependent thalassemia and patients with nontransfusion-dependent thalassemia and can lead to complications in various organ systems, especially the liver.
- Splenectomy is a risk factor for the development of some complications such as pulmonary hypertension and hypercoagulability and vascular disease.
- Advancing age is another risk factor for the emergence of complications at a higher incidence such as malignancy.
- β-Thalassemia is a disease of multiple complications and risk factors, necessitating the need for a multidisciplinary management team.

INTRODUCTION

Thalassemia syndromes are complex systemic disorders. Clinical complications are related to the underlying pathophysiological mechanisms, namely ineffective erythropoiesis, chronic hemolytic anemia, and iron overload (**Fig. 1**). Some complications are present in both patients with transfusion-dependent thalassemia (TDT) and patients with nontransfusion-dependent thalassemia (NTDT); however, some others can be more prevalent in one or the other form. The authors herein present different complications seen in patients with β-thalassemia, the pathophysiology underlying these complications, and their management.

[a] Department of Clinical Sciences and Community Health, University of Milan, Milan, Italy;
[b] UOC General Medicine, Fondazione IRCCS Ca' Granda Ospedale Maggiore Policlinico, Milan, Italy; [c] Division of Hematology-Oncology, Department of Internal Medicine, American University of Beirut Medical Center, Beirut, Lebanon
* Corresponding author.
E-mail address: ataher@aub.edu.lb

Hematol Oncol Clin N Am 37 (2023) 365–378
https://doi.org/10.1016/j.hoc.2022.12.007
0889-8588/23/© 2022 Elsevier Inc. All rights reserved.

hemonc.theclinics.com

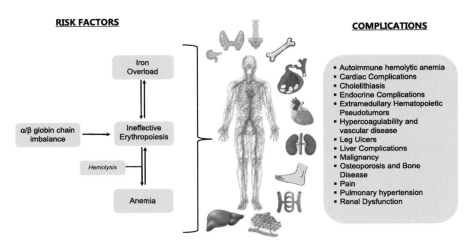

Fig. 1. Underlying pathophysiology and subsequent risk factors for the development of complications in β-thalassemia.

AUTOIMMUNE HEMOLYTIC ANEMIA

Increasing number of reports suggest an association between β-thalassemia and autoimmune diseases.[1] Autoimmune hemolytic anemia (AIHA) is a common entity among patients with β-thalassemia. A recent study from the authors' group estimated that AIHA has a prevalence of 1% in adult patients with congenital hemolytic anemias. Previous splenectomy, recent transfusions, infections, and pregnancy represent risk factors.[2] The diagnosis of AIHA may be challenging in chronic hemolytic patient. Besides the importance of assigning the best matched red blood cell unit to the patient, the recognition of a "true" AIHA is pivotal for a proper therapy. Most of the patients respond to steroids; however, one forth requires further treatment that include recombinant human erythropoietin and hydroxyurea.[3]

CARDIAC COMPLICATIONS

A wide range of cardiovascular abnormalities are seen in patients with β-thalassemia. Despite significant improvement in the clinical management of thalassemia, cardiovascular involvement remains the primary cause of mortality and one of the major causes of morbidity in patients with thalassemia.[4–7] Among arrhythmias, atrial fibrillation (AF) is the most frequent, and its prevalence has increased in recent times probably because of longer survival of patients with thalassemia due to improvement in treatments.[8] Notably, the prevalence of AF in TDT reported in most studies is higher than the one in the general population. The combination of iron infiltration and dilatation of the left atrium creates a unique environment for AF. Atrial or multifocal atrial tachycardia can also be seen. AF may be a consequence of heart failure, it may cause heart failure, and it may be found in aging but well-controlled and chelated individuals. Atherogenic vascular complications and myocardial parenchymal damage have also been described in patients with β-thalassemia. Patients with TDT can also be at increased risk for sudden cardiac death.[9]

The regular assessment of cardiac status in patients with β-thalassemia should first include regular controls of electrocardiogram (ECG). Transthoracic echocardiography is also recommended to be done as part of the annual basic cardiovascular assessment.[10] An evaluation of cardiac iron content with cardiac MRI T2* should be performed as well.[11,12] These noninvasive tools may help to identify those patients who are at high risk of heart failure, AF onset, or sudden cardiac death, even when cardiac function is conserved. For the subgroup of patients at high risk of developing cardiac arrhythmias, 24-hour ECG Holter monitoring or cardiac loop recordings is suggested to detect early atrial fibrillation or malignant arrhythmias and to evaluate the opportunity of prophylactic treatment.[13] Prevention of iron loading with an appropriate and regular iron chelation therapy is mandatory to prevent or to control heart dysfunction, and intensive chelation strategies should be implemented in case of heart failure. Impaired myocardial function may also require specific cardiac treatment, including the use of angiotensin-converting enzyme inhibitors, βblockers, and diuretics (furosemide and/or aldosterone antagonists). The initiation of all the aforementioned modalities for the management of cardiovascular disease should be done in accordance with the corresponding guidelines published by cardiology societies or associations.

CHOLELITHIASIS

The presence of cholelithiasis and gallstones has been reported to be higher in NTDT patients compared with TDT.[14–18] There are many contributing factors to the pathogenesis of cholelithiasis, including the precipitation of bilirubin in the bile as a result of increased hemolysis. Iron deposition within gallbladder and ineffective erythropoiesis have also been shown to play a role in the development of cholelithiasis and subsequent formation of gallstones. Ultrasonography is the most helpful tool to monitor cholelithiasis. Clinically cholelithiasis results in gastrointestinal symptoms, leading frequently to a cholecystectomy. Removal of the gallbladder during splenectomy is a common practice, especially if stones are symptomatic; this is particularly important, as acute cholecystitis can have serious consequences in the splenectomized patients.[19]

ENDOCRINE COMPLICATIONS
Hypogonadotropic Hypogonadism

Hypogonadotropic hypogonadism (HH) is the most frequent form of endocrinopathy in patients with TDT and is the main cause of infertility in these patients.[20] HH in β-thalassemia is caused by iron deposits in the pituitary gland and gonads at an early age. The prevalence and clinical presentations of HH varies considerably between sexes and between regions around the world. Routine testing of the hypothalamic-pituitary gonadal axis should be conducted in close collaboration with the endocrinologists. Hormone replacement therapy must be introduced in absence of clinical contraindications to alleviate symptoms of sexual hormone deficiency and in the cases of delayed or arrested puberty. Assisted reproductive techniques may also be needed.[13]

Growth and Pubertal Delay

The pathogenesis of the growth disorders is multifactorial and dependent on age at presentation.[21–23] In early childhood, growth retardation is mainly due to hypoxia, anemia, ineffective erythropoiesis, and nutritional factors. During late childhood, iron overload affecting the growth hormone (GH)-insulin-like growth factor 1 (IGF-1) axis in addition to the presence of other endocrine complications are the main factors affecting growth. After 11 years of age, delayed or arrested puberty is an important contributing factor to growth failure. Assessment of GH secretion should be performed in case of strong clinical suspicion and in patients with at least one other pituitary hormone deficiency and very low IGF-1 level and in cases of severe osteoporosis.[24,25] Treatment of GH deficiency, when established, is substitutive therapy with subcutaneous recombinant GH.

Hypothyroidism

The existing evidence of the prevalence of hypothyroidism among patients with TDT and NTDT has been recently summarized in a systematic review and meta-analysis of cross-sectional studies.[26] Hypothyroidism in β-thalassemia is strongly correlated with both anemia and iron overload. Assessment of thyroid function should be performed annually, beginning at the age of 9 years.[27] Free T4 and TSH are also key investigations. Additional tests may include the thyroid autoantibodies and hypothalamic-pituitary MRI, especially in patients with central hypothyroidism. In terms of management options, overt and central hypothyroidisms are treated with levothyroxine (L-thyroxine). In patients with subclinical hypothyroidism, a regular follow-up is recommended with an intensification of iron chelation therapy and careful monitoring.[13]

Impaired Glucose Tolerance and Insulin-Dependent Diabetes Mellitus

Impaired glucose tolerance (IGT) and insulin-dependent diabetes mellitus (IDDM) are also relatively common complications in patients with β-thalassemia. Both liver and pancreatic β-cell siderosis and glucose toxicity can impair glucose tolerance. Moreover, the interplay between liver siderosis and chronic hepatitis C infection facilitates and accelerates the progression to IDDM.[28] The risk of developing IGT/IDDM depends on the efficacy of iron chelation, family predisposition, and risk factors such as poor compliance to therapy. The diagnostic criteria for glucose intolerance and subsequent management of IGT and IDDM in these patients should be done as per the established guidelines.[13]

Hypoparathyroidism

Hypoparathyroidism is one of the less frequent endocrinopathies in patients with β-thalassemia.[29,30] Its incidence is variable and seems to affect men more frequently.[31–33] Most patients show a mild form of the disease accompanied by paresthesia and prolonged QTC interval. Laboratory data of patients show hypocalcemia, hyperphosphatemia, low levels of PTH, and 1,25 dihydroxy calcifediol. An increase in FGF23, which controls serum I,25(OH)2D3 levels and phosphate homeostasis, has also been reported in patients with TDT with hypoparathyroidism.[34] Treatment of hypoparathyroidism aims to prevent acute and chronic complications of hypocalcemia. Therapy includes oral administration of vitamin D or one of its analogues in addition to calcitriol to normalize plasma calcium and phosphate levels. If hyperphosphatemia persists, a therapy with phosphate binders can be considered.[13]

Adrenal Insufficiency

Published data on adrenal insufficiency in adult patients with β-thalassemia are scarce.[35–38] Iron toxicity can affect the hypothalamic-pituitary-adrenal axis at different levels. The presence of high serum adrenocorticotropic hormone (ACTH) levels is consistent with direct damage to the adrenal glands, which can be confirmed by MRI.[39] Adrenal insufficiency develops gradually, and symptoms, such as fatigue, may be nonspecific and overlapping with those of chronic anemia. An evaluation of basal adrenal function (ACTH and cortisol basal levels) must be performed every year in adult patients with β-thalassemia, and an ACTH stimulation test should be performed in selected cases. In case of a confirmed diagnosis, replacement therapy with cortisone acetate must be initiated, and for patients with subclinical adrenal impairment, replacement therapy should be implemented in case of stressful events.

EXTRAMEDULLARY HEMATOPOIETIC PSEUDOTUMORS

Ineffective erythropoiesis can lead to medullary expansion and subsequent bone deformities and low bone mass.[40] Beyond the bone marrow, compensatory hemopoietic points can also be activated anywhere in the body, leading to the formation of extramedullary pseudotumours in different organs and locations in the body such as the spinal canal.[41] The paraspinal involvement, which accounts for approximately 11% to 15% of the manifestations requires special attention due to the severe clinical consequences secondary to spinal cord compression. Hypertransfusion, radiation, and surgery have been suggested as common management approaches to control these extramedullary hematopoietic masses. One recent study showed that in patients with NTDT with extramedullary hematopoiesis, hydroxyurea may lead to independence from regular transfusion therapy without further expansion of ectopic hematopoietic tissue.[42]

HYPERCOAGULABILITY AND VASCULAR DISEASE

Several factors that lead to the hypercoagulable state in patients with β-thalassemia have been identified and described. These are presented in detail in Chapter XXX.

LEG ULCERS

Leg ulcers are more commonly seen in patients with NTDT.[43,44] Severe anemia, ineffective erythropoiesis, splenectomy, and hypercoagulability are all risk factors for the development of leg ulcers.[44,45] This risk is even higher in patients with NTDT with iron overload.[46–48] Observational studies have shown that blood transfusion or hydroxyurea therapy with or without erythropoietin may have a beneficial role in managing these leg ulcers.[49,50] Pentoxifylline, which alters the rheological properties of the red blood cell, was also shown to accelerate the healing process of leg ulcers.[51] Additional therapeutic modalities that have been used for leg ulcers include the use of an oxygen chambers, the use of the vasodilator dilazep, skin grafts, and platelet-derived wound healing factors and granulocyte macrophage colony-stimulating factors.[52,53] There is limited evidence on the benefit of anticoagulation for the management of leg ulcers in patients with NTDT.[54]

LIVER COMPLICATIONS

Iron overload and viral hepatitis are the 2 main causes of liver disease in patients with β-thalassemia, leading to chronic inflammation, fibrosis and cirrhosis, and ultimately hepatocellular carcinoma.

In the case of hepatic iron overload, free or nontransferrin-bound iron mediates the hepatic and extrahepatic tissue damage.[55] Their accumulation in the liver and specifically in the hepatocytes and the other liver cells lead to severe oxidative stress and overproduction of toxic reactive oxygen species (ROS), which cause lipid peroxidation and protein damage. The subsequent hepatic inflammation and necrosis lead to fibrosis and cirrhosis.[56] More information on the evaluation and management of iron overload is available in Chapter XXX.

Chronic infection with hepatitis B virus (HBV) or hepatitis C virus (HCV) in combination with iron load hepatotoxicity remains a major risk factor for acceleration of liver fibrosis in patients with β-thalassemia. Prevalence of patients with thalassemia with hepatitis B surface antigen–positive ranges from 0.3% to 5.7%, with higher prevalence of HBV chronic infection in Asia and Southeast Asia countries.[57] Anti-HBV drugs include interferon and nucleos(t)ide analogues (lamivudine, adefovir, entecavir, telbivudine, and tenofovir). The prevalence of hepatitis C in patients with β-thalassemia on the other hand is variable depending on local disease prevalence but can be as high as 85.4%.[58] Emerging evidence has confirmed the efficacy and safety of DAAs in patients with inherited blood disorders, including β-thalassemia.[59,60] Sofosbuvir/velpatasvir (SOF/VEL) is the first once-daily single fixed-dose pangenotypic regimen approved for treatment of HCV infection. Its use in β-thalassemia was shown in a recent study on 7 HCV-RNA-positive patients with TDT who received SOF/VEL treatment (at 400 mg/100 mg daily) for 24 weeks. Results demonstrated that SVR12 was confirmed in all 7 (100%), with significant change in means of ALT and AST levels between baseline and week 24.[61]

Increased iron burden in the liver is a major risk factor for hepatocellular carcinoma (HCC) in patients with β-thalassemia, especially in those in the older age group. A thorough review of the prevalence and incidence of HCC in patients with β-thalassemia has been previously described by the authors' group.[62] Many mechanisms and risk factors for HCC development have also been described assessing the roles of hepatitis viruses, cirrhosis, transfusions, and, most importantly, iron overload in liver carcinogenesis.[62] Prevention of HCC essentially relies on the early management of the risk factors, namely, iron overload and hepatitis infections. Treatment options for HCC in patients with β-thalassemia are largely based on data extrapolated from the general population. The reported therapeutic modalities include surgical resection, chemoembolization, sorafenib, and percutaneous radioablation.[63–66] Liver transplantation is another proposed modality for the management of HCC in the general population.[67]

MALIGNANCY

Many epidemiological and survival studies have described the prevalence of malignancy in β-thalassemia.[68–72] There exists an increase in the incidence of malignancy development in β-thalassemia, especially in the older patient population. Among solid cancers, HCC is the most commonly described type, followed by renal cell carcinoma, thyroid carcinoma, and breast cancer. As for hematologic malignancies, both lymphomas and leukemias have been commonly diagnosed in patients with β-thalassemia in addition to cases of multiple myeloma and myeloproliferative neoplasms. Different risk factors put these patients at greater risk of developing solid and hematological malignancies compared with the general population. These factors include iron overload–induced oxidative damage and immunologic aberrancies, immunomodulation caused by transfusions, viral infections (oncogenic viruses' transmission from blood transfusions), hydroxyurea use (affecting both DNA synthesis and repair), and bone marrow stimulation due to chronic anemia (JAK2/STAT5 erythropoietin-driven erythroid hyperplasia).[73] Screening for several malignancies in patients with β-thalassemia through routine laboratory testing and imaging should be performed based on the type of cancer and the symptoms present in order to achieve early diagnosis and prompt treatment.

OSTEOPOROSIS AND BONE DISEASE

Osteopenia and osteoporosis with a consequent increased risk of fractures are well known and frequently seen in patients with β-thalassemia.[8] The physiopathology of osteopenia/osteoporosis is multifactorial. Direct iron toxicity on bone can impair osteoid maturation and inhibit mineralization. Nutritional imbalances or hormonal alterations due to other endocrinopathies can also be a risk factor. The presence of vitamin D deficiency and hypercalciuria are also contributors to low bone mass density and/or fragility fractures.[74] The gold standard for the classification of bone conditions is bone mineral density (BMD). Assessment of BMD by bone densitometry should be performed every 18 to 24 months, accompanied by vertebral fracture assessment. The current treatment of patients with bone disease includes vitamin D and calcium supplementation and bisphosphonates (oral or intravenous) therapy; this has been associated with reduction of bone reabsorption, increase of BMD, reduction of back pain, and improved quality of life overtime.[75-78] Recently also denosumab and anabolic therapy with teriparatide have been used in treatment of osteoporosis in patients with thalassemia.[79-81]

PAIN

Pain represents a significant issue in patients with β-thalassemia. Indeed, most of patients older than 35 years report chronic pain of moderate-to-severe intensity, and its severity increases with age, contributing to the decline of quality of life and the development of depression and anxiety. Chronic pain is more frequent in patients with NTDT and those who started regular transfusions later. The most common site of chronic pain is the lower back, and the most frequent pain trigger is low hemoglobin.[82] Its management should follow the guidelines for the general population. However, given the polypharmacotherapy and liver and renal involvement, caution is required for therapy prescription.

PULMONARY HYPERTENSION

Pulmonary hypertension is more commonly seen in patients with NTDT, and when it manifests, it is often associated with functional limitation and can lead to right-sided heart failure.[83-86] Its development in β-thalassemia syndromes is multifactorial and includes anemia, hemolysis, endothelial dysfunction, increased vascular tone, inflammation, hypercoagulability, and vascular remodeling.[87,88] Data regarding the use of pulmonary vasodilator therapies in β-thalassemia are limited. For management of pulmonary hypertension, the use of sildenafil citrate, bosentan (endothelin receptor antagonist), and epoprostenol (prostacyclin analogue) were shown to be effective in some cases.[89-94]

RENAL DYSFUNCTION

Renal manifestations in patients with β-thalassemia are becoming more common.[95,96] Evidence of proximal tubular damage and increased urinary secretion of markers such as N-acetyl-β-D-glucosaminidase and β2-microglobulin, calcium, phosphate and magnesium, uric acid, and amino acids has been observed and reported in TDT patients.[97,98] Renal dysfunction is also evident in patients with NTDT and is associated with anemia, hemolysis, and iron overload. Many of these patients with NTDT also showed evidence of abnormally elevated estimated glomerular filtration rate and creatinine clearance, in addition to proteinuria.[99] Renal dysfunction has been shown to progress to end-stage renal disease in these patients.[100] Both iron overload and chronic anemia could explain renal and tubular dysfunction in patients with β-thalassemia. Renal manifestations attributed to iron chelating agents are rare yet possible. For example, cases of deferasirox-induced proximal tubulopathy and Fanconi syndrome in addition to cases of acute renal failure necessitating dialysis following intravenous deferoxamine overdose have been described in some patients. The management of serum creatinine elevation should be individualized based on the magnitude of increase and the presence for additional risk factors for renal disease or comorbid conditions. Dose modifications and monitoring in patients who experience renal adverse events secondary to iron chelating agents should follow the currently available guidelines. There is a need for close monitoring and follow-up of renal function through laboratory and urine tests both in TDT and NTDT patients, as their life expectancy has increased, and this puts them at increased risk of developing severe renal disease.

SUMMARY

In conclusion, the risk factors for the development of complications in patients with β-thalassemia are multifactorial. Moreover, there are similarities and differences between TDT and NTDT patients in terms of disease-related complications and their subsequent management. Early screening and management for specific disease-related complications should be considered in all patients with β-thalassemia according to their clinical risk factors.

CLINICS CARE POINTS

- To have a better understanding of the complications associated with β-thalassemia, it is important to be familiar with the underlying pathophysiology.
- Patient compliance and adherence to treatment are essential factors for the prevention of complications and for the improvement of health and quality-of-life outcomes in βpatients with β-thalassemia.

DISCLOSURE

The authors have nothing to disclose.

REFERENCES

1. El Hasbani G, Musallam KM, Uthman I, et al. Thalassemia and autoimmune diseases: absence of evidence or evidence of absence? Blood Rev 2022;52: 100874.
2. Motta I, Giannotta J, Ferraresi M, et al. Autoimmune hemolytic anemia as a complication of congenital anemias. A case series and review of the literature. J Clin Med 2021;10(15):3439.
3. Roumenina LT, Chadebech P, Bodivit G, et al. Complement activation in sickle cell disease: dependence on cell density, hemolysis and modulation by hydroxyurea therapy. Am J Hematol 2020;95(5):456–64.
4. Borgna-Pignatti C, Cappellini MD, De Stefano P, et al. Survival and complications in thalassemia. Ann N Y Acad Sci 2005;1054:40–7.
5. Russo V, Rago A, Papa AA, et al. Electrocardiographic presentation, cardiac arrhythmias, and their management in β-thalassemia major patients. Ann Noninvasive Electrocardiol 2016;21(4):335–42.
6. Detterich J, Noetzli L, Dorey F, et al. Electrocardiographic consequences of cardiac iron overload in thalassemia major. Am J Hematol 2012;87(2):139–44.

7. Barbero U, Fornari F, Guarguagli S, et al. Atrial fibrillation in beta-thalassemia major patients: diagnosis, management and therapeutic options. Hemoglobin 2018;42(3):189–93.
8. Manolopoulos PP, Lavranos G, Mamais I, et al. Vitamin D and bone health status in beta thalassemia patients-systematic review. Osteoporos Int 2021;32(6): 1031–40.
9. Russo V, Melillo E, Papa AA, et al. Arrhythmias and sudden cardiac death in beta-thalassemia major patients: noninvasive diagnostic tools and early markers. Cardiol Res Pract 2019;2019:9319832.
10. Di Odoardo LAF, Giuditta M, Cassinerio E, et al. Myocardial deformation in iron overload cardiomyopathy: speckle tracking imaging in a beta-thalassemia major population. Intern Emerg Med 2017;12(6):799–809.
11. Carpenter JP, He T, Kirk P, et al. On T2* magnetic resonance and cardiac iron. Circulation 2011;123(14):1519–28.
12. Pennell DJ, Udelson JE, Arai AE, et al. Cardiovascular function and treatment in beta-thalassemia major: a consensus statement from the American Heart Association. Circulation 2013;128(3):281–308.
13. Farmakis D, Porter J, Taher A, et al. Thalassaemia International Federation Guidelines for the Management of Transfusion-dependent Thalassemia. HemaSphere 2021;6(8):e732.
14. Shahramian I, Behzadmehr R, Afshari M, et al. Cholelithiasis in thalassemia major patients: a report from the south-east of iran. Int J Hematol Oncol Stem Cell Res 2018;12(2):117–22.
15. Khavari M, Hamidi A, Haghpanah S, et al. Frequency of cholelithiasis in patients with Beta-thalassemia intermedia with and without hydroxyurea. Iran Red Crescent Med J 2014;16(7):e18712.
16. Maulana MB, Fuadi MR. Clinical pathology aspect on diagnosis cholelithiasis in beta-Thalassemia patient: a case report. Ann Med Surg (Lond) 2022;81: 104454.
17. Lotfi M, Keramati P, Assdsangabi R, et al. Ultrasonographic assessment of the prevalence of cholelithiasis and biliary sludge in beta-thalassemia patients in Iran. Med Sci Monit 2009;15(8):CR398–402.
18. Galanello R, Piras S, Barella S, et al. Cholelithiasis and Gilbert's syndrome in homozygous beta-thalassaemia. Br J Haematol 2001;115(4):926–8.
19. Borgna-Pignatti C, Rigon F, Merlo L, et al. Thalassemia minor, the Gilbert mutation, and the risk of gallstones. Haematologica 2003;88(10):1106–9.
20. Vidal A, Dhakal C. Association of beta-thalassaemia and hypogonadotropic hypogonadism. Case Rep Obstet Gynecol 2022;2022:4655249.
21. Soliman AT, Khalafallah H, Ashour R. Growth and factors affecting it in thalassemia major. Hemoglobin 2009;33(Suppl 1):S116–26.
22. Dhouib NG, Ben Khaled M, Ouederni M, et al. Growth and endocrine function in tunisian thalassemia major patients. Mediterr J Hematol Infect Dis 2018;10(1): e2018031.
23. Skordis N, Kyriakou A. The multifactorial origin of growth failure in thalassaemia. Pediatr Endocrinol Rev 2011;8(Suppl 2):271–7.
24. Soliman A, De Sanctis V, Elsedfy H, et al. Growth hormone deficiency in adults with thalassemia: an overview and the I-CET recommendations. Georgian Med News 2013;(222):79–88.
25. Soliman A, De Sanctis V, Yassin M, et al. Growth hormone–insulin-like growth factor-I axis and bone mineral density in adults with thalassemia major. Indian J Endocrinol Metab 2014;18(1):32.

26. Haghpanah S, Hosseini-Bensenjan M, Sayadi M, et al. The prevalence of hypothyroidism among patients with β-thalassemia: a systematic review and meta-analysis of cross-sectional studies. Hemoglobin 2021;45(5):275–86.

27. Rindang C, Batubara JR, Amalia P, et al. Some aspects of thyroid dysfunction in thalassemia major patients with severe iron overload. Paediatr Indonesiana 2011;51(2):66–72.

28. De Sanctis V, Soliman AT, Elsedfy H, et al. The ICET-A recommendations for the diagnosis and management of disturbances of glucose homeostasis in thalassemia major patients. Mediterr J Hematol Infect Dis 2016;8(1):e2016058.

29. Bazi A, Harati H, Khosravi-Bonjar A, et al. Hypothyroidism and hypoparathyroidism in thalassemia major patients: a study in sistan and baluchestan province, iran. Int J Endocrinol Metab 2018;16(2):e13228.

30. Majid H, Jafri L, Ahmed S, et al. Unique classification of parathyroid dysfunction in patients with transfusion dependent thalassemia major using Nomogram-A cross sectional study. Ann Med Surg 2019;45:22–6.

31. De Sanctis V, Soliman AT, Canatan D, et al. An ICET-A survey on hypoparathyroidism in patients with thalassaemia major and intermedia: a preliminary report. Acta Bio Med Atenei Parmensis. 2017;88(4):435.

32. Sleem GA, Al-Zakwani IS, Almuslahi M. Hypoparathyroidism in adult patients with Beta-thalassemia major. Sultan Qaboos Univ Med J 2007;7(3):215–8.

33. Vogiatzi MG, Macklin EA, Trachtenberg FL, et al. Differences in the prevalence of growth, endocrine and vitamin D abnormalities among the various thalassaemia syndromes in North America. Br J Haematol 2009;146(5):546–56.

34. Saki F, Salehifar A, Kassaee SR, et al. Association of vitamin D and FGF23 with serum ferritin in hypoparathyroid thalassemia: a case control study. BMC Nephrol 2020;21(1):482.

35. Matin S, Jahromi MG, Karemizadeh Z, et al. The Frequency of Adrenal Insufficiency in Adolescents and Young Adults with Thalassemia Major versus Thalassemia Intermedia in Iran. Mediterr J Hematol Infect Dis 2015;7(1):e2015005.

36. Huang KE, Mittelman SD, Coates TD, et al. A significant proportion of thalassemia major patients have adrenal insufficiency detectable on provocative testing. J Pediatr Hematol Oncol 2015;37(1):54.

37. Poggi M, Samperi I, Mattia L, et al. New insights and methods in the approach to thalassemia major: the lesson from the case of adrenal insufficiency. Front Mol Biosci 2019;6:162.

38. Baldini M, Mancarella M, Cassinerio E, et al. Adrenal insufficiency: an emerging challenge in thalassemia? Am J Hematol 2017;92(6):E119–21.

39. Guzelbey T., Gurses B., Ozturk E., et al., Evaluation of iron deposition in the adrenal glands of β thalassemia major patients using 3-tesla MRI, Iranian J Radiol, 13 (3), 2016, e36375.

40. Rivella S. The role of ineffective erythropoiesis in non-transfusion-dependent thalassemia. Blood Rev 2012;26(Suppl 1):S12–5.

41. Haidar R, Mhaidli H, Taher AT. Paraspinal extramedullary hematopoiesis in patients with thalassemia intermedia. Eur Spine J 2010;19(6):871–8.

42. Cario H, Wegener M, Debatin KM, et al. Treatment with hydroxyurea in thalassemia intermedia with paravertebral pseudotumors of extramedullary hematopoiesis. Ann Hematol 2002;81(8):478–82.

43. Musallam KM, Rivella S, Vichinsky E, et al. Non-transfusion-dependent thalassemias. Haematologica 2013;98(6):833–44.

44. Taher AT, Musallam KM, Karimi M, et al. Overview on practices in thalassemia intermedia management aiming for lowering complication rates across a region of endemicity: the OPTIMAL CARE study. Blood 2010;115(10):1886–92.

45. Musallam KM, Taher AT, Duca L, et al. Levels of growth differentiation factor-15 are high and correlate with clinical severity in transfusion-independent patients with beta thalassemia intermedia. Blood Cells Mol Dis 2011;47(4):232–4.

46. Musallam KM, Cappellini MD, Daar S, et al. Serum ferritin levels and morbidity in β-thalassemia intermedia: a 10-year cohort study. Blood 2012;120(21):1021.

47. Musallam KM, Cappellini MD, Taher AT. Evaluation of the 5mg/g liver iron concentration threshold and its association with morbidity in patients with beta-thalassemia intermedia. Blood Cells Mol Dis 2013;51(1):35–8.

48. Musallam KM, Cappellini MD, Wood JC, et al. Elevated liver iron concentration is a marker of increased morbidity in patients with β thalassemia intermedia. Haematologica 2011;96(11):1605.

49. Gamberini MR, Fortini M, De Sanctis V. Healing of leg ulcers with hydroxyurea in thalassaemia intermedia patients with associated endocrine complications. Pediatr Endocrinol Rev 2004;2(Suppl 2):319–22.

50. al-Momen AK. Recombinant human erythropoietin induced rapid healing of a chronic leg ulcer in a patient with sickle cell disease. Acta Haematol 1991; 86(1):46–8.

51. Dettelbach HR, Aviado DM. Clinical pharmacology of pentoxifylline with special reference to its hemorrheologic effect for the treatment of intermittent claudication. J Clin Pharmacol 1985;25(1):8–26.

52. Opartkiattikul N, Sukpanichnant S, Wanachiwanawin W, et al. A double-blind placebo control trial of dilazep in beta-thalassemia/hemoglobin E patients. Southeast Asian J Trop Med Public Health 1997;28(Suppl 3):167–71.

53. Josifova D, Gatt G, Aquilina A, et al. Treatment of leg ulcers with platelet-derived wound healing factor (PDWHFS) in a patient with beta thalassaemia intermedia. Br J Haematol 2001;112(2):527–9.

54. Levin C, Koren A. Healing of refractory leg ulcer in a patient with thalassemia intermedia and hypercoagulability after 14 years of unresponsive therapy. Isr Med Assoc J 2011;13(5):316–8.

55. Taher A, Musallam KM, El Rassi F, et al. Levels of non-transferrin-bound iron as an index of iron overload in patients with thalassaemia intermedia. Br J Haematol 2009;146(5):569–72.

56. Sikorska K, Bernat A, Wroblewska A. Molecular pathogenesis and clinical consequences of iron overload in liver cirrhosis. Hepatobiliary Pancreat Dis Int 2016;15(5):461–79.

57. Singh H, Pradhan M, Singh RL, et al. High frequency of hepatitis B virus infection in patients with beta-thalassemia receiving multiple transfusions. Vox Sang 2003;84(4):292–9.

58. Mehta R, Kabrawala M, Nandwani S, et al. Safety and Efficacy of Sofosbuvir and Daclatasvir for Hepatitis C Virus Infection in Patients with beta-Thalassemia Major. J Clin Exp Hepatol 2018;8(1):3–6.

59. Mangia A, Sarli R, Gamberini R, et al. Randomised clinical trial: sofosbuvir and ledipasvir in patients with transfusion-dependent thalassaemia and HCV genotype 1 or 4 infection. Aliment Pharmacol Ther 2017;46(4):424–31.

60. Hezode C, Colombo M, Bourliere M, et al. Elbasvir/Grazoprevir for Patients With Hepatitis C Virus Infection and Inherited Blood Disorders: A Phase III Study. Hepatology 2017;66(3):736–45.

61. Sharara AI, Rustom LBO, Marrache M, et al. Sofosbuvir/velpatasvir for chronic hepatitis C infection in patients with transfusion-dependent thalassemia. Am J Hematol 2019;94(2):E43–5.

62. Finianos A, Matar CF, Taher A. Hepatocellular carcinoma in β-thalassemia patients: review of the literature with molecular insight into liver carcinogenesis. Int J Mol Sci 2018;19(12):4070.

63. Mancuso A, Rigano P, Renda D, et al. Hepatocellular carcinoma on cirrhosis-free liver in a HCV-infected thalassemic. Am J Hematol 2005;78(2):158–9.

64. Mancuso A, Sciarrino E, Renda MC, et al. A prospective study of hepatocellular carcinoma incidence in thalassemia. Hemoglobin 2006;30(1):119–24.

65. Mancuso A. Hepatocellular carcinoma in thalassemia: a critical review. World J Hepatol 2010;2(5):171–4.

66. Rampone B, Schiavone B, Martino A, et al. Current management strategy of hepatocellular carcinoma. World J Gastroenterol 2009;15(26):3210–6.

67. Mancuso A, Perricone G. Time to define a new strategy for management of hepatocellular carcinoma in thalassaemia? Br J Haematol 2015;168(2):304–5.

68. Karimi M, Giti R, Haghpanah S, et al. Malignancies in patients with beta-thalassemia major and beta-thalassemia intermedia: a multicenter study in Iran. Pediatr Blood Cancer 2009;53(6):1064–7.

69. Chung WS, Lin CL, Lin CL, et al. Thalassaemia and risk of cancer: a population-based cohort study. J Epidemiol Community Health 2015;69(11):1066–70.

70. Borgna-Pignatti C, Rugolotto S, De Stefano P, et al. Survival and complications in patients with thalassemia major treated with transfusion and deferoxamine. Haematologica 2004;89(10):1187–93.

71. Modell B, Khan M, Darlison M, et al. Improved survival of thalassaemia major in the UK and relation to T2* cardiovascular magnetic resonance. J Cardiovasc Magn Reson 2008;10:42.

72. Voskaridou E, Kattamis A, Fragodimitri C, et al. National registry of hemoglobinopathies in Greece: updated demographics, current trends in affected births, and causes of mortality. Ann Hematol 2019;98(1):55–66.

73. Hodroj MH, Bou-Fakhredin R, Nour-Eldine W, et al. Thalassemia and malignancy: An emerging concern? Blood Rev 2019;37:100585.

74. Voskaridou E, Terpos E. New insights into the pathophysiology and management of osteoporosis in patients with beta thalassaemia. Br J Haematol 2004; 127(2):127–39.

75. Voskaridou E, Terpos E, Spina G, et al. Pamidronate is an effective treatment for osteoporosis in patients with beta-thalassaemia. Br J Haematol 2003;123(4): 730–7.

76. El-Hawy MA, Saleh NY. Effect of cyclic pamidronate administration on osteoporosis in children with beta-thalassemia major: a single-center study. Clin Exp Pediatr 2022;65(8):405–9.

77. Voskaridou E, Anagnostopoulos A, Konstantopoulos K, et al. Zoledronic acid for the treatment of osteoporosis in patients with beta-thalassemia: results from a single-center, randomized, placebo-controlled trial. Haematologica 2006; 91(9):1193–202.

78. Naithani R, Seth T, Tandon N, et al. Zoledronic Acid for Treatment of Low Bone Mineral Density in Patients with Beta Thalassemia Major. Indian J Hematol Blood Transfus 2018;34(4):648–52.

79. Yassin MA, Abdel Rahman MO, Hamad AA, et al. Denosumab versus zoledronic acid for patients with beta-thalassemia major-induced osteoporosis. Medicine (Baltimore) 2020;99(51):e23637.

80. Yassin MA, Soliman AT, De Sanctis V, et al. Effects of the anti-receptor activator of nuclear factor kappa B ligand denusomab on beta thalassemia major-induced osteoporosis. Indian J Endocrinol Metab 2014;18(4):546–51.

81. Gagliardi I, Celico M, Gamberini MR, et al. Efficacy and safety of teriparatide in beta-thalassemia major associated osteoporosis: a real-life experience. Calcif Tissue Int 2022;111(1):56–65.

82. Piga A. Impact of bone disease and pain in thalassemia. Hematol Am Soc Hematol Educ Program 2017;2017(1):272–7.

83. Derchi G, Galanello R, Bina P, et al. Prevalence and risk factors for pulmonary arterial hypertension in a large group of β-thalassemia patients using right heart catheterization: a Webthal study. Circulation 2014;129(3):338–45.

84. Grisaru D, Rachmilewitz EA, Mosseri M, et al. Cardiopulmonary assessment in beta-thalassemia major. Chest 1990;98(5):1138–42.

85. Aessopos A, Stamatelos G, Skoumas V, et al. Pulmonary hypertension and right heart failure in patients with beta-thalassemia intermedia. Chest 1995;107(1):50–3.

86. Machado RF, Gladwin MT. Pulmonary hypertension in hemolytic disorders: pulmonary vascular disease: the global perspective. Chest 2010;137(6 Suppl):30S–8S.

87. Farmakis D, Aessopos A. Pulmonary hypertension associated with hemoglobinopathies: prevalent but overlooked. Circulation 2011;123(11):1227–32.

88. Morris CR, Vichinsky EP. Pulmonary hypertension in thalassemia. Ann N Y Acad Sci 2010;1202:205–13.

89. Littera R, La Nasa G, Derchi G, et al. Long-term treatment with sildenafil in a thalassemic patient with pulmonary hypertension. Blood 2002;100(4):1516–7.

90. Derchi G, Forni GL, Formisano F, et al. Efficacy and safety of sildenafil in the treatment of severe pulmonary hypertension in patients with hemoglobinopathies. Haematologica 2005;90(4):452–8.

91. Derchi G, Balocco M, Bina P, et al. Efficacy and safety of sildenafil for the treatment of severe pulmonary hypertension in patients with hemoglobinopathies: results from a long-term follow up. Haematologica 2014;99(2):e17–8.

92. Anthi A, Tsangaris I, Hamodraka ES, et al. Treatment with bosentan in a patient with thalassemia intermedia and pulmonary arterial hypertension. Blood 2012;120(7):1531–2.

93. Ussavarungsi K, Burger CD. Pulmonary arterial hypertension in a patient with beta-thalassemia intermedia and reversal with infusion epoprostenol then transition to oral calcium channel blocker therapy: review of literature. Pulm Circ 2014;4(3):520–6.

94. Karami H, Darvishi-Khezri H, Kosaryan M, et al. The improvement of pulmonary artery pressure after bosentan therapy in patients with beta-thalassemia and Doppler-defined pulmonary arterial hypertension. Int Med Case Rep J 2019;12:1–7.

95. Quinn CT, Johnson VL, Kim HY, et al. Renal dysfunction in patients with thalassaemia. Br J Haematol 2011;153(1):111–7.

96. Musallam KM, Taher AT. Mechanisms of renal disease in beta-thalassemia. J Am Soc Nephrol 2012;23(8):1299–302.

97. Ponticelli C, Musallam KM, Cianciulli P, et al. Renal complications in transfusion-dependent beta thalassaemia. Blood Rev 2010;24(6):239–44.

98. Bhandari S, Galanello R. Renal aspects of thalassaemia a changing paradigm. Eur J Haematol 2012;89(3):187–97.

99. Ziyadeh FN, Musallam KM, Mallat NS, et al. Glomerular hyperfiltration and proteinuria in transfusion-independent patients with beta-thalassemia intermedia. Nephron Clin Pract 2012;121(3–4):c136–43.
100. Mallat NS, Musallam KM, Mallat SG, et al. End stage renal disease in six patients with beta-thalassemia intermedia. Blood Cells Mol Dis 2013;51(3): 146–8.

Clinical Challenges with Iron Chelation in Beta Thalassemia

Janet L. Kwiatkowski, MD, MSCE

KEYWORDS

- Iron chelation • Deferasirox • Deferiprone • Deferoxamine • Adherence
- Adverse effects

KEY POINTS

- Inadequate iron chelation is associated with increased morbidity and mortality in patients with transfusion-dependent beta-thalassemia.
- Poor adherence to iron chelation is a major challenge to adequate iron chelation, and the regular assessment of adherence is important.
- Individual pharmacokinetics may impact the efficacy of iron chelation.
- Adverse effects vary among the iron chelators and impact dose tolerance and adherence.

INTRODUCTION

Conventional therapy for severe thalassemia includes regular red cell transfusions along with administration of iron chelation therapy to prevent and treat complications of iron overload. Three iron chelators currently are clinically available: deferoxamine, given subcutaneously; deferasirox, taken orally once daily as a dispersible tablet, film-coated tablet, or sprinkle formulation; and deferiprone, taken orally three times a day in liquid or tablet form or twice daily with a newer modified-release formulation. Iron chelation is very effective and when appropriately used, it can control iron burden and prevent or even reverse many of the complications of iron overload. Iron-associated cardiac complications, once the predominant cause of mortality in individuals with transfusion-dependent beta thalassemia (TDT),[1] have declined recently in resourced countries.[2] This improvement has been attributed to several factors including the availability of oral iron chelation and to regular monitoring of iron overload with cardiac and liver magnetic resonance imaging (MRI) with adjustments in iron chelation to manage iron burden effectively. Nonetheless, iron-related morbidity remains common,[3] and premature deaths still occur in individuals with thalassemia,[4] often due

Division of Hematology, Department of Pediatrics, Perelman School of Medicine, University of Pennsylvania, 3501 Civic Center Boulevard, Clinical Hub Building, Room 13547, Philadelphia, PA 19104, USA
E-mail address: kwiatkowski@chop.edu

Hematol Oncol Clin N Am 37 (2023) 379–391
https://doi.org/10.1016/j.hoc.2022.12.013
0889-8588/23/© 2022 Elsevier Inc. All rights reserved.

to ineffective control of iron burden. Many factors contribute to suboptimal iron chelation, including challenges with adherence, interpatient variations in chelator bioavailability, adverse effects of iron chelation that limit optimal dosing, and difficulties with precise monitoring of response. These factors will be discussed in the sections below.

ADHERENCE

Poor adherence represents one of the greatest challenges to effective iron chelation. Adherence rates vary widely and depend on many factors, including the method of measurement, the definition of appropriate adherence, the patient population, and the chelator agent being assessed. In a review of 18 studies conducted between 1985 and 2006, adherence rates to iron chelation ranged from 59% to 98%.[5] In a more recent report from a longitudinal registry of the Thalassemia Clinical Research Network (TCRN), between 81% and 88% of patients were reported to have good adherence, receiving at least three-quarters of prescribed doses during the follow-up period.[6]

Adherence to iron chelation correlates strongly with patient outcomes including the degree of iron burden, organ dysfunction, and survival.[5] Adherence inversely correlates with serum ferritin and non-transferrin bound iron (NTBI) levels and with liver iron concentration.[7–10] In one study of 52 patients with TDT, the mean serum ferritin level was 1454 ± 1242 µg/L in patients with good compliance, defined as receiving subcutaneous deferoxamine four to five times per week, compared with 4686 ± 2866 µg/L in those taking the medication less frequently ($P < .001$).[8] Levels of NTBI also were significantly lower in the good compliance group.[8] In another study of 126 patients with TDT receiving deferoxamine monotherapy, serum ferritin level was significantly lower among patients with good compliance than those with poor compliance (3081 ± 891 vs 3751 ± 1368 µg/L, $P = .0043$).[9] Adherence with oral iron chelation also has been shown to impact control of transfusional iron overload in TDT and other blood disorders.[11,12] Among 154 patients who participated in the ECLIPSE study comparing the deferasirox film-coated tablet with the dispersible tablet form, the average patient-reported adherence score mediated 66.6% ($P = .012$) of the association between treatment and change in serum ferritin.[12] Better adherence to iron chelation also is associated with lower liver iron levels. In one study of 76 patients with TDT, a significant correlation between decreased compliance and liver iron concentration was found ($r = 0.67, P < .001$).[7]

Importantly, poor adherence with iron chelation is associated with an increased risk of developing iron-associated complications. In one study, patients with fair compliance with deferoxamine were 10.7 times more likely to develop heart disease than patients with optimal compliance.[7] In another study of 45 patients with TDT, poor compliance with deferoxamine was associated with left ventricular restrictive filling pattern ($P = .007$) and cardiac mortality ($P = .003$).[13] Similarly, a reduced risk of cardiac disease was found among patients with good compliance with deferoxamine, defined as ability to perform more than 265 infusions per year.[14] Poor adherence with chelation also is associated with an increased risk of developing iron-associated endocrinopathies such as diabetes mellitus, hypothyroidism, and hypogonadotropic hypogonadism. In one retrospective study of 145 adult patients with TDT, 8 of 11 (72.7%) patients who developed multiple endocrine complications had poor adherence with iron chelation defined as receiving 50% or fewer of prescribed doses, compared with only 4 of 24 (16.6%) of patients without multiple endocrinopathies ($P = .002$).[15]

Survival also is impacted by adherence to iron chelation.[16,17] In a retrospective study of patients with beta-thalassemia followed at Italian centers between 1997 and 2001, only 21% of patients who died had good compliance with iron chelation compared with 67% of patients who were alive.[18] Moreover, in a longitudinal study of 45 patients with TDT, the 15-year cumulative survival rate was 52% in patients with poor, 93% in patients with moderate, and 100% in patients with excellent compliance with chelation therapy.[13] Similarly, among 447 Egyptian patients with a mean age of 14.2 years, mortality was higher among individuals with poor compliance ($P < .05$).[19]

Factors Impacting Adherence to Iron Chelation

Adherence is influenced by both patient-related factors and properties of the iron chelators (**Table 1**). Age consistently has been shown to impact adherence. Adherence rates typically are higher in young children, likely due to parental supervision of medication administration, compared with older patients.[20,21] Conversely, adolescence is a particularly challenging time for medication adherence in thalassemia, similar to other chronic health conditions.[20,22] In an international survey of deferoxamine use, patients ages 10 to 18 were more likely to have missed at least one medication dose in the past month compared with patients older than 18 years.[20]

Patients' feelings and beliefs about iron chelation also impact adherence and in an international survey of deferoxamine use, this was the most common category of reasons for missed doses.[20] Iron overload in its early stages is asymptomatic, and the benefits of chelation therapy are not readily appreciable to patients, which may hinder motivation to take the medication. The inconvenience of treatment and unwanted effects add to this challenge. Patient-perceived adverse effects of iron chelation are associated with reduced adherence rates.[20] Among 371 patients in the TCRN ages 5 to 58 year old, perceived sensitivity to deferoxamine and side effects of oral chelation both correlated negatively with patient-reported adherence.[23]

The presence of a strong support system is important to promote adherence. The lack of support of family, friends, or professional caregivers negatively impacts adherence,[20] whereas the presence of family support positively influences adherence.[4] Socioeconomic factors such as lower family income also are potential barriers to optimal adherence.[4,24] Patient forgetfulness also has been reported as a cause of poor adherence.[25] In a study of the TCRN, lower physical quality of life also predicted poor adherence.[26] Adherence to iron chelation may also reflect overall health choices, as one study showed lower adherence rates to deferoxamine in smokers compared with

Table 1
Factors that impact adherence to iron chelation

Factor	Comment
Patient-related	
Age	Young children > adults > adolescents
Forgetfulness	
Quality of life	Lower quality of life associated with reduced adherence
Presence of support system	Support system/positive reinforcement facilitates adherence
Patient feelings and beliefs	
Medication-related	
Route of administration	Oral > subcutaneous/intravenous
Chelator schedule	Fewer doses per day and days per week facilitate adherence
Chelator formulation	Film-coated tablet > dispersible tablet
Chelator adverse effects	Adverse effects reduce adherence

nonsmokers.[21] Finally, depression and anxiety disorders also have been shown to negatively impact adherence with iron chelation.[21,27,28]

Properties of the individual iron chelators also impact adherence rates. The route of administration is important, with adherence to oral chelation generally being superior to the subcutaneous route. In a review of 18 studies of iron chelation, compliance with deferoxamine ranged from 59% to 78%, whereas for deferiprone, rates were higher at 79% to 98%.[5] In the longitudinal registry study of the TCRN, adherence was higher with deferasirox (88%–90%) than with deferoxamine (70%–81%).[6] Patients who reported difficulty sticking themselves and problems wearing the infusion pump had lower adherence with deferoxamine.[21] Deferoxamine must be mixed and drawn up in a syringe, which is time-consuming and adds complexity to the treatment regimen and problems with mixing deferoxamine negatively impact adherence.[26] Changing from deferoxamine to oral deferasirox also is associated with improved adherence.[26]

The drug formulation, itself, impacts adherence. The first formulation of deferasirox available was a dispersible tablet, which is dissolved in a glass of water or juice. Subsequently, film-coated tablet and sprinkle formulations became available, simplifying treatment. In addition, gastrointestinal adverse effects may be lower with the newer formulations, which do not contain lactose that is present in the dispersible tablet. In the ECLIPSE study, patient-reported outcomes showed greater adherence and satisfaction, better palatability, and fewer concerns with the film-coated tablet compared with the dispersible tablet.[29] In a study of 606 patients using claims data, the medication possession ratio, a measure of adherence, improved with a switch to the deferasirox film-coated tablet in patients with a variety of underlying diagnoses, including 107 with thalassemia.[30] Similarly, in a study of 20 children and adults with sickle cell disease and TDT, a significant improvement in adherence using medication possession ratio was noted with the switch from the dispersible tablet to the film-coated tablet.[31]

The medication schedule also may impact adherence. Deferasirox is administered once daily, as compared with deferiprone, which is given two to three times a day, depending on the formulation. Studies directly comparing adherence rates between the two oral chelators are limited. However, in the DEEP-2 study, mean compliance with deferiprone was 92% and with deferasirox, 95%, which was not statistically different.[32] In a study of the modified-release formulation of deferiprone, which is administered twice daily, compared with the three times a day dosing, patients reported a strong preference for the twice daily schedule.[33] Given that forgetfulness is a major barrier to adherence,[34] twice daily dosing might promote better adherence. Higher complexity treatment regimens also may negatively impact adherence. Adherence with monotherapy generally is better than with combination chelation.[26] The presence of additional comorbidities such as diabetes, hypothyroidism, or cardiac disease also adds additional medications to the treatment regimen, which may reduce adherence.

Adverse effects vary between different iron chelators (**Table 2**). For a patient experiencing adverse effects, switching to a different iron chelator may improve adherence. In the TCRN, switching chelators resulted in increased adherence regardless of the agent to which the switch was made, though a switch from deferoxamine to deferasirox was more common.[21]

Assessing and Improving Adherence with Iron Chelation in Clinical Practice

Unfortunately, assessment of adherence is difficult, and a standard method is lacking. Different methods to measure adherence have been used across studies including patient or family report, health care provider assessment, pill or vial counts, Medication

Table 2
Adverse effects of iron chelators

Deferoxamine	Deferasirox[64]	Deferiprone[54]
Local reactions	Gastrointestinal: nausea, vomiting, abdominal pain, diarrhea	Gastrointestinal: nausea, vomiting, abdominal pain
Ophthalmologic changes	Hepatic transaminitis; rare hepatic failure	Hepatic transaminitis
High-frequency hearing loss, tinnitus	Renal: increased creatinine, proteinuria, Fanconi syndrome; rare renal failure	Arthralgia
Bone abnormalities	Skin rash	Neutropenia
Allergic reactions	Ulcers/gastrointestinal bleeding	Agranulocytosis
Pulmonary at high doses[78]	Cytopenias (rare)	Lowered plasma zinc levels
Neurologic at high doses[79]		
Increased risk of Yersinia and Klebsiella infections[76,77]		

Event Monitor System caps, and, for deferoxamine, review of electronic pump records.[5] Filled pharmacy prescriptions or specialty pharmacy deliveries can be assessed but will only indicate that the patient received the medication and not that they took it. Given the limitations in the methodology of adherence assessment, it is essential to discuss adherence with patients on a regular basis. The health care provider serves as an important support for patients to promote adherence.[20] In clinical practice, patient or family report typically is used, or surrogate markers of iron chelation such as ferritin levels or liver iron concentration are used to infer adherence. Given the impact of chelator adverse effects on adherence, it is essential to ask patients about these unwanted effects and to consider adjusting the dose or switching iron chelators to improve adherence. Providers should work with the patient and family to determine the most acceptable and effective chelation regimen, taking into account schedules and preferences.

Studies addressing the impact of interventions to improve adherence to iron chelation are limited. Given that forgetfulness is a common reason for reduced adherence, methods to remind the patient to take the medication, such as setting alarms, using medication phone applications, or drug use calendars, may promote adherence. In one study of 86 children with TDT in Thailand, using a calendar along with medication counseling by a pharmacist improved adherence, and for deferiprone-containing regimens, was superior to counseling alone.[25] In a study of 23 patients with TDT, behavioral contracting with positive reinforcement also improved adherence.[27] Unfortunately, controlled studies assessing the impact of computer and mobile technology on adherence to iron chelation have not been conducted.[35]

Methods to promote adherence in adolescent patients are needed, given the decline in adherence in this age group. In one retrospective study, the impact of a transition navigator on adherence rates to hydroxyurea or iron chelation was assessed among adolescents with hemoglobinopathies. Improved adherence rates were seen after implementation of the transition navigator.[36] Eighty-eight percent (22/25) of patients in the post-transition navigator cohort maintained or improved their self-reported adherence to at least 4 days a week compared with only 57% (8/14) in the pre-transition navigator cohort ($P = .048$).[36]

VARIABLE PHARMACOKINETICS

Some patients have inadequate control of iron burden despite receiving the highest recommended dose of an individual chelator.[37] This may occur in the setting of poor adherence or with a very high transfusional iron intake, as ongoing transfusion requirements impact the dose of chelator needed.[38] Interpatient pharmacokinetic variability also may impact the response to iron chelation, which has been best demonstrated with deferasirox,[37] with less variability reported with deferiprone.[39,40]

In one study, patients with TDT and inadequate response to a 30 mg/kg dose of deferasirox dispersible tablet had significantly lower systemic drug exposure compared with those with adequate response ($P < .00001$), likely due to differences in bioavailability.[37] Deferasirox pharmacokinetics vary substantially between the patients[41] and may be influenced by lean body mass, body weight, and hepatic and renal functions.[42]

The role of pharmacogenetics on deferasirox pharmacokinetics has varied across studies, possibly due to differences in sample size and population characteristics. In the study by Chirnomas and colleagues, no association of single-nucleotide polymorphisms (SNPs) in UGT1A1, UGT1A3, BCRP, and MRP2 with deferasirox pharmacokinetics was found.[37] In a study of healthy Chinese subjects who received a single dose of deferasirox, the presence of the c.-24T allele of ABCC2 gene that encodes a multidrug resistance protein was associated with 65% increase in clearance and 42% lower area under the curve.[72] Deferasirox undergoes glucuronidation in the liver and is eliminated in the feces. In a study of 60 adults with TDT, SNPs in UGT1A1 and UGT1A3 genes involved in metabolism and elimination of the drug, significantly influenced pharmacokinetic parameters.[75] In another study, the trough levels of deferasirox were influenced by SNPs in UGT1A1, CYP1A1, CYP1A2, and MRP2G.[43] Furthermore, in a study of children with TDT, certain UGT1A1, CYP1A1, and CYP1A2 SNPs were associated with ferritin and/or liver iron levels, suggesting an impact on the drug's efficacy.[44] The use of pharmacogenetics and/or monitoring of drug levels could improve treatment response, although this is not routinely done in clinical practice.

The drug formulation also may impact the effectiveness of treatment, with one study showing higher bioavailability with deferasirox film-coated tablet compared with the dispersible tablet form.[45] Better adherence with the film-coated tablet than the dispersible tablet may lead to better improvement in ferritin trajectory.[46] In addition, dosing schedule may be important as patients who respond poorly to maximal once daily deferasirox dosing may have an improved response by dividing the dose into twice daily dosing.[47–50] In a study of 22 patients with inadequate response to once daily treatment, 18 (81.8%) had improved response, with reduction in serum ferritin levels and liver iron concentration with the divided dosing.[47] In a more recent study that randomized 50 patients with TDT to continue once daily deferasirox or to switch to twice daily dosing at the same total daily dose, reduction in serum ferritin after 6 months of treatment was superior in the twice daily dosing group.[49] Interestingly, 7 of 25 in the twice-daily dosing group discontinued the study for nonadherence compared with 2 of 25 in the control group, which, although not significantly different, may reflect a negative impact of more frequent dosing on adherence.

ADVERSE EFFECTS OF IRON CHELATORS

Adverse effects may limit the ability to use a specific iron chelator or to treat with an effective dose. Local infusion site reactions may limit acceptability of deferoxamine to patients. Other adverse effects including ophthalmologic and audiological as well as bone effects can be limited by appropriate dose titration to avoid overchelation.[73,74] Severe allergic reactions may preclude use of the drug, but sensitization protocols may enable restarting the drug if alternatives are not available.[51,52]

Agranulocytosis, defined as an absolute neutrophil count less than 500/mcL, occurs in 1% to 2% of individuals treated with deferiprone, most commonly in the first 6 to 12 months of treatment, and does not seem to be dose related.[53] In postmarketing surveillance, where regular blood count monitoring and education are not as robust as within clinical trials, the agranulocytosis case fatality rate was 11%.[53] Thus, weekly blood count monitoring for at least the first 6 months of treatment is recommended along with ongoing counseling about the importance of holding the drug and checking the neutrophil count in the setting of fevers or significant illness. These requirements are difficult for patients and can limit the acceptability of the drug and adherence with monitoring, potentially placing patients at risk of adverse outcomes. Furthermore, the risk of recurrence among individuals who develop agranulocytosis is high at 75%.[53] Therefore, it is not recommended to restart deferiprone in a patient with a history of this complication. Nausea, vomiting, and abdominal pain with deferiprone also may limit acceptability. These symptoms most commonly occur early in therapy, and a gradual increase in dose may help prevent the problem. In addition, taking the medication with food may alleviate the gastrointestinal symptoms. Finally, hepatic transaminitis has been reported in 7.5% of patients taking the drug.[54] This adverse effect seems to be dose-related, so lowering the drug dose may lead to improvement.

Adverse effects with deferasirox also may limit its use. Serious adverse effects include gastric and duodenal ulcers, which may perforate and can occur in children as well as adults.[55–58] Careful questioning about abdominal symptoms, limiting concomitant nonsteroidal anti-inflammatory drug use, and use of acid blockers if indicated may help to prevent serious outcomes. Other gastrointestinal symptoms including abdominal pain, nausea, and diarrhea are common, occurring in 19.4% in one study of TDT patients and leading to discontinuation in 4.1%.[59] Gastrointestinal symptoms may be lower with the newer film-coated tablet and granule formulations and may improve with reducing the drug dose.

A rise in serum creatinine occurs in about a third of patients with TDT treated with deferasirox,[60] but reaches the abnormal range in only 3.6% and is dose-related.[61] More serious occurrences of Fanconi syndrome with normal anion gap metabolic acidosis, hypokalemia, hypophosphatemia, hypouricemia, glucosuria, phosphaturia, and/or aminoaciduria, which may progress to multiorgan failure, have been reported, typically in the setting of low iron burden or rapidly declining iron burden.[62,63] Elevations in hepatic transaminases to five times the upper limit of normal or higher are reported in 6% of patients with TDT and are dose-dependent.[64] Fulminant hepatic failure is a rare but severe complication reported in both children and adults treated with deferasirox.[64]

Many of the adverse effects of iron chelation are dose-related, including the gastrointestinal effects and hepatic transaminitis with deferiprone and deferasirox and renal effects with deferasirox. In clinical practice, the patient can be managed with reducing the chelator dose, but the lower dose may not be adequate to control iron burden and match ongoing transfusional iron intake.[38] One option is to switch to another iron chelator altogether but if the alternative requires subcutaneous infusion, this may not be acceptable and/or may impede adherence. Alternatively, adding a second iron chelator, such as deferoxamine a few days a week, may control iron burden, limiting toxicity with the lower chelator dose and promoting adherence with fewer days of painful infusions.

CHALLENGES WITH ASSESSING CHELATION RESPONSE USING SERUM FERRITIN LEVELS

Monitoring of iron burden and assessment of adequacy of iron chelation is accomplished through hepatic and cardiac MRI; however, these studies usually are obtained only annually. Interval response typically is assessed through trends in the serum ferritin level, which can be obtained with each transfusion. Ferritin levels have been shown to correlate with the body iron burden, but the correlation is not precise and limitations exist.[65,66] Ferritin levels are increased in the setting of infection and inflammation[67] and decreased with vitamin C deficiency,[68] which complicates the accurate assessment of iron overload and appropriate chelation modifications.

With iron chelation, the change in serum ferritin does not always correlate well with the change in liver iron concentration, the gold standard measurement of iron burden. In one study, among 38 patients with TDT who were receiving a variety of chelator regimens, change in ferritin accurately predicted liver iron response in only 46% of assessments.[69] The direction of change in ferritin was opposite that of the liver iron concentration in 21% and was in the same direction but the degree of change differed more than twofold in 36% of patients. Similarly, in a post hoc analysis of data from the EPIC trial, an open label trial of deferasirox in patients with TDT, 85 of 311 patients (27.3%) had either no change or an increase in serum ferritin after 1 year of treatment.[70] Among these ferritin nonresponders, approximately half showed improvement in liver iron concentration. Conversely, among ferritin responders, about 20% did not show a corresponding improvement in liver iron concentration. Thus, appropriate adjustments in iron chelation to control iron burden may be difficult when using serum ferritin levels. Generally, improvements in ferritin levels predicted a reduction in liver iron concentration but rising ferritin levels less reliably predicted worsening liver iron concentration, which could lead to overchelation. Routine monitoring of the liver and cardiac iron by MRI can overcome this challenge, but practically, these assessments can be obtained at most twice a year.

COST AND ACCESS

Finally, a well-identified, but difficult to quantify challenge with iron chelation is the cost and availability of the iron chelators, which vary worldwide. A recent retrospective analysis using the U.S. MarketScan Commercial and Medicaid Multi-State Database estimated that on average, chelation therapy costs $52,718 per patient annually,[71] a substantial economic burden. Patient co-pays may strain personal finances, impair adherence, and worsen outcomes. Moreover, in poor resourced countries, chelator availability is often limited and the cost to patients may be prohibitive. Improved access to iron chelation globally is needed to enable appropriate iron chelation for patients.

CLINICS CARE POINTS

- Iron chelation regimens should be tailored to the patient/family, taking into account preferences, adverse effects and lifestyle.

- Efficacy of iron chelation should be regularly assessed with serial serum ferritin levels and magnetic resonance imaging of the liver and heart, with appropriate changes in iron chelation to maintain optimal control of iron burden.

- Methods to improve iron burden include addressing adherence, increasing the chelator dose (not to exceed the maximum recommended dose), changing the iron chelator or its formulation, and adding a second iron chelating agent.

- Adherence should be regularly aseessed, obstacles to adherence should be addressed, and ongoing support should be provided to promote adherence.

DISCLOSURE

J.L. Kwiatkowski has consulted for Chiesi, Forma, Biomarin, Agios, Regeneron, Imara, and Bristol Myers Squibb.

REFERENCES

1. Borgna-Pignatti C, Rugolotto S, DeStefano P, et al. Survival and disease complications in thalassemia major. Ann N Y Acad Sci 1998;850:227–31.
2. Modell B, Khan M, Darlison M, Westwood MA, Ingram D, Pennell DJ. Improved survival of thalassaemia major in the UK and relation to T2* cardiovascular magnetic resonance. J Cardiovasc Magn Reson 2008;10:42.
3. Jobanputra M, Paramore C, Laird SG, McGahan M, Telfer P. Co-morbidities and mortality associated with transfusion-dependent beta-thalassaemia in patients in England: a 10-year retrospective cohort analysis. Br J Haematol 2020;191(5):897–905.
4. Lee WS, Toh TH, Chai PF, Soo TL. Self-reported level of and factors influencing the compliance to desferrioxamine therapy in multitransfused thalassaemias. J Paediatr Child Health 2011;47(8):535–40.
5. Delea TE, Edelsberg J, Sofrygin O, et al. Consequences and costs of noncompliance with iron chelation therapy in patients with transfusion-dependent thalassemia: a literature review. Transfusion 2007;47(10):1919–29.
6. Kwiatkowski JL, Kim HY, Thompson AA, et al. Chelation use and iron burden in North American and British thalassemia patients: a report from the Thalassemia Longitudinal Cohort. Blood 2012;119(12):2746–53. Research Support, N.I.H., Extramural Research Support, Non-U.S. Gov't.
7. Richardson ME, Matthews RN, Alison JF, et al. Prevention of heart disease by subcutaneous desferrioxamine in patients with thalassaemia major. Aust N Z J Med 1993;23(6):656–61.
8. al-Refaie FN, Wickens DG, Wonke B, Kontoghiorghes GJ, Hoffbrand AV. Serum non-transferrin-bound iron in beta-thalassaemia major patients treated with desferrioxamine and L1. Br J Haematol 1992;82(2):431–6.
9. Elalfy MS, Abdin IA, El Safy UR, Ibrahim AS, Ebeid FS, Salem DS. Cardiac events and cardiac T2* in Egyptian children and young adults with beta-thalassemia major taking deferoxamine. Hematol Oncol Stem Cell Ther 2010;3(4):174–8.
10. Payne KA, Desrosiers MP, Caro JJ, et al. Clinical and economic burden of infused iron chelation therapy in the United States. Transfusion 2007;47(10):1820–9.
11. Escudero-Vilaplana V, Garcia-Gonzalez X, Osorio-Prendes S, Romero-Jimenez RM, Sanjurjo-Saez M. Impact of medication adherence on the effectiveness of deferasirox for the treatment of transfusional iron overload in myelodysplastic syndrome. J Clin Pharm Ther 2016;41(1):59–63.
12. Taher AT, Origa R, Perrotta S, et al. Influence of patient-reported outcomes on the treatment effect of deferasirox film-coated and dispersible tablet formulations in the ECLIPSE trial: A post hoc mediation analysis. Am J Hematol 2019;94(4):E96–9.
13. Efthimiadis GK, Hassapopoulou HP, Tsikaderis DD, et al. Survival in thalassaemia major patients. Circ J 2006;70(8):1037–42.

14. Gabutti V, Piga A. Results of long-term iron chelating therapy. Acta Haematol 1996;95:26–36.

15. De Sanctis V, Elsedfy H, Soliman AT, et al. Clinical and biochemical data of adult thalassemia major patients (TM) with multiple endocrine complications (MEC) versus TM patients with normal endocrine functions: a long-term retrospective study (40 years) in a tertiary care center in Italy. Mediterr J Hematol Infect Dis 2016;8(1):e2016022.

16. Ballas SK, Zeidan AM, Duong VH, DeVeaux M, Heeney MM. The effect of iron chelation therapy on overall survival in sickle cell disease and beta-thalassemia: a systematic review. Am J Hematol 2018;93(7):943–52.

17. Triantos C, Kourakli A, Kalafateli M, et al. Hepatitis C in patients with beta-thalassemia major. A single-centre experience. Ann Hematol 2013;92(6):739–46.

18. Ceci A, Baiardi P, Catapano M, et al. Risk factors for death in patients with beta-thalassemia major: results of a case-control study. Haematologica 2006;91(10):1420–1.

19. Mokhtar GM, Gadallah M, El Sherif NH, Ali HT. Morbidities and mortality in transfusion-dependent Beta-thalassemia patients (single-center experience). Pediatr Hematol Oncol 2013;30(2):93–103.

20. Ward A, Caro JJ, Green TC, et al. An international survey of patients with thalassemia major and their views about sustaining life-long desferrioxamine use. BMC Clin Pharmacol 2002;2:3.

21. Trachtenberg F, Vichinsky E, Haines D, et al. Iron chelation adherence to deferoxamine and deferasirox in thalassemia. Am J Hematol 2011;86(5):433–6.

22. Burkhart PV, Sabate E. Adherence to long-term therapies: evidence for action. J Nurs Scholarsh 2003;35(3):207.

23. Trachtenberg FL, Mednick L, Kwiatkowski JL, et al. Beliefs about chelation among thalassemia patients. Research Support. Extramural Health Qual Life Outcomes 2012;10:148.

24. Mohamed R, Abdul Rahman AH, Masra F, Abdul Latiff Z. Barriers to adherence to iron chelation therapy among adolescent with transfusion dependent thalassemia. Front Pediatr 2022;10:951947.

25. Chawsamtong S, Jetsrisuparb A, Kengkla K, Jaisue S. Effect of drug use calendar on adherence to iron chelation therapy in young thalassemia patients. Pharm Pract (Granada) 2022;20(1):2570.

26. Trachtenberg FL, Gerstenberger E, Xu Y, et al. Relationship among chelator adherence, change in chelators, and quality of life in thalassemia. Qual Life Res 2014;23(8):2277–88.

27. Koch DA, Giardina PJ, Ryan M, MacQueen M, Hilgartner MW. Behavioral contracting to improve adherence in patients with thalassemia. J Pediatr Nurs 1993;8(2):106–11.

28. Mednick L, Yu S, Trachtenberg F, et al. Symptoms of depression and anxiety in patients with thalassemia: prevalence and correlates in the thalassemia longitudinal cohort. Am J Hematol 2010;85(10):802–5.

29. Taher AT, Origa R, Perrotta S, et al. Patient-reported outcomes from a randomized phase II study of the deferasirox film-coated tablet in patients with transfusion-dependent anemias. Health Qual Life Outcomes 2018;16(1):216.

30. Cheng WY, Said Q, Hao Y, et al. Adherence to iron chelation therapy in patients who switched from deferasirox dispersible tablets to deferasirox film-coated tablets. Curr Med Res Opin 2018;34(11):1959–66.

31. Oyedeji CI, Crawford RD, Shah N. Adherence to iron chelation therapy with deferasirox formulations among patients with sickle cell disease and beta-thalassemia. J Natl Med Assoc 2021;113(2):170–6.

32. Maggio A, Kattamis A, Felisi M, et al. Evaluation of the efficacy and safety of deferiprone compared with deferasirox in paediatric patients with transfusion-dependent haemoglobinopathies (DEEP-2): a multicentre, randomised, open-label, non-inferiority, phase 3 trial. Lancet Haematol 2020;7(6):e469–78.

33. Badawy SM, Kattamis A, Ezzat H, et al. The safety and acceptability of twice-daily deferiprone for transfusional iron overload: A multicentre, open-label, phase 2 study. Br J Haematol 2022;197(1):e12–5.

34. Theppornpitak K, Trakarnsanga B, Lauhasurayotin S, et al. A study to assess and improve adherence to iron chelation therapy in transfusion-dependent thalassemia patients. Hemoglobin 2021;45(3):171–4.

35. Badawy SM, Morrone K, Thompson A, Palermo TM. Computer and mobile technology interventions to promote medication adherence and disease management in people with thalassemia. Cochrane Database Syst Rev 2019;6(6):CD012900.

36. Allemang B, Allan K, Johnson C, et al. Impact of a transition program with navigator on loss to follow-up, medication adherence, and appointment attendance in hemoglobinopathies. Pediatr Blood Cancer 2019;66(8):e27781.

37. Chirnomas D, Smith AL, Braunstein J, et al. Deferasirox pharmacokinetics in patients with adequate versus inadequate response. Blood 2009;114(19):4009–13.

38. Cohen AR, Glimm E, Porter JB. Effect of transfusional iron intake on response to chelation therapy in {beta}-thalassemia major. Blood 2008;111(2):583–7.

39. Bellanti F, Danhof M, Della Pasqua O. Population pharmacokinetics of deferiprone in healthy subjects. Br J Clin Pharmacol 2014;78(6):1397–406.

40. Bellanti F, Del Vecchio GC, Putti MC, et al. Population pharmacokinetics and dosing recommendations for the use of deferiprone in children younger than 6 years. Br J Clin Pharmacol 2017;83(3):593–602.

41. Nisbet-Brown E, Olivieri NF, Giardina PJ, et al. Effectiveness and safety of ICL670 in iron-loaded patients with thalassaemia: a randomised, double-blind, placebo-controlled, dose-escalation trial. Lancet 2003;361(9369):1597–602.

42. Galeotti L, Ceccherini F, Fucile C, et al. Evaluation of pharmacokinetics and pharmacodynamics of deferasirox in pediatric patients. Pharmaceutics 2021;13(8):1238.

43. Cusato J, Allegra S, Massano D, De Francia S, Piga A, D'Avolio A. Influence of single-nucleotide polymorphisms on deferasirox C trough levels and effectiveness. Pharmacogenomics J 2015;15(3):263–71.

44. Allegra S, De Francia S, Cusato J, et al. Deferasirox pharmacogenetic influence on pharmacokinetic, efficacy and toxicity in a cohort of pediatric patients. Pharmacogenomics 2017;18(6):539–54.

45. Piolatto A, Berchialla P, Allegra S, et al. Pharmacological and clinical evaluation of deferasirox formulations for treatment tailoring. Sci Rep 2021;11(1):12581.

46. Taher AT, Weber S, Han J, Bruederle A, Porter JB. Predicting serum ferritin levels in patients with iron overload treated with the film-coated tablet of deferasirox during the ECLIPSE study. Am J Hematol 2019;94(1):E15–7.

47. Buaboonnam J, Takpradit C, Viprakasit V, et al. Long-term effectiveness, safety, and tolerability of twice-daily dosing with deferasirox in children with transfusion-dependent thalassemias unresponsive to standard once-daily dosing. Mediterr J Hematol Infect Dis 2021;13(1):e2021065.

48. Karimi M, Haghpanah S, Bahoush G, et al. Evaluation of efficacy, safety, and satisfaction taking deferasirox twice daily versus once daily in patients with transfusion-dependent thalassemia. J Pediatr Hematol Oncol 2020;42(1):23–6.

49. Panachiyil GM, Babu T, Sebastian J, Ravi MD. Efficacy and tolerability of twice-daily dosing schedule of deferasirox in transfusion-dependent paediatric beta-thalassaemia patients: a randomized controlled study. J Pharm Pract 2022;27. 8971900211038301.

50. Pongtanakul B, Viprakasit V. Twice daily deferasirox significantly improves clinical efficacy in transfusion dependent thalassaemias who were inadequate responders to standard once daily dose. Blood Cells Mol Dis 2013;51(2):96–7.

51. La Rosa M, Romeo MA, Di Gregorio F, Russo G. Desensitization treatment for anaphylactoid reactions to desferrioxamine in a pediatric patient with thalassemia. J Allergy Clin Immunol 1996;97(1 Pt 1):127–8.

52. Surapolchai P, Poachanukoon O, Satayasai W, Silapamongkonkul P. Modified desensitization protocols for a pediatric patient with anaphylactic reaction to deferoxamine. J Med Assoc Thai 2014;97(Suppl 8):S217–22.

53. Tricta F, Uetrecht J, Galanello R, et al. Deferiprone-induced agranulocytosis: 20 years of clinical observations. Am J Hematol 2016;91(10):1026–31.

54. Ferriprox Prescribing Information. 2021.

55. Zahra A, Ragab A, Al-Abboh H, Ismaiel A, Adekile AD. Perforated duodenal ulcer associated with deferasirox in a child with beta-thalassemia major. Hemoglobin 2021;45(5):335–7.

56. Shakir FTZ, Sultan R, Siddiqui R, Shah MZ, Javed A, Maryam N. Drug-induced duodenal perforation in the paediatric patient with thalassemia major, an unreported side effect of iron- chelating agent: A case report. J Pak Med Assoc 2022;72(7):1441–3.

57. Yadav SK, Gupta V, El Kohly A, Al Fadhli W. Perforated duodenal ulcer: a rare complication of deferasirox in children. Indian J Pharmacol 2013;45(3):293–4.

58. Bauters T, Mondelaers V, Robays H, Hunninck K, de Moerloose B. Gastric ulcer in a child treated with deferasirox. Pharm World Sci 2010;32(2):112–3.

59. Zengin Ersoy G, Aycicek A, Odaman Al I, et al. Safety and efficacy of deferasirox in patients with transfusion-dependent thalassemia: A 4-year single-center experience. Pediatr Hematol Oncol 2021;38(6):555–63.

60. Cappellini MD, Cohen A, Piga A, et al. A phase 3 study of deferasirox (ICL670), a once-daily oral iron chelator, in patients with beta-thalassemia. Blood 2006; 107(9):3455–62.

61. Cappellini MD, Porter J, El-Beshlawy A, et al. Tailoring iron chelation by iron intake and serum ferritin: the prospective EPIC study of deferasirox in 1744 patients with transfusion-dependent anemias. Haematologica 2010;95(4):557–66.

62. Baum M. Renal Fanconi syndrome secondary to deferasirox: where there is smoke there is fire. J Pediatr Hematol Oncol 2010;32(7):525–6.

63. Yui JC, Geara A, Sayani F. Deferasirox-associated Fanconi syndrome in adult patients with transfusional iron overload. Vox Sang 2021;116(7):793–7.

64. Jadenu Prescribing Information. 7/2020 2020.

65. Brittenham GM, Cohen AR, McLaren CE, et al. Hepatic iron stores and plasma ferritin concentration in patients with sickle cell anemia and thalassemia major. Am J Hematol 1993;42(1):81–5.

66. Telfer PT, Prestcott E, Holden S, Walker M, Hoffbrand AV, Wonke B. Hepatic iron concentration combined with long-term monitoring of serum ferritin to predict complications of iron overload in thalassaemia major. Br J Haematol 2000; 110(4):971–7.

67. Rujeerapaiboon N, Tantiworawit A, Piriyakhuntorn P, et al. Correlation Between Serum Ferritin and Viral Hepatitis in Thalassemia Patients. Hemoglobin 2021; 45(3):175–9.
68. Chapman RW, Hussain MA, Gorman A, et al. Effect of ascorbic acid deficiency on serum ferritin concentration in patients with beta-thalassaemia major and iron overload. J Clin Pathol 1982;35(5):487–91.
69. Puliyel M, Sposto R, Berdoukas VA, et al. Ferritin trends do not predict changes in total body iron in patients with transfusional iron overload. Am J Hematol 2014; 89(4):391–4.
70. Porter JB, Elalfy M, Taher A, et al. Limitations of serum ferritin to predict liver iron concentration responses to deferasirox therapy in patients with transfusion-dependent thalassaemia. Eur J Haematol 2017;98(3):280–8.
71. Paramore C, Vlahiotis A, Moynihan M, Cappell K, Ramirez-Santiago A. Treatment patterns and costs of transfusion and chelation in commercially-insured and Medicaid patients with transfusion-dependent beta thalassemia. Blood 2017; 130(1):5635.
72. Cao K, Ghuanghui R, Chengcan L, et al. ABCC2 c.-24 C>T single-nucleotide polymorphism was associated with the pharmacokinetic variability of deferasirox in Chinese subjects. Eur J Clin Pharmacol 2020;76:51–9.
73. Porter JB, Jaswon MS, Huens ER, et al. Desferrioxamine ototoxicity:evaluation of risk factors in thalassaemic patients and guidelines for safe dosage. Br J Haematol 1989;73:403–9.
74. Olivieri NF, Koren G, Harris J, et al. Growth failure and bony changes induced by deferoxamine. Am J Pediatr Hematol Oncol 1992;14:48–56.
75. Cusato J, Allegra S, De Francia S, et al. Role of pharmacogenetics on deferasirox AUC and efficacy. Pharmacogenetics 2016;17(6):571–82.
76. Adamkiewicz TV, Berkovitch M, Krishnan C, et al. Infection due to Yersinia enterocolitica in a series of patients with beta-thalassemia:incidnec and predisposing factors. Clin Infect Dis 1998;27:1362–6.
77. Chan GC, Chan S, Ho PL, et al. Effects of chelators (deferoxamine, deferiprone and deferasirox) on the growth of Klebsiella pneumoniae and Aeromonas hydrophila isolated from transfusion-dependent thalassemia patients. Hemoglobin 2009;33:352–60.
78. Freedman MH, Grisaru D, Olivieri N, et al. Pulmonary syndrome in patients with thalassemia major recieiving intravenous deferoxamine infusions. Am J Dis Child 1990;144:565–9.
79. Levine JE, Cohen A, MacQueen M, et al. Sensorimotor neurotoxicity associated with high-dose deferoxamine treatment. J Pediatr Hematol Oncol 1997;19: 139–41.

Fertility and Pregnancy in Women with Transfusion-Dependent Thalassemia

Farzana A. Sayani, MD[a],*, Sylvia T. Singer, MD[b],
Katie T. Carlberg, MD[c], Elliott P. Vichinsky, MD[b]

KEYWORDS

- Transfusion-dependent thalassemia • Thalassemia major • Fertility • Pregnancy
- Iron chelation

KEY POINTS

- Iron-associated hypogonadotropic hypogonadism and compromised ovarian reserve, commonly affect fertility in women with transfusion-dependent thalassemia, and hence discussions of optimization of chelation therapy and fertility preservation should start early with the prepubescent girl and her family.
- Multidisciplinary evaluation of a woman with transfusion-dependent thalassemia wishing to become pregnant should include preconception counseling, partner testing, fertility evaluation, and preconception clinical evaluation.
- Preconception clinical evaluation should include assessment of iron burden, cardiac and liver function, thyroid function, glucose tolerance, thrombotic risk, infection screening, detection of alloantibodies and extended red blood cell phenotyping, and a medication review.
- Since pregnancy in women with transfusion-dependent thalassemia is considered high risk, multidisciplinary care in the antepartum, peripartum, and postpartum periods are important for successful pregnancies, and emphasize the importance of maintaining pre-transfusion hemoglobin more than 10 g/dL, monitoring of cardiac and endocrine function, reevaluation of iron burden and chelation, and psychosocial support.
- Prenatal screening and preimplantation genetic testing offer options for couples at high risk for having an affected child.

[a] Division of Hematology/Oncology, Hospital of the University of Pennsylvania, Perelman School of Medicine, 3400 Civic Center Boulevard, Philadelphia, PA 19104, USA; [b] Division of Hematology/Oncology, UCSF Benioff Children's Hospital, 747 52nd Street, Oakland, CA 94609, USA; [c] Division of Cancer and Blood Disorders, University of Washington, Seattle Children's Hospital, 4800 Sand Point Way NE, Seattle, WA 98105, USA
* Corresponding author.
E-mail address: farzana.sayani@pennmedicine.upenn.edu

Hematol Oncol Clin N Am 37 (2023) 393–411
https://doi.org/10.1016/j.hoc.2022.12.008
0889-8588/23/© 2022 Elsevier Inc. All rights reserved.

INTRODUCTION

Survival of individuals with transfusion-dependent thalassemia (TDT) has significantly increased during the years due to improvement in multidisciplinary comprehensive care, improved transfusion practices, advances in iron load monitoring and increased availability of oral chelators.[1] In the past, pregnancy for women with TDT was considered very high risk primarily due to the cardiac iron overload and was often not recommended. As care has evolved alongside many advances in reproductive technologies (ARTs), pregnancy has proved not only possible but also increasingly safe with marked improvements in maternal and fetal survival. However, a high rate of fertility problems mostly attributed to hypogonadism, affects 40% to 90% of patients with TDT.[2–5] Despite an increased understanding of the pathophysiology of reproductive issues in these women, and improved outcomes, the general perception and even official obstetric recommendations have lagged behind the clinical evidence.[6] Advances in reproductive medicine have led to expanding options for conception, which have often not been accessible to women with TDT. Women with TDT have a wide arrange of complications beyond the reproductive axis that can affect infertility and pregnancy outcomes. These are best addressed by a multidisciplinary approach with early introduction and discussion of family planning. This article reviews these topics and highlights clinical recommendations for optimizing pregnancy outcomes for women with TDT.

PATHOPHYSIOLOGY OF SUBFERTILITY
Mechanisms: Iron Effect on the Reproductive System

The natural physiologic decline in female fertility, follicle aging, and early menopause result from mechanisms that include an increase in oxidative stress due to reactive oxygen species production, reduced enzymatic antioxidant defense mechanisms, a compromised microenvironment, and a decline in granulosa cell production of estradiol.[7] In women with TDT, disruption of reproductive tissue is thought to occur through similar mechanisms, alongside iron-induced cumulative damage to the endocrine system. Transfusion-induced hemosiderosis through damage to the pituitary and the hypothalamic-pituitary axis can cause hypogonadotrophic hypogonadism (HH) and subsequent subfertility. However, there is also data that iron-induced ovarian damage impairs oocyte number and function. Studies showed increased levels of redox activity in the follicular fluid and deposition of hemosiderin in endometrial glandular epithelium of women with thalassemia major (TM) and severe iron overload.[8–10]

Additionally, extensive iron deposition impairing oocyte function has been implicated as a cause of premature ovarian insufficiency and failure of in vitro fertilization (IVF) attempts.[9,11] Significantly reduced ovarian volume in TM women (mean age 30.3 years) to the range of that seen in postmenopausal women was also shown and could be a result of iron toxicity within ovarian tissue.[12] Several studies assessed ovarian function in TDT and attempted to determine the relation between iron overload and ovarian function determined by ovarian reserve. Ovarian reserve, assessed by anti-Mullerian hormone (AMH) and antral follicle counts (AFC) were lower in TM women when compared with normal controls (**Figs. 1**).[2,13] In another study, AMH was in the low-normal range but dropped in TM women in mid 30s and older. AMH correlated with non-transferrin-bound-iron (NTBI) suggesting a role of labile iron in lowering oocyte quality.[12] A 10-year longitudinal study found low AMH correlating with AFC in TM women, as compared with matched control women and to patients with HH due to other causes, concluding that iron overload is an independent cause of ovarian damage.[14]

However, despite this data, multiple reports on successful ovulation induction and pregnancies, even in those suffering from primary or secondary amenorrhea, suggest that some ovarian function is preserved. This is supported by recent studies showing that despite significantly low ovarian reserve in TM women undergoing IVF, as measured by AMH and AFC, oocyte quality was not affected and they achieved high fertilization rates.[15] Another study also suggested that primordial follicles may not be affected by iron overload because they found no difference in their characteristics in cryopreserved ovarian tissue. However, these were young patients (<17 years old) who may have not yet developed a more severe tissue iron overload. Data on the incidence of ovulation induction failure, and its relation to iron overload and ovarian reserve is limited and requires more study.

Given the frequent successful results of ovulation induction, infertility is generally attributed to pituitary siderosis disrupting the pituitary-gonadal axis.[16] The anterior pituitary has increased transferrin receptor expression, perhaps making it particularly vulnerable to siderosis, and significant loading has been suggested secondary to increased gland activity during puberty.[17] The high sensitivity of anterior pituitary to iron is also thought to result from the presence of L-type Ca^{2+} channels providing a major pathway for iron influx (as also shown to occur in the myocardium and pancreas).[18]

Iron-induced damage to the anterior pituitary and HH is a known endocrinopathy in patients with iron overload.[19] Standard iron burden measures and intensity of chelation have been used for association with gonadal dysfunction; however, they cannot reliably assess pituitary hormone secretion capacity and reproductive potential.[16,20] MRI technology for pituitary iron quantitation may help in determining the intensity

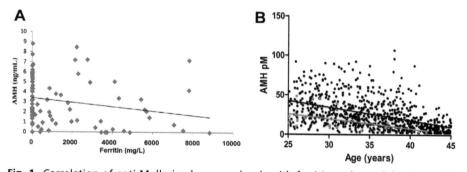

Fig. 1. Correlation of anti-Mullerian hormone levels with ferritin and age. (A) Serum AMH and ferritin levels in women with TM (n = 43) and normal controls (n = 44). AMH levels were significantly lower in women with TM (median = 1.77 ng/mL) compared with those in controls (median = 3.52 ng/mL; P = .002). Ferritin levels for women with TM were significantly higher (median = 2287 mg/L) than in controls (median = 13.0 mg/L; P ≤ .001). (B) AMH levels in TM women, 25 years and older (n = 23, red circles) were compared with normo-ovulatory controls (n = 759, black circles) showing that the slopes of the regression lines against age were not statistically different (P = .56). The slope was significant for the normal controls and for the patients with thalassemia, implying an association with age. The levels in the women with thalassemia were in the low normal range and dropped less than the normal levels in women aged older than 30 years. (*Adapted from* [A] Uysal A, Alkan G, Kurtoglu A, et al. Diminished ovarian reserve in women with transfusion-dependent beta-thalassemia major: is iron gonadotoxic? Eur J Obstet Gynecol Reprod Biol 2017;216:72; with permission. [B] Singer S, Vichinsky E, et al. Reproductive capacity in iron overloaded women with thalassemia major. Blood 2011;118:2878; with permission.)

of pituitary siderosis, the relation to total body iron, and detection of early-stage endocrinopathies.[21] Pituitary iron deposition was observed in TDT patients younger than 10 years of age whereas clinically significant effects and pituitary volume loss were observed during the second decade of life. Both pituitary iron overload and gland shrinkage were independently predictive of hypogonadism.[22]

The progressive nature of pituitary iron loading and difficulty of reversing it has been shown in a longitudinal study with prior splenectomy accelerating pituitary iron loading.[23] Increased chelation resulted in decrease in ferritin, liver and cardiac iron, and a parallel decrease in pituitary iron but only in those with a less severe pituitary iron burden. However, the decrease in iron load did neither result in the reversal of the low anterior pituitary volume nor improve gonadotrophin levels and AMH levels. In this study, the deleterious changes in the pituitary appeared a decade later (third and fourth decades of life) compared with a prior study[22] possibly due to improved iron chelation (adherence and perhaps higher efficacy) because patients used mostly oral deferasirox.[22] There was a strong correlation with cardiac iron and a cardiac T2* of 20 ms or lesser, predicted significant pituitary iron overload. Because pituitary MRI is often not clinically available, cardiac T2* data can be used for clinical management and in discussions of reproductive status, chelation optimization, and planning fertility preservation.

Evaluation of Hypogonadism and Ovarian Reserve

Although luteinizing hormone/follicle-stimulating hormone and estradiol along with pubertal development can define hypogonadism in thalassemia, they have poor predictive values of female reproductive potential.[4] AMH and AFC have been suggested as alternatives. AMH is produced by the granulosa cells of the preantral and antral follicles and has little gonadotropin-induced intercycle and intracycle variability, making it an ideal biomarker for this patient population. In a study of 36 TDT women, 60% (n = 22) showed diminished reserve as assessed by AFC and AMH levels.[24] Both AMH and AFC have an inverse relationship to ferritin levels in women with TDT and decline more rapidly in this patient population than in normal age-matched women.[2,12,13]

Beyond the severity and duration of iron overload affecting fertility, the age at which a woman attempts pregnancy is another important consideration. Early introduction of the topic and clinical evaluation, even before young women are contemplating having a child, is important and can assist in attaining pregnancy when relevant. Education programs and counseling for fertility preservation are scarce. Still, physicians taking care of patients with thalassemia must address reproduction and family planning early.

PREGNANCIES IN WOMEN WITH TRANSFUSION-DEPENDENT THALASSEMIA

During the years, there have been an increasing number of publications reporting successful pregnancies in women with TDT.[5,7,25–39] In one series, a review of 17 publications in a 17-year period identified 417 reported pregnancies, with only 2 maternal deaths.[40] As evidenced from these publications, maternal and fetal outcomes can be optimized when the pregnancy is managed by a multidisciplinary team, with preconception counseling, optimization of maternal health, and close monitoring during pregnancy. In a recent report of 30 TDT patients (37 pregnancies) who received multidisciplinary care, 80% had single pregnancies, 17% had 2 pregnancies, 46% were spontaneous, and 64% needed gonadotrophin-inducted ovulation and/or ARTs.[38] All pregnancies resulted in live births with no newborn complications. The median ferritin increased during pregnancies, and the cardiac T2* remained more than

20 milliseconds; however, the liver iron content increased from a mean of 3.37 to 9.06 mg/g dry weight, with recommendations for prompt chelation after delivery.

Fetal complications in pregnant women with TDT include a 2-fold increased risk of intrauterine growth restriction and prematurity, low birth weight, and multiple gestations. If only accounting for the singleton gestations, the rate of intrauterine growth restriction in pregnancies of women with thalassemia is similar to the rate of 8% within the general Italian population.[5] Hormonal stimulation or IVF accounts for the higher rates of multiples, ranging from 1.6% to 18.9%.[5,27,30,32,38,41] In a large Italian study, the rate of miscarriages in women with TDT was comparative to that of the general population.[5] The main risks to the mother are related to cardiac complications, which can be reduced by ensuring optimal cardiac function and liver and cardiac iron control before conception. The risks of pregnancy-specific complications including preeclampsia and hemorrhage are similar to the background population. Cesarean section is most often the chosen delivery method due to concerns of cephalo-pelvic disproportion resulting from maternal short stature and skeletal deformities. Overall, pregnancy does not alter the natural course of thalassemia. Despite pregnancy in women with thalassemia being considered high risk, coordinated multidisciplinary care with close monitoring and optimization of maternal cardiac iron and function, results in generally favorable outcomes.

Early introduction of family planning, counseling, partner testing, fertility evaluation, and clinical evaluation of the woman with TDT in a multidisciplinary setting is key to improving outcomes. For those with subfertility, early discussion of options with psychosocial support can help reduce the stress and anxiety around starting a family. Once pregnancy is achieved, close multidisciplinary monitoring can help increase the likelihood of a healthy mother and baby. **Fig. 2** highlights the overall approach to optimizing pregnancy outcomes in women with TDT.

PREGNANCIES IN WOMEN WITH NON–TRANSFUSION-DEPENDENT THALASSEMIA AND ALPHA-THALASSEMIA

The treatment of non–transfusion-dependent thalassemia (NTDT) includes occasional or more frequent blood transfusions for certain indications such as pregnancy, and similar

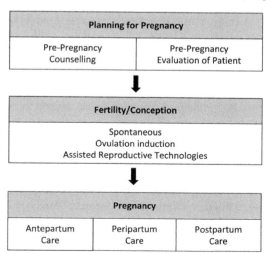

Fig. 2. Overview of approach to successful pregnancy in women with TDT.

standards and guidelines as those for TDT are followed. NTDT patients need to be monitored and treated for risk of thrombosis in pregnancy especially in splenectomized and infrequently transfused patients. In a large study, transfusion was required in 80% and pregnancies were associated with a 20.5% incidence of spontaneous abortion, 31.8% preterm delivery, 24.2% IUGR, and 72.7% cesarean section.[42] Others showed safe and favorable outcomes in patients with NTDT receiving multidisciplinary care.[43]

The approach to pregnancies in alpha-thalassemia, deletional hemoglobin H disease (HbH), or nondeletional, in particular hemoglobin H-constant spring (HbH-CS), varies based on the country where patients reside. In the United States, patients with HbH-CS are often regularly or frequently transfused when they reach adulthood and as common practice during pregnancy.[44] When regular transfusion were less often applied, mean gestational age at delivery and birthweight were significantly lower,[45] in particular for women with HbH-CS, suggesting the importance of close monitoring of fetal growth and transfusion support.

PLANNING FOR PREGNANCY
Considerations Before Pregnancy

Counseling and early planning are essential to minimize risk to the mother and fetus (**Table 1**). Testing the partner for significant thalassemia gene mutations and genetic counseling as appropriate is imperative. Cardiac disease, liver disease, endocrinopathies, and infections, increase the overall risk of complications during pregnancy. Ideally, a multidisciplinary team composed of a hematologist, reproductive medicine specialist, obstetrician, cardiologist, endocrinologist, and psychologist should be involved.

Cardiac iron and function

The maternal cardiovascular system undergoes dramatic adjustments during a pregnancy secondary to increased metabolic demand and blood volume. These include myocardial hypertrophy, chamber enlargement, and mild functional multivalvular regurgitation. Benign arrhythmias are also common. These changes are typically transient, with parameters returning to baseline within weeks of delivery. In a large report of TDT pregnancies, minimal transient cardiac function changes were noted.[5] The increase in left ventricular end-diastolic diameter and left-ventricular end-systolic diameter in TDT women is more pronounced than seen in normal pregnancies.[26,30,35] Additional observable changes include fall in ejection and shortening fractions. Chronic anemia and increased systemic vascular resistance can lead to left ventricular dysfunction, and right-sided strain may be present due to pulmonary hypertension. Patients with TDT, however, may have decreased cardiac reserve due to myocyte injury due to iron deposition, particularly NTBI.[46] Cardiac complications remain the primary cause of death in TDT, making close cardiac monitoring throughout pregnancy imperative. Pregnant women with TDT may experience complications such as dysrhythmia, right ventricular dysfunction, and cardiac failure, reported in 1.1% to 15.6%.[30,47] The common practice of withholding chelation therapy during pregnancy, may worsen cardiac function in patients with marginal myocardial function or siderosis. Two cases of overt heart failure and subsequent death have been reported.[28] In a recent study, 2 of 17 women (12%) who had normal prepregnancy global heart T2* values (>20 ms) showed the development of myocardial iron on their postpartum imaging.[48] In another study, 3 of 16 patients (19%) had evidence of new iron overload on postpregnancy imaging.[38] Importantly, 2 of the 3 patients that showed cardiac iron overload after pregnancy had moderate liver iron burden before pregnancy, suggesting hepatic iron predisposes to developing cardiac iron. Because liver iron

Table 1
Recommendations for the evaluation of women with transfusion-dependent thalassemia who desire pregnancy

Prepregnancy Counseling	
Partner testing	• Genetic testing for thalassemia/hemoglobinopathies • Genetic counseling if at risk
Fertility evaluation	• Hypothalamic-pituitary-gonadal axis evaluation • Ovarian reserve assessment (AMH and/or AFC) • Ultrasound of uterus and ovaries • Hysterosalpingography • Postcoital test
Prepregnancy Clinical Evaluation of the Patient	
Assessment of iron burden	• Serum ferritin. Target <1000 µg/L • Liver MRI. Target LIC <7 mg/g dry weight • Cardiac MRI. Target T2* >20 ms
Cardiology	• Echocardiogram • ECG • 24-h Holter monitor
Hepatology	• Liver enzymes and function tests • Abdominal ultrasound
Endocrinology	• Thyroid function • Oral glucose tolerance test/fructosamine • Adrenal function • Vitamin D level, calcium homeostasis • Bone evaluation with DEXA
Infection screening	• HIV, HCV, HBV, rubella, toxoplasmosis, syphilis
Transfusion medicine	• Screen for red cell alloantibodies and autoantibodies • Extended red cell phenotyping/genotyping
Thrombotic risk assessment	• History of venous thromboembolic event • Splenectomy • Family history of thrombophilia
Medication review	• Discuss stopping: chelators, bisphosphonates, ACE inhibitor, hydroxyurea, oral hypoglycemic agents • Discuss starting: folic acid, vitamin D

Abbreviations: AFC, antral follicle counts; AMH, anti-Mullerian hormone; ECG, electrocardiogram; HBV, hepatitis B virus; HCV, hepatitis C virus; HIV, human immunodeficiency virus; LIC, liver iron content; MRI, magnetic resonance imaging.

concentration (LIC) increased significantly in most of these studies, optimizing iron chelation and reducing liver and cardiac iron burden before conception is key.

All women with TDT should have a thorough evaluation of their cardiac function before pursuing a pregnancy. This includes an electrocardiogram (ECG), echocardiogram, 24-hour Holter monitor, T2* MRI, and evaluation by a cardiologist. Ideally a prepregnancy T2* of greater than or equal to 20 milliseconds should be achieved. Patients with evidence of significant cardiac iron overload (T2* MRI <20 ms) or left ventricular dysfunction or arrhythmias should be discouraged from planning a pregnancy at that time. Such individuals should be started on aggressive chelation to restore cardiac function and a T2* greater than 20 milliseconds.[49]

Liver iron and function
Before pregnancy, all women should have liver function evaluated by biochemical tests and liver iron load assessed by MRI. Goal LIC should be less than 7 mg/g dry

weight.[50,51] If significantly elevated, intensified chelation should be administered to optimize liver health before conception. Ultrasound (US) should be obtained of the gallbladder given increased risk of gallstones.[38] In patients with evidence of sludge or stones, cholecystectomy should be considered before pregnancy.

Endocrine status

Before pregnancy, women should be thoroughly evaluated and managed for thalassemia-associated endocrinopathies. Osteopenia and osteoporosis are common in TDT.[4,52] Assessment of bone mineral density with dual-energy x-ray absorptiometry (DEXA) should occur when planning pregnancy and regular supplementation with vitamin D before and during pregnancy is recommended to optimize bone health.[51,53] The level of 25-hydroxyvitamin D and dose of vitamin D to be targeted and used during pregnancy are not yet clear. Vitamin D is recommended not only for bone health but also to minimize risk of gestational diabetes.[54]

For patients with diabetes, optimal glucose control should be stressed to improve chances of conception. Because hemoglobin A_{1C} cannot be used for transfusion-dependent patients, fructosamine concentrations can be followed with a goal of less than 300 nmol/L for a minimum of 3 months before conception.[53,55] Because hypothyroidism is common in TDT, thyroid function should be evaluated and optimized preconception.[49]

Infection

The immune system of pregnant women with thalassemia is compromised due to the elevated estrogen levels of pregnancy, the variable state of iron overload, and absence of a spleen in some. All patients should be screened for human immunodeficiency virus (HIV), hepatitis B (HBV), hepatitis C (HCV), rubella and other pathogens that may affect pregnancy. Therapy should be recommended for women with HIV and/or hepatitis C virus (HCV).[38,49,53]

Medication review

Before conception or induction of ovulation, medications should be reviewed because some will need optimization, whereas others may need to be discontinued.[38,40,49] Folic acid, calcium, and vitamin D should be optimized. One study describes a higher rate of neural tube defects in this population and subsequent recommendations include a higher dose of folic acid than is typically recommended for pregnancy (5 mg daily rather than 1 mg daily).[29,47,56] Oral chelators are known to be harmful to the fetus and thus should be switched to deferoxamine (DFO) before conception or induction of ovulation.[57,58] Bisphosphonates are contraindicated during pregnancy and thus should be stopped 6 months before conception. Antiviral agents including interferon and ribavirin should also be stopped 6 months before conception or fertility treatments. Other medications including hydroxyurea, angiotensin converting enzyme (ACE) inhibitors or oral hypoglycemic agents should also be reviewed and discontinued preconception.

FERTILITY
Achieving Pregnancy

Spontaneous pregnancy is possible in the well-transfused and well-chelated patient who has had normal pubertal development and a normal menstrual cycle. This is more common among younger women who have had the advantages of the advances in overall thalassemia care including improved transfusions, iron load monitoring, and iron chelation. Despite improvements in management of iron overload, abnormalities of ovulation occur for 30% to 80% of adult women primarily due to hypogonadotropic hypogonadism in the setting of pituitary transfusional-iron overload.[59-62] For women who cannot achieve pregnancy spontaneously, ovulation induction alone or in combination with assisted ARTs may be an option.[3,38,49]

Although most patients with HH no longer have pulsatile gonadotropins, induction of ovulation in women has been highly successful. In a study with 36 patients, ages 20 years to 39 years, ovulation was achieved for 80% of patients.[24] The high success rate suggests a degree of ovarian protection from damage resulting in sufficient reserve.[10] A variety of ovulation induction regimens exist, including gonadotropins (FSH and LH) and clomiphene citrate, which stimulates the development of follicles, and human chorionic gonadotropin, which triggers ovulation after follicle development. The protocols include close monitoring of the induced cycles with biochemical testing and transvaginal US scans to assess follicle development for tailored drug dosing.[38] The protocols are associated with increased risk of twin or triplet pregnancies and ovarian hyperstimulation syndrome, and thus ovulation-induction procedures should be undertaken by an experienced reproductive team. Some women may require ART involving ovulation induction, oocyte retrieval, and oocyte or embryo manipulation in vitro. Since these evaluations and procedures can take time, are psychologically taxing, and have variable outcomes, early referral to an experienced reproductive team is encouraged especially in women in their 30s or those with comorbidities.

There are no data on harmful effects of iron chelation therapy during hormonal stimulation therapy; however, oral chelators should be changed to DFO.[49] Some choose to hold iron chelation despite lack of data.

Given the risk for ovarian insufficiency, especially in older women with TDT, elective cryopreservation of oocytes or ovarian tissue should be considered while these tissues are still attainable.[63] Such methods are also relevant to TDT women planning hematopoietic stem cell transplant (HSCT) or gene therapy, which involves hematotoxic treatment and has shown to be successful.[41,63,64]

MANAGEMENT DURING PREGNANCY
Antepartum, Peripartum, and Postpartum Care

Comprehensive, multidisciplinary care by a team including an obstetrician, cardiologist, endocrinologist, hematologist, and psychologist are important in ensuring a safe pregnancy with positive outcomes for both mother and baby. **Table 2** summarizes the recommendations for the management of the pregnant woman with TDT.

Antepartum Care

Transfusions
For women who were transfusion-dependent before pregnancy, regular transfusions should continue with a pretransfusion hemoglobin goal of greater than 10 g/dL. Overall, transfusion requirements are increased during pregnancy.[5,42] Some patients require more frequent low-volume transfusions due to the increased metabolic stress of pregnancy as well as to support adequate fetal oxygenation. Women with thalassemia intermedia (TI) may develop a transfusion requirement during pregnancy due to the dilutional drop in hemoglobin, which occurs naturally.[65] Caution should be used when considering the initiation of transfusions given the potential risk of alloimmunization and hemolysis leading to worsening anemia in the fetus.

All women with thalassemia should have extended phenotyping and in some cases genotyping at the outset of pregnancy if they have not had such testing in the past. If initiation of transfusions is deemed necessary, phenotypically matched units should be used. If unavailable, matching for Rh and Kell has been shown to decrease alloimmunization by 53%.[47]

Iron chelation

The use of chelation therapy and choice of best chelation agent during pregnancy have not been addressed in clinical studies and remain controversial. The current standard of practice is to discontinue chelation therapy as soon as pregnancy is established and hold throughout the course of pregnancy due to the concern of teratogenicity.[49] Fetal malformations, including skeletal anomalies, were reported in the offspring of rats after DFO exposure.[66] Decreased offspring viability and increased renal anomalies were reported in animal studies after deferasirox exposure. Case reports of women who had become pregnant while taking deferasirox; however, all of whom discontinued chelation on discovery of pregnancy at various time points report no teratogenicity.[57] Similarly, reports depicting the use of DFO during the second and third trimesters did not report any fetal toxicities.[39,58,67] Holding chelation for 9 months might have deleterious long-term consequences on cardiac function especially in those with previous myocardial deposition. Myocardial iron deposition and worsening of cardiac function with fatal heart failure have been described.[26,68] Some investigators support chelation, mostly with DFO, in the third trimester, when the benefits outweigh the risks especially in women with previous myocardial iron deposition or borderline cardiac function.[38,49,53,58] DFO has been the agent of choice during pregnancy because its larger molecular size prohibits it from crossing the placenta. Even

Table 2	
Recommendations for the clinical management of the pregnant woman with transfusion-dependent thalassemia	
Antepartum Care	
Maternal	
Transfusion support	• Maintain pretransfusion hemoglobin >10 g/dL
Iron burden assessment	• Serum ferritin monthly
Chelation	• May consider deferoxamine if worsening cardiac function in third trimester
Cardiac function	• Echocardiogram each trimester
Liver function	• Liver enzymes and function each trimester
Endocrine function	• Thyroid function each trimester • Oral glucose tolerance test: 16 wk, and 18–24 wk
Blood pressure	
Thrombotic risk assessment	• Consider prophylaxis in high-risk women
Fetal	
Fetal growth	• Serial ultrasound: Routine plus serial starting at 24 wk
Peripartum Care	
Mode of delivery	• Caesarean section vs vaginal
Anesthesia	• Epidural preferred
Thrombotic risk assessment	• Consider prophylaxis in high-risk women
High cardiac iron	• Consider deferoxamine infusion through labor
Postpartum Care	
Thrombotic risk assessment	• Consider prophylaxis: 7 d after vaginal delivery, 6 wk after C-section
Breastfeeding	• Encouraged
Contraception counseling	
Reinitiation of chelation	• Discuss on case-by-case basis
Psychosocial support	• Through all stages

though there have been no human reports of fetal anomalies with DFO, the woman should be counseled before its administration during pregnancy. In the event of new onset cardiac dysfunction during pregnancy, DFO may be used in earlier trimesters, weighing risks and benefits, and in close collaboration with a cardiologist. No clinical trials have addressed this topic, and specific recommendations are needed.

Cardiac, endocrine, and liver evaluation
Close monitoring by subspecialists including a cardiologist and endocrinologist during pregnancy is important to identify early subtle changes that may require intervention.[49] ECGs, echocardiograms, and laboratory tests to assess thyroid and liver function should be obtained once each trimester. Because this population is at higher risk of developing gestational diabetes, screening for gestational diabetes with an oral glucose tolerance test should occur at 16 weeks gestation and again at 28 weeks if the initial check at 16 weeks is normal. For women who develop diabetes, regular serum fructosamine levels should be monitored and managed in close collaboration with an endocrinologist.

Thrombotic risk
Pregnancy induces a hypercoagulable state with physiologic increases in fibrin and coagulation factors, and concomitant decreases in fibrinolytic activity and protein S levels. Additionally, there is reduction in venous flow velocity during gestation. Thalassemia is a hypercoagulable state, especially in nontransfused and splenectomized individuals.[69] The pathophysiology has been well described and involves interactions of disrupted thalassemic red blood cell membrane surfaces, platelets, and endothelium.[47,70,71]

No thrombotic events were noted in women receiving low molecular weight heparin during pregnancy.[5] The recommendations, therefore, are to keep women who are at higher thrombotic risk (prior splenectomy, non–transfusion-dependent TI, and prior recurrent miscarriages) on prophylaxis with low molecular weight heparin during pregnancy and during the postpartum period.[49,72] Women with postsplenectomy thrombocytosis may already be on low dose aspirin, which should be continued despite the addition of low molecular weight heparin.[5,38]

Peripartum Care

There is no general consensus on the timing and mode of delivery for women with thalassemia. Generally, for noncomplicated pregnancies, spontaneous onset of labor is reasonable. An individualized assessment by a multidisciplinary team is recommended when determining the best approach to delivery.

For women with prior evidence of cardiac iron overload or dysfunction, continuous infusion of DFO (2 g intravenous during 24 hours) during labor may be considered to minimize the risk of cardiac decompensation or arrhythmias in the setting of acidosis associated with prolonged labor.[53]

Skeletal pathologic conditions common in women with TDT have significant implications during childbirth. Approximately 80% of these women require cesarean section, often due to cephalopelvic disproportion. There are, however, case series consisting of well-transfused and chelated women that report cesarean section rates as low as 19%.[30]

For anesthesia, regional blockade is preferred to general anesthesia given the prevalence of maxillofacial deformities. The anatomic changes associated with marrow expansion can complicate intubation and securing the airway. Placement of a spinal epidural must also be carefully considered because scoliosis and osteoporosis are common. Osteoporosis, present in 40% to 50% of patients with TDT, can lead to reduced height of the vertebral bodies displacing the conus caudally.[73]

Due to the possibility of alloantibodies and prolonged time to acquire crossmatched units, the request for packed red blood cells should be placed early in the perinatal period.

Postpartum Care

In the procoagulant states of pregnancy and thalassemia, cesarean section and ART add to the risk of venous thromboembolism. No clinical trials have addressed the role of postpartum thromboprophylaxis. However, guidelines recommend low-molecular-weight heparin prophylaxis while in the hospital, and for 7 days after a vaginal delivery or for 6 weeks after a cesarean section.[49,53] Antibiotic treatment is recommended after delivery due to the higher risk of infections, particularly in splenectomized patients.[38,42] Initiation of chelation therapy shortly after delivery is critical. Reports suggest that use of DFO during breastfeeding is safe but study on its transmission through breast milk is limited.[74] Breastfeeding should be encouraged in all women except in those who are at risk of vertical transmission: women who are HIV or hepatitis C RNA positive and/or are hepatitis B surface antigen positive.

All patients should receive contraception counseling in the postnatal period. Options for contraception are limited in patients with TDT. Intrauterine devices should be avoided given the increased risk of infection. Estrogen-containing oral contraception may further increase the risk of thromboembolism. Progestin-only oral contraceptive pills or barrier methods are most commonly recommended.

Psychological support for the mother and new family is important in the postnatal period, with special attention to signs of anxiety and depression.

Social, Psychological, and Ethical Consideration

The ability to create a family, traditionally by bearing children, has a significant impact on and is often seen as a measurement of an individual's quality of life. The approach to counseling a couple regarding the maternal and fetal risks for a woman with TDT may vary based on culture. In some regions, the influence of a strong societal expectation for family development may play a significant role in a provider's decision to support a couple because they pursue a pregnancy. In the United States, the conversation may place more weight on couples to decide based on their own beliefs and goals, with a medical team providing information to help inform a couple's decision. One topic that is difficult but important to discuss is that of shortened life span. Although the projected life expectancy for individuals with TDT has improved, studies depict that it remains significantly shorter than expected for the general population.[75] How this may have an impact on a couple's decision cannot be known until the conversation is had. Evaluation and counseling prepregnancy and during gestation as part of a multidisciplinary approach are strongly recommended.

Careful planning of care before and during pregnancy, involving various specialists, can result in a good outcome for a pregnant woman with TDT. Strict monitoring of the parameters listed previously is crucial, in particular, cardiac function and considerations of initiation of chelation.

OPTIONS TO ATTAINING A FAMILY

For women with TDT with severe cardiac iron overload who are considered high risk to carry a pregnancy, options include delaying pregnancy until after aggressive chelation and cardiac risk reduction, adoption, or surrogacy.

For couples at risk of having an affected child, as in the case where one parent has TI or TM and the partner is a carrier, options include pregnancy with prenatal screening after conception, including the recently developed method of noninvasive prenatal testing (NIPT) for beta globin mutations,[76] preimplantation genetic testing (PGT) before pregnancy, third-party reproduction, or adoption. Third-party reproduction involves IVF using donor games and allows a couple to have offspring genetically related to one of the partners. The use of either a donor egg or donor sperm is a viable option, although sperm may be preferred given the cost and ease of collection. The feasibility of gamete donation varies between countries.[77] Adoption may be a feasible option; however, access to and eligibility for adoption vary. The various options for a couple are personal and will vary within the context of the accepted social, religious, political, and ethical practices of their community or society.

Prenatal Diagnosis

The motivations for determining disease status once a pregnancy is established range from termination of an affected pregnancy, providing information to help family and providers prepare for a child's needs, and in the case of alpha-thalassemia, therapeutic options including intrauterine transfusions, and recently in utero HSCT. Early diagnosis by sampling of a fetal sample is key. Current methods of prenatal screening involve invasive procedures to acquire fetal DNA from chorionic villus sampling or amniocentesis, which are offered after 10 weeks and 15 weeks gestation, respectively. These procedures pose risks including miscarriage, limb reduction, infection, and Rh sensitization.[78,79] Prior information through NIPT will likely also become more widely used in the coming years.[76]

Preimplantation Genetic Testing

For at-risk couples, PGT is a method for reducing the risk of having an affected fetus, and overcomes the need to terminate an affected pregnancy.

PGT involves close collaboration between geneticists, gynecologists, and embryologists. PGT involves couple counseling of the genetic diagnosis, PGT, IVF, and associated risks. The PGT cycle involves ovarian stimulation, oocyte retrieval and fertilization by intracytoplasmic sperm injection, embryo culture and biopsy, followed by genetic analysis using a combination of PCR based protocols, whole genome amplification, and next-generation sequencing.[80,81] Unaffected embryos are then selected for implantation. PGT is highly specialized and involves technical expertise and skill at all levels. One study assessed the implantation rates for 20 couples in which both partners were beta-thalassemia carriers who underwent PGT with biopsies of the blastomere or blastocyte stage. The rate of implantation was found to be slightly increased when biopsies were taken at the blastocyte stage: 26.7% and 47.6%, respectively.[82] The rate of successful pregnancy after PGT in thalassemia carriers is similar to the general rate of 30%.[83] PGT to select embryos that are free of thalassemia and are also an HLA match for a couple's affected child considering HSCT is now an option. The likelihood of finding an unaffected embryo that is also an HLA-matched significantly drops to 18.8%.[80] This procedure however is associated with multiple procedural and technical challenges, bone marrow transplantation, psychological impact, and ethical considerations, stressing the importance of comprehensive counseling of the at-risk couple.

Overall, both prenatal diagnosis and PGT offer at-risk couples options in their goal to have an unaffected child, however, are challenging both diagnostically, but also with respect to the infrastructure and resources needed (**Table 3**).

Table 3
Comparison between prenatal diagnosis and preimplantation genetic testing

	Conventional Prenatal Diagnosis	Preimplantation Genetic Testing	Non-invasive Prenatal Testing
Timing of genetic analysis	During pregnancy: • CVS: from 11 weeks, • Amniocentesis: from 15 weeks	Before initiation of pregnancy	From 9 weeks of pregnancy (by maternal blood draw)
Risk to fetus, pregnancy or baby	Miscarriage <2%	Similar to conventional ART	None
Accuracy of genetic analysis	> 99%	> 99%	Yet to be validated
Chance of healthy delivery	75% (based on genetic risk per disease transmission)	30% per embryo transfer (limited by embryo implantation and outcomes)	75% (based on genetic risk per disease transmission)
Major disadvantages	Consideration of termination of affected pregnancy	• Technically advanced, multiple steps, labor intensive • Unpredictable pregnancy and birth rate • More expensive	Extensive validation pending
Major advantages	Well-validated procedure	Avoids need to consider therapeutic termination	• Early diagnosis • Limited risks in pregnancy

Abbreviations: ART, assisted reproductive technologies; CVS, chorionic villus sampling.
Adapted from Vrettou C, Kakourou G, Mamas T, Traeger-Synodinos. Prenatal and preimplantation diagnosis in hemoglobinopathies. International Journal of Laboratory Medicine 2018;40(Suppl. 1):74-82; with permission.

SUMMARY

As women with TDT are seeking pregnancy, ensuring the best outcomes for both mother and baby require concerted and collaborative efforts between the hematologist, obstetrician, cardiologist, hepatologist, and genetic counselor among others. Active engagement and support of the patient and partner through this often personal and emotionally charged process is imperative. Proactive counseling, early fertility evaluation, optimal management of iron overload and organ function, and application of advances in ART and prenatal screening are important in ensuring a healthy outcome. Many unanswered questions remain requiring further study, including fertility preservation and best timing to implement it, in light of advances in curative options, chelation therapy during pregnancy, and indications and duration of anticoagulation.

DISCLOSURE

FA Sayani: Grant/Research/Clinical Trial Support: Agios Pharmaceuticals, Celgene, Novartis, Imara, Protagonist.

EP Vichinsky: Grant/Research/Clinical Trial Support: Agios Pharmaceuticals, Blue-bird Bio, Global Blood Therapeutics, Novartis, Novo Nordisk. Consultant/Advisory Boards: BioMarin Pharmaceuticals, Bluebird bio, Chiesi Corp, Forma Therapeutics, Global Blood Therapeutics. All of the relevant financial relationships listed have been mitigated.

REFERENCES

1. Modell B, Khan M, Darlison M, et al. Improved survival of thalassaemia major in the UK and relation to T2* cardiovascular magnetic resonance. J Cardiovasc Magn Reson 2008;10:42.
2. Uysal A, Alkan G, Kurtoğlu A, et al. Diminished ovarian reserve in women with transfusion-dependent beta-thalassemia major: Is iron gonadotoxic? Eur J Obstet Gynecol Reprod Biol 2017;216:69–73.
3. Galanello R, Origa R. Beta-thalassemia. Orphanet J Rare Dis 2010;5:11.
4. Borgna-Pignatti C, Rugolotto S, De Stefano P, et al. Survival and complications in patients with thalassemia major treated with transfusion and deferoxamine. Hae-matologica 2004;89(10):1187–93.
5. Origa R, Piga A, Quarta G, et al. Pregnancy and beta-thalassemia: an Italian multicenter experience. Haematologica 2010;95(3):376–81.
6. ACOG Committee on Obstetrics ACOG Practice Bulletin No. 78: hemoglobinop-athies in pregnancy. Obstet Gynecol 2007;109(1):229–37.
7. Pafumi C, Leanza V, Coco L, et al. The reproduction in women affected by cooley disease. Hematol Rep 2011;3(1):e4.
8. Birkenfeld A, Goldfarb AW, Rachmilewitz EA, et al. Endometrial glandular haemo-siderosis in homozygous beta-thalassaemia. Eur J Obstet Gynecol Reprod Biol 1989;31(2):173–8.
9. Roussou P, Tsagarakis NJ, Kountouras D, et al. Beta-thalassemia major and fe-male fertility: the role of iron and iron-induced oxidative stress. Anemia 2013; 2013:617204.
10. Castaldi MA, Cobellis L. Thalassemia and infertility. Hum Fertil (Camb) 2016; 19(2):90–6.
11. Reubinoff BE, Simon A, Friedler S, et al. Defective oocytes as a possible cause of infertility in a beta-thalassaemia major patient. Hum Reprod 1994;9(6):1143–5.
12. Singer ST, Vichinsky EP, Gildengorin G, et al. Reproductive capacity in iron over-loaded women with thalassemia major. Blood 2011;118(10):2878–81.
13. Chang H-H, Chen M-J, Lu M-Y, et al. Iron overload is associated with low anti-müllerian hormone in women with transfusion-dependent β-thalassaemia. BJOG 2011;118(7):825–31.
14. Talaulikar VS, Bajoria R, Ehidiamhen AJ, et al. A 10-year longitudinal study of evaluation of ovarian reserve in women with transfusion-dependent beta thalas-saemia major. Eur J Obstet Gynecol Reprod Biol 2019;238:38–43.
15. Mensi L, Borroni R, Reschini M, et al. Oocyte quality in women with thalassaemia major: insights from IVF cycles. Eur J Obstet Gynecol Reprod Biol X 2019;3: 100048.
16. Papadimas J, Goulis DG, Mandala E, et al. beta-thalassemia and gonadal axis: a cross-sectional, clinical study in a Greek population. Hormones (Athens) 2002; 1(3):179–87.
17. Çetinçakmak MG, Hattapoğlu S, Menzilcioğlu S, et al. MRI-based evaluation of the factors leading to pituitary iron overload in patients with thalassemia major. J Neuroradiol 2016;43(4):297–302.

18. Oudit GY, Sun H, Trivieri MG, et al. L-type Ca2+ channels provide a major pathway for iron entry into cardiomyocytes in iron-overload cardiomyopathy. Nat Med 2003;9(9):1187–94.

19. Olivieri NF, Brittenham GM. Management of the thalassemias. Cold Spring Harb Perspect Med 2013;3(6):a011767.

20. Farmaki K, Tzoumari I, Pappa C, et al. Normalisation of total body iron load with very intensive combined chelation reverses cardiac and endocrine complications of thalassaemia major. Br J Haematol 2010;148(3):466–75.

21. Lam WWM, Au WY, Chu WCW, et al. One-stop measurement of iron deposition in the anterior pituitary, liver, and heart in thalassemia patients. J Magn Reson Imaging 2008;28(1):29–33.

22. Noetzli LJ, Panigrahy A, Mittelman SD, et al. Pituitary iron and volume predict hypogonadism in transfusional iron overload. Am J Hematol 2012;87(2):167–71.

23. Singer ST, Fischer R, Allen I, et al. Pituitary iron and factors predictive of fertility status in transfusion dependent thalassemia. Haematologica 2021;106(6): 1740–4.

24. Bajoria R, Chatterjee R. Hypogonadotrophic hypogonadism and diminished gonadal reserve accounts for dysfunctional gametogenesis in thalassaemia patients with iron overload presenting with infertility. Hemoglobin 2011;35(5–6): 636–42.

25. Walker EH, Whelton MJ, Beaven GH. Successful pregnancy in a patient with thalassaemia major. J Obstet Gynaecol Br Commonw 1969;76(6):549–53.

26. Perniola R, Magliari F, Rosatelli MC, et al. High-risk pregnancy in beta-thalassaemia major women. Report of three cases. Gynecol Obstet Invest 2000; 49(2):137–9.

27. Skordis N, Petrikkos L, Toumba M, et al. Update on fertility in thalassaemia major. Pediatr Endocrinol Rev 2004;2(Suppl 2):296–302.

28. Tuck SM. Fertility and pregnancy in thalassemia major. Ann N Y Acad Sci 2005; 1054:300–7.

29. Butwick A, Findley I, Wonke B. Management of pregnancy in a patient with beta thalassaemia major. Int J Obstet Anesth 2005;14(4):351–4.

30. Ansari S, Azarkeivan A, Kivan AA, et al. Pregnancy in patients treated for beta thalassemia major in two centers (Ali Asghar Children's Hospital and Thalassemia Clinic): outcome for mothers and newborn infants. Pediatr Hematol Oncol 2006; 23(1):33–7.

31. Mancuso A, Giacobbe A, De Vivo A, et al. Pregnancy in patients with beta-thalassaemia major: maternal and foetal outcome. Acta Haematol 2008; 119(1):15–7.

32. Toumba M, Kanaris C, Simamonian K, et al. Outcome and management of pregnancy in women with thalassaemia in Cyprus. East Mediterr Health J 2008;14(3): 628–35.

33. Anastasi S, Lisi R, Abbate G, et al. Absence of teratogenicity of deferasirox treatment during pregnancy in a thalassaemic patient. Pediatr Endocrinol Rev 2011; 8(Suppl 2):345–7.

34. Vini D, Servos P, Drosou M. Normal pregnancy in a patient with β-thalassaemia major receiving iron chelation therapy with deferasirox (Exjade®). Eur J Haematol 2011;86(3):274–5.

35. Thompson AA, Kim H-Y, Singer ST, et al. Pregnancy outcomes in women with thalassemia in North America and the United Kingdom. Am J Hematol 2013; 88(9):771–3.

36. Al-Riyami N, Al-Khaduri M, Daar S. Pregnancy Outcomes in Women with Homozygous Beta Thalassaemia: A single-centre experience from Oman. Sultan Qaboos Univ Med J 2014;14(3):e337–41.

37. Akıncı B, Yaşar AŞ, Özdemir Karadaş N, et al. Fertility in Patients with Thalassemia and Outcome of Pregnancies: A Turkish Experience. Turk J Haematol 2019;36(4):274–7.

38. Cassinerio E, Baldini IM, Alameddine RS, et al. Pregnancy in patients with thalassemia major: a cohort study and conclusions for an adequate care management approach. Ann Hematol 2017;96(6):1015–21.

39. Takhviji V, Zibara K, Azarkeivan A, et al. Fertility and pregnancy in Iranian thalassemia patients: An update on transfusion complications. Transfus Med 2020;30(5):352–60.

40. Carlberg KT, Singer ST, Vichinsky EP. Fertility and Pregnancy in Women with Transfusion-Dependent Thalassemia. Hematol Oncol Clin North Am 2018;32(2):297–315.

41. Santarone S, Natale A, Olioso P, et al. Pregnancy outcome following hematopoietic cell transplantation for thalassemia major. Bone Marrow Transpl 2017;52(3):388–93.

42. Nassar AH, Naja M, Cesaretti C, et al. Pregnancy outcome in patients with beta-thalassemia intermedia at two tertiary care centers, in Beirut and Milan. Haematologica 2008;93(10):1586–7.

43. Lee BS, Sathar J, Sivapatham L, et al. Pregnancy outcomes in women with non-transfusion dependent thalassaemia (NTDT): A haematology centre experience. Malays J Pathol 2018;40(2):149–52.

44. Singer ST, Kim H-Y, Olivieri NF, et al. Hemoglobin H-constant spring in North America: an alpha thalassemia with frequent complications. Am J Hematol 2009;84(11):759–61.

45. Ake-Sittipaisarn S, Sirichotiyakul S, Srisupundit K, et al. Outcomes of pregnancies complicated by haemoglobin H-constant spring and deletional haemoglobin H disease: A retrospective cohort study. Br J Haematol 2022;199(1):122–9.

46. Tsironi M, Karagiorga M, Aessopos A. Iron overload, cardiac and other factors affecting pregnancy in thalassemia major. Hemoglobin 2010;34(3):240–50.

47. Lao TT. Obstetric care for women with thalassemia. Best Pract Res Clin Obstet Gynaecol 2017;39:89–100.

48. Meloni A, Gamberini MR, Neri MG, et al. Changes of cardiac iron and function during pregnancy in trasfusion-dependent thalassemia patients. J Cardiovasc Magn Reson 2016;18(S1):P270.

49. Skordis N. Fertility and pregnancy. 2021 guidelines for the management of transfusion dependent thalassemia (TDT). 4th Edition. Nicosia, Cyprus: Thalassaemia International Federation; 2021. p. 214–29 Version 2.0.. .

50. Davies JM, Lewis MPN, Wimperis J, et al. Review of guidelines for the prevention and treatment of infection in patients with an absent or dysfunctional spleen: prepared on behalf of the British Committee for Standards in Haematology by a working party of the Haemato-Oncology task force. Br J Haematol 2011;155(3):308–17.

51. Cappellini MD, Farmakis D, Porter J, et al. Guidelines for the management of transfusion dependent thalassemia (TDT). 4th edition. n.d: Thalassaemia International Federation; 2021.

52. Vogiatzi MG, Macklin EA, EFJ B, et al. Bone disease in thalassemia: a frequent and still unresolved problem. J Bone Miner Res 2009;24(3):543–57.

53. Petrakos G, Andriopoulos P, Tsironi M. Pregnancy in women with thalassemia: challenges and solutions. Int J Womens Health 2016;8:441–51.

54. Triunfo S, Lanzone A, Lindqvist PG. Low maternal circulating levels of vitamin D as potential determinant in the development of gestational diabetes mellitus. J Endocrinol Invest 2017;40(10):1049–59.

55. Spencer DH, Grossman BJ, Scott MG. Red cell transfusion decreases hemoglobin A1c in patients with diabetes. Clin Chem 2011;57(2):344–6.

56. Ibba RM, Zoppi MA, Floris M, et al. Neural tube defects in the offspring of thalassemia carriers. Fetal Diagn Ther 2003;18(1):5–7.

57. Diamantidis MD, Neokleous N, Agapidou A, et al. Iron chelation therapy of transfusion-dependent β-thalassemia during pregnancy in the era of novel drugs: is deferasirox toxic? Int J Hematol 2016;103(5):537–44.

58. Singer ST, Vichinsky EP. Deferoxamine treatment during pregnancy: is it harmful? Am J Hematol 1999;60(1):24–6.

59. Allegra A, Capra M, Cuccia L, et al. Hypogonadism in beta-thalassemic adolescents: a characteristic pituitary-gonadal impairment. The ineffectiveness of long-term iron chelation therapy. Gynecol Endocrinol 1990;4(3):181–91.

60. Chatterjee R, Katz M, Cox TF, et al. Prospective study of the hypothalamic-pituitary axis in thalassaemic patients who developed secondary amenorrhoea. Clin Endocrinol (Oxf) 1993;39(3):287–96.

61. Bronspiegel-Weintrob N, Olivieri NF, Tyler B, et al. Effect of age at the start of iron chelation therapy on gonadal function in beta-thalassemia major. N Engl J Med 1990;323(11):713–9.

62. Skordis N, Gourni M, Kanaris C, et al. The impact of iron overload and genotype on gonadal function in women with thalassaemia major. Pediatr Endocrinol Rev 2004;2(Suppl 2):292–5.

63. Dolmans M-M, Donnez J. Fertility preservation in women for medical and social reasons: Oocytes vs ovarian tissue. Best Pract Res Clin Obstet Gynaecol 2021; 70:63–80.

64. Chung K, Donnez J, Ginsburg E, et al. Emergency IVF versus ovarian tissue cryopreservation: decision making in fertility preservation for female cancer patients. Fertil Steril 2013;99(6):1534–42.

65. Taylor DJ, Lind T. Red cell mass during and after normal pregnancy. Br J Obstet Gynaecol 1979;86(5):364–70.

66. Bosque MA, Domingo JL, Corbella J. Assessment of the developmental toxicity of deferoxamine in mice. Arch Toxicol 1995;69(7):467–71.

67. Tsironi M, Ladis V, Margellis Z, et al. Impairment of cardiac function in a successful full-term pregnancy in a homozygous beta-thalassemia major: does chelation have a positive role? Eur J Obstet Gynecol Reprod Biol 2005;120(1):117–8.

68. Jensen CE, Tuck SM, Wonke B. Fertility in beta thalassaemia major: a report of 16 pregnancies, preconceptual evaluation and a review of the literature. Br J Obstet Gynaecol 1995;102(8):625–9.

69. Taher AT, Otrock ZK, Uthman I, et al. Thalassemia and hypercoagulability. Blood Rev 2008;22(5):283–92.

70. Leung TY, Lao TT. Thalassaemia in pregnancy. Best Pract Res Clin Obstet Gynaecol 2012;26(1):37–51.

71. Ambroggio S, Peris C, Picardo E, et al. β-thalassemia patients and gynecological approach: review and clinical experience. Gynecol Endocrinol 2016;32(3):171–6.

72. Nassar AH, Usta IM, Taher AM. Beta-thalassemia intermedia and pregnancy: should we anticoagulate? J Thromb Haemost 2006;4(6):1413–4.

73. Voskaridou E, Kyrtsonis MC, Terpos E, et al. Bone resorption is increased in young adults with thalassaemia major. Br J Haematol 2001;112(1):36–41.
74. Surbek DV, Glanzmann R, Nars PW, et al. Pregnancy and lactation in homozygous beta-thalassemia major. J Perinat Med 1998;26(3):240–3.
75. Modell B, Khan M, Darlison M, et al. Improved survival of thalassaemia major in the UK and relation to T2* cardiovascular magnetic resonance. J Cardiovasc Magn Reson 2008;10:42.
76. Erlich HA, López-Peña C, Carlberg KT, et al. Noninvasive Prenatal Test for β-Thalassemia and Sickle Cell Disease Using Probe Capture Enrichment and Next-Generation Sequencing of DNA in Maternal Plasma. J Appl Lab Med 2022; 7(2):515–31.
77. Gianaroli L, Ferraretti AP, Magli MC, et al. Current regulatory arrangements for assisted conception treatment in European countries. Eur J Obstet Gynecol Reprod Biol 2016;207:211–3.
78. Tabor A, Alfirevic Z. Update on procedure-related risks for prenatal diagnosis techniques. Fetal Diagn Ther 2010;27(1):1–7.
79. Meleti D, De Oliveira LG, Araujo Júnior E, et al. Evaluation of passage of fetal erythrocytes into maternal circulation after invasive obstetric procedures. J Obstet Gynaecol Res 2013;39(9):1374–82.
80. Mamas T, Kakourou G, Vrettou C, et al. Hemoglobinopathies and preimplantation diagnostics. Int J Lab Hematol 2022;44(Suppl 1):21–7.
81. Vrettou C, Kakourou G, Mamas T, et al. Prenatal and preimplantation diagnosis of hemoglobinopathies. Int J Lab Hematol 2018;40(Suppl 1):74–82.
82. Kokkali G, Traeger-Synodinos J, Vrettou C, et al. Blastocyst biopsy versus cleavage stage biopsy and blastocyst transfer for preimplantation genetic diagnosis of beta-thalassaemia: a pilot study. Hum Reprod 2007;22(5):1443–9.
83. Cao A, Kan YW. The prevention of thalassemia. Cold Spring Harb Perspect Med 2013;3(2):a011775.

Hematopoietic Stem Cell Transplantation in Thalassemia

Mattia Algeri, MD[a,1,*], Mariachiara Lodi, MD[a,1],
Franco Locatelli, MD, PhD[a,b,1]

KEYWORDS

- Hematopoietic stem cell transplantation • Thalassemia • Hemoglobinopathies
- Sibling donor transplantation • Unrelated donor transplantation
- Cord blood transplantation • Haploidentical transplantation

KEY POINTS

- Allogeneic hematopoietic stem-cell transplantation (allo-HSCT) still remains the only consolidated, potentially curative treatment of thalassemia major (TM).
- With modern transplant protocols, in children with TM transplanted from an HLA-identical sibling donor, allo-HSCT offers disease-free survival rates exceeding 90%.
- Using stringent criteria of donor/recipient compatibility (ie, high-resolution molecular typing for HLA class I and II loci), outcomes after allo-HSCT from a matched unrelated donor now approach those of HLA-identical sibling allo-HSCT recipients.
- The experience of the last decade has shown that HLA-haploidentical HSCT is a safe and feasible approach in young patients with TM lacking a fully-matched donor.
- Although long-term thalassemia-free survivors display a quality of life similar to that of the general population, the importance of potential long-term complications after allo-HSCT has increasingly been recognized in recent years.

INTRODUCTION

In the last half-century, the life expectancy of thalassemia major (TM) patients has dramatically improved and, with the proper administration of supportive care, consisting of chronic blood transfusions and regular iron chelation therapy, now exceeds 50 years in high-income countries.[1–3] However, the need for a life-long treatment poses a significant burden on patients' quality of life, as virtually all of them have to

[a] Department of Hematology/Oncology, Cell and Gene Therapy – IRCCS, Bambino Gesù Children's Hospital, Rome, Italy; [b] Department of Life Sciences and Public Health, Catholic University of the Sacred Heart, Rome, Italy
[1] These authors contributed equally.
* Corresponding author.
E-mail address: mattia.algeri@opbg.net

hemonc.theclinics.com

plan their lives around transfusions and even subjects receiving optimal care are exposed to a non-negligible risk of complications, arising from either transfusion therapy or as a consequence of iron overload.[4–8] In recent years, the development of new agents that improve red blood cell (RBC) maturation has offered the opportunity to alleviate disease phenotype, but the achievement of transfusion independence is obtained at best in a small fraction of patients and, in any case, bound to chronic drug administration.[9] Finally, it must be highlighted that most of the patients with TM reside in developing countries, where access to safe and adequate transfusion therapy as well as regular chelation is often available only for a minority of subjects.[10] Allogeneic hematopoietic stem cell transplantation (allo-HSCT) still remains the more consolidated, potentially curative treatment of Beta-TM. Indeed, although exciting results have been obtained with novel approaches of gene-addition therapy, their widespread application is limited by affordability challenges due to the high costs, which recently led to the arrest of commercialization in Europe.[11] Gene-editing strategies based on re-induction of HbF production have also consistently shown promising results in terms of safety and efficacy, but are currently available only within clinical trials.[12,13] In parallel with the development of these innovative therapies, the advances in high-resolution donor HLA-typing, choice of conditioning regimen, graft-versus-host disease (GvHD) prophylaxis and supportive care measures have continuously improved overall HSCT outcome in TM. This article provides an overview of the current state of art, as well as of future perspectives, of allo-HSCT in TM.

PRETRANSPLANT RISK STRATIFICATION

The goal of HSCT in TM is to replace the patient's marrow with healthy functional hematopoietic stem cells (HSCs), capable of supporting effective erythropoiesis before major organ dysfunction and complications arise. In this perspective, HSCT should be performed as early as possible, ideally in early childhood, to avoid the burden of comorbidities associated with chronic transfusions (**Fig. 1**). Several studies have shown that patients transplanted at a young age have a better overall (OS) and event-free survival (EFS) as compared with late adolescents and adults and the

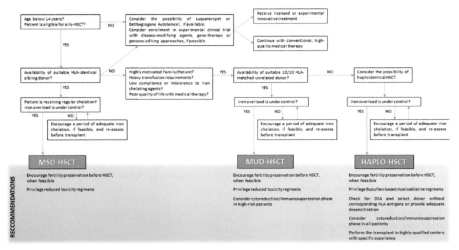

Fig. 1. Proposed algorithm to guide decisions on HSCT in TM patients with regular access to adequate supportive care

age of 14 years has been proposed as cutoff for achieving optimal outcomes in HSCT for TM in a large European Group for Blood and Marrow Transplant (EBMT) registry analysis. To predict the risk of transplant-related complications and the likelihood of successful HSCT outcome in TM,[14,15] in the late 1980s the Pesaro group developed a well-recognized scoring system based on three different variables: (1) quality of chelation therapy (regular versus non-regular), (2) any hepatomegaly and its severity (palpable liver edge more than 2 cm below the costal margin), (3) presence of any degree of liver fibrosis on pretransplant liver biopsy examination.[16] The absence of any of these risk factors identified patients belonging to the risk class 1, whereas the presence of all these factors qualified a patient as belonging to class 3 (**Fig. 2**).

The data collected through the long experience of the Pesaro group showed an estimated thalassemia-free survival (TFS) probability of 85% to 90%, 80%, and 65% to 70% for patients in risk classes 1, 2, and 3, respectively, with the risk of transplant-related mortality (TRM) increasing progressively from class 1 to class 3 and with the age of the subjects.[16–18]

The Pesaro classification has several limitations. First, it applies only to the pediatric population and it's not validated in adults.[19] In addition, two of the three variables, chelation quality, and hepatomegaly, are subjected to intra- and interobserver variabilities. Although a scoring system based on the precise, quantitative, determination of iron overload would offer increased accuracy and applicability, all attempts to identify such criteria have failed so far.[20]

Another limitation of the Pesaro's risk stratification is that it did not include a very high-risk subgroup of class III more prevalent in developing countries. As HSCT has been increasingly offered in these countries as well, recognizing this high-risk group is extremely important to adequately modify HSCT protocols.[21–23] In this regard, it has been suggested that patients above 7 years of age and with liver sizes of 5 cm represent a very high risk subgroup within the conventional Class III group (Class III Vellore high risk or Class III VHR).[23]

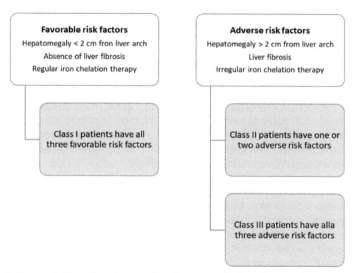

Fig. 2. Predictive variables of outcome after hematopoietic cell transplantation in patients with thalassemia

Despite these limitations, the Pesaro classification has the indisputable merit to provide a powerful demonstration of how the quality of medical care that patients have received before transplantation is a critical determinant of post-allo-HSCT outcome.

ADVANCES IN CONDITIONING REGIMEN

Similarly to other nonmalignant conditions, the aim of allo-HSCT for TM is not to eradicate a malignant clone and to benefit from the graft-versus-leukemia effect, but rather to achieve a level of engraftment capable of sustaining long-term effective erythropoiesis.[24] However, achievement of this goal is anything but trivial and several peculiar clinical and biological aspects of TM needs to be considered in the tailoring of conditioning regimen. First, the rejection/recurrence rate of thalassemia is significantly higher than that of other non-malignant diseases or acute leukemias.[25] At the time of transplantation and in contrast to leukemia patients, the immune system of patients with TM is not heavily impaired by previous cytotoxic agent therapy and, in this setting, the increased risk of primary and secondary graft failure is further exacerbated by sensitization to RBC antigens and development of anti-HLA antibodies, as a consequence of prolonged RBC transfusions.[26]

In addition, TM is characterized by ineffective erythropoiesis and variable erythroid expansion, which may further contribute to an increase in the risk of graft failure (GF).[27] Finally, iron overload and related hyper-production of reactive oxygen species, resulting from ineffective erythropoiesis and chronic transfusions, is associated with short- and long-term complications after HSCT.[28]

Thus, the ideal conditioning regimen should be capable of eradicating an expanded bone marrow (BM) and providing adequate immunosuppression to achieve sustained engraftment while avoiding excessive toxicity on chronically iron-damaged tissues. For many years, the predominant conditioning regimen was based on the combination of busulfan (BU) at 14 to 16 mg/kg and cyclophosphamide (CY) at 160 to 200 mg/kg. Unfortunately, such regimen, although capable of eradicating thalassemia hyperplastic BM, has been associated with a high incidence of hepatic complications, in particular sinusoidal obstruction syndrome (SOS), and heart toxicity.[29] Attempts to optimize this preparative backbone by reducing the dose of CY were associated with a significant increase in graft rejection rate.[30] In the last two decades, new conditioning strategies for patients with TM have been introduced with improved results, such as intravenous BU, or treosulfan (TREO) combined with thiotepa (TT) and fludarabine (FLU).[31,32]

In a recent, multicenter retrospective analysis conducted by the Center for International Blood and Bone Marrow Transplantation Research (CIBMTR) in conjunction with several Asian Centers of 1100 patients transplanted for TM, the use of busulfan (BU)/cyclophosphamide (CY)/fludarabine (FLU) conditioning was associated with better OS and EFS and reduced incidence of GF as compared with BU/CY alone. In the same study, excellent outcomes were documented also in patients transplanted with a conditioning regimen based on the combination of CY, intravenous BU, FLU, TT, and ATG.[15] This type of conditioning was reported for the first time in a Chinese study conducted on 82 children with TM who received peripheral blood stem cell (PBSC) transplantation from either a matched unrelated donor (MUD) or a Matched Sibling Donor (MSD) after a conditioning regimen based on the combination of CY, intravenous BU, FLU, TT and ATG. With this protocol, named the "NF-08-TM", the estimated 3-year OS and TFS were 92.3% and 90.4% in the MUD group and 90.0% and 83.3% in the MSD group.[32]

Although historically associated with high rates of Graft Failure, reduced-intensity conditioning (RIC) has been increasingly investigated in patients with TM, to reduce not only short-term toxicities but also long-term comorbidities, such as growth impairment, endocrine dysfunction, and infertility.[33] TREO, a structural analog of BU with strong myeloablative and immunosuppressive activity and limited extramedullary toxicity, has been used to replace BU by several groups, in view of its favorable toxicity profile.[34–36] Bernardo and colleagues[31] reported the outcome of 60 patients with TM (including 12 adults), who were transplanted either from MSDs or MUDs, after conditioning with a combination of TREO, TT, and FLU. The 5-year overall survival and DFS were 93% and 84%, respectively, for the whole cohort, without the occurrence of SOS.[31] The use of TREO/TT/FLU was capable of reducing the risk of SOS and early TRM also in a cohort of patients with high-risk TM, although it was also associated with a high incidence of early mixed chimerism and graft loss when BM cells were used as a source of stem cells.[37] In a recent retrospective analysis of 722 patients transplanted for TM after either a BU-FLU or TREO-FLU-based conditioning regimen, no differences in OS and acute (aGvHD) and chronic GvHD (cGVHD) incidence were observed between the two groups. However, an increased incidence of second HSCT was recorded in the TREO-FLU cohort (HR 2.24 [95% CI: 1.21 to 4.13%]; $P = 0.01$) and, although indications for second procedures were not reported, the most common reason was likely primary or secondary graft failure or graft loss.[38] Another RIC regimen based on the combination of hydroxyurea (HU), alemtuzumab, FLU, melphalan (MEL), and TT has been investigated in a recent phase 2 prospective trial conducted in 33 Patients with TM receiving unrelated BM or umbilical cord blood (UCB) grafts. The OS and TFS in this cohort were 82% and 79%, respectively.[39] An attractive strategy adopted by different groups to increase the engraftment rate of patients with TM is represented by the introduction of a preconditioning cytoreduction/immunosuppression phase combined with a pretransplant hypertransfusion regimen aimed at reducing the degree of BM erythroid tissue hyperplasia. One approach, pioneered by Lucarelli and colleagues,[40] is based on HU and azathioprine administration from day -45 to -11 and a course of FLU approximately 2 weeks before transplantation. Another effective strategy, developed by Anurathapan and colleagues[41,42] in the haploidentical setting, consists of a prolonged pretransplant pharmacologic immunosuppression phase with FLU and dexamethasone, which has been further implemented with the addition of Bortezomib and Rituximab in highly alloimmunized patients.

DONOR SELECTION AND STEM CELL SOURCE
Hemopoietic Stem Cell Transplantation from HLA-Matched Sibling Donor

In the past 30 years, more than 2000 patients with TM have undergone HSTC from HLA-matched related donors. In reports published in the first decade of the 2000s, OS and TFS rates above 90% and 80%, respectively, have been consistently reported in class I patients by several groups.[43,44] These results were also confirmed in a retrospective EBMT survey, which included 1061 patients treated with MSD transplantation. The OS and TFS were 91% and 83%, respectively. Thanks to additional refinements in patients preparation and the introduction of RIC regimens, in low-risk subjects transplanted in more recent years, the TFS rates have further improved and now stably approach or even exceed 90%.[15,45] For this reason, for subjects with an available MSD allo-HSCT is now considered a standard-care of procedure and is increasingly offered at a young age, to avoid the development of organ damage. Indeed, although with the adoption of RIC regimens survival has increased above 90% also in high-risk patients, TFS still remains suboptimal, ranging from 66% to 81%.

Although the use of BM-derived HSCs as a source for transplantation is a rather standardized practice in MSD transplantation, other stem sources have been investigated. The feasibility of using cord blood (CB) from HLA-identical siblings for HSCT in patients with TM has been shown since 2003. This type of transplantation was associated with a reduced risk of aGvHD and cGvHD and transplant-related mortality (TRM), provided the CB unit had an adequate number of nucleated cells (ie, > 3.5×10^7/kg).[46] In a large retrospective analysis published in 2013 OS, TFS, aGvHD, and cGVHD were 95%, 88%, 20%, and 12% for BM recipients ($n = 389$) and 96%, 81%, 10%, and 5% for CB recipients ($n = 70$), respectively.[45]

Promising results have been observed also after co-transplantation of UCB and BM-derived HSCs harvested from the same MFD. The combined infusion resulted in better hematopoietic recovery, with preservation of the CB-related protective effect on the occurrence of GvHD.[47]

The use of PBSCs from MSD has been evaluated by several groups to overcome the risk of graft failure in TM.[37,48,49] PBSC grafts have been associated with faster engraftment[37,49] and with a low incidence of graft rejection.[49] However, this beneficial effect is counterbalanced by an increased risk of cGvHD, which is a particularly detrimental complication in nonmalignant disease.[48–50] In the large retrospective analysis performed by EBMT, the use of PBSC was associated with significantly lower OS and EFS as compared with BM and UCB grafts.[51] However, in the updated results of 193 MSD-HSCTs performed after "NF-08-TM" conditioning, an impressive OS and TFS of 97.4% was reported, with a remarkably low incidence of grade II-IV aGvHD (5.4%) and moderate/severe cGVHD (3.9%) despite the use of PBSC grafts.[52] Ethical concerns on the mobilization of minor donors have to be considered when analyzing the results obtained with this approach.

Hemopoietic stem cell transplantation from HLA-matched unrelated donor

Less than 20% of patients with TM have a suitable HLA-identical, and not affected, sibling donor. Thanks to the introduction of high-resolution molecular techniques for HLA typing and the increased availability of voluntary donors in the international registries, the percentage of patients who benefited from an allo-HSCT using an MUD has increased significantly in recent decades.[53] Currently, the likelihood of finding an 8/8 MUD varies among racial and ethnic groups, with the highest probability, around 75%, observed among whites of European descent, whereas the likelihood of finding a suitable donor for patients belonging to ethnic minorities is significantly more limited, due the under-representation of non-Caucasian donors in the registries.[54]

The first clinical reports of MUD-HSCT in TM date back to the early 1990s (**Table 1**). In 2002, the Italian cooperative group for Bone Marrow Transplantation (GITMO) reported the outcomes of the first large series of 32 consecutive Patients with TM (aged 2 to 28 years) given MUD-HSCT.[55] The OS and TFS estimates were 79% and 66%, with rejection and TRM rates of 12.5% and 19%, respectively. The incidences of grade II to IV aGvHD and cGvHD were 41% and 25%, respectively.

In a more recent study, the same group reported the results of 68 patients with TM transplanted from an MUD selected by high-resolution HLA molecular typing, after a BU-based conditioning regimen, combined with either CY, TT, or TT and FLU. The OS and TFS in the whole cohort were 79% and 66%, respectively. Grade II to IV aGvHD and cGVHD occurred in 40% and 18% of patients, respectively, and the graft failure rate was 14.4%. In the Class I and II group, OS and TFS were 97% and 80%, respectively, whereas in the Class III group they were 65% and 54%, respectively.[56] RIC regimens have been successfully used also in the MUD setting. In a study involving 60 children, adolescents, and young adults transplanted after a TT-based conditioning regimen, a TFS of 82% was observed in the 40 subjects who received the allograft from a MUD, with a cumulative incidence of grade II-IV aGvHD in the whole cohort (including also

Table 1
Clinical outcome of the alternative donor in children and young adults with thalassemia major

N	Source	Conditioning	GvHD Prophylaxis	Median Age (Years)	OS %	TFS %	TRM %	GF%	aGVHD %	cGVHD %	Refs
Matched Unrelated Donors or Unrelated Cord Blood											
68	BM	BU-CY 25% BU-TT/CY 62% BU-TT-FLU 13%	CSA, MTX,	15 (2 to 37)	79.3	65.8	20	13	40	18	La Nasa et al,[56] 2005
122	BM	BU/TREO-TT-CY/FLU	CSA, MTX,	10.5 (1 to 35)	84	75	16.4	13.1	28	13	Locatelli et al,[58] 2011
40	BM	TREO-TT-FLU	ATG, CSA,MTX	7(1 to 37) *including 20 MSD	93	84	7	9	14	2	Bernardo et al,[31] 2021
52	PB	CY-BU-TT-FLU	ATG, CSA,MTX,MMF,	6 (2 to 15)	92.3	90.4	7.7	1.9	9.6	0	Li et al,[52] 2012
48	PBSC	CY-BU-FLU	ATG, CSA,MTX,MMF,	4 (2 to 11)	100	100	0	0	8.3	8.3	Sun et al,[57] 2019
16	BM	FLU-BU-TT-CY (+pre-conditioning)	ATG, CSA,MTX,MMF, Methylprednisolone	9.6 (1.4 to 24)	94	94	6	0	19	13	Gaziev et al,[40] 2013
33	BM/UCB	FLU-TT-MELPHALAN (+pre-conditioning)	BM: Tacrolimus/CSA, MTX, Methylprednisolone UCB: Tacrolimus/CSA, MMF	8.5 (1 to 17)	82	79	NR	1 (UCB)	BM 24 UCB 44	BM 29 UCB 21	Shenoy et al,[39] 2018
173	PBSC	CY-BU-TT-FLU (+pre-conditioning)	ATG CSA-MTX-MMF	6 (2 to 23) *whole cohort of 486 HSCT	93.6	90.4	4.4	4.8	23.6 (II-IV)	6.9 severe	He et al,[32]
26	BM/PBSC	BU-CY-FLU	ATG CSA/Tacrolimus	8 (2 to 10)	94	82	7	0	28	15	Anarathapan et al,[42] 2014

(continued on next page)

Table 1
(continued)

N	Source	Conditioning	GvHD Prophylaxis	Median Age (Years)	OS %	TFS %	TRM %	GF%	aGVHD %	cGVHD %	Refs
35	CB	BU/CY	ATG CSA/Tacrolimus ± Prednisone	4 (0.5 to 14)	62	21	34	57	23	16	Ruggeri et al,[63] 2011
35	CB	BU/CY	ATG, CSA, Methylprednislone	5.5 (1.2 to 14)	88.5	73.9	11.4	0	47	34	Jaing et al,[64] 2012
9	CB	BU/CY/FLU	ATG, CSA, Methylprednisolone	3.8 (1.5 to 7)	100	56	0	44	33	11	Shah et al,[66] 2015
Haploidentical donors											
22	BM/PB	BU-TT-CY (+pre-conditioning)	ATG, CSA, CD34+ sel. (n = 14) CD34 + sel & CD3/19+ depl. (n = 8)	7.5 (3 to 14)	90	61	14	29	NR	NR	Sodani et al,[68] 2010
11	BM/PB	BU-TT-CY (+pre-conditioning)	ATG, CSA, Methilprednosolone	7(3 to 15.2)	90	80	14		28	6	Gaziev et al,[76] 2018
8	PB	CY-BU-FLU	ATG, CSA, MTX	5.5 (3 to 14)	100	100	0	0	25 (III-IV)	12.5	Sun et al,[83] 2018
83	PB	BU-FLU (+pre-conditioning)	ATG Post-transplant CY Tacrolims/MMF	12 (1 to 28)	96	96	–	0	36	6	Anurathapan et al,[41] 2020

Abbreviations: BM, bone marrow; BU, busulfan; CSA, Cyclosporin A; CY, Cyclophosphamide; MMF, Mycophenolate Mofetil; MTX, Methotrexate; PBSC, peripheral blood stem cells; Treo, Treosulfan; TT, Thiotepa; UCB, umbilical cord blood.

*, It refers to the fact that the median age and range is related to a whole group of 60 patients, including also 20 who received HSCT from MSD.

20 MSD) of 21%.[31] In the URTH trial, evaluating another RIC regimen based on the combination of FLU, MEL, and TTin 33 children with TM, a similar TFS probability of 82% was recorded. The cumulative incidence (CI) of grade II–IV aGVHD was 24%, whereas the 2-year CI of extensive cGVHD was 29%. Although generally BM is the preferred stem cell source for HSCT in TM and other nonmalignant disorders to reduce the risk of GvHD in a setting in which it does not provide any relevant benefit, several Asian groups reported promising results with PBSC transplantation from MUD in TM.[42,57] The updated results of the "NF-08-TM" conditioning protocol in 173 patients with TM who received PSBC grafts from 10/10 MUD, reported an OS and a TFS of 93.6% and 90.4%, respectively. The incidence of grade II-IV aGVHD and moderate/severe cGVHD in this cohort was 23.6% and 6.9%, respectively. Less satisfactory results were obtained with mismatched unrelated donor HSCT.[32] Another Chinese group reported an OS and EFS of 100% in 48 children with TM transplanted after a conditioning regimen combining CY, intravenous BU, FLU, and ATG, with a CI of grade II-IV aGVHD and cGVHD of 8.3% and 8.3%, respectively.[57]

A recent, large, multicenter retrospective analysis showed that, in the modern era, with the adoption of strict immunogenetic compatibility criteria, comparable OS and EFS after MSD and MUD transplantation can be achieved.[15] Despite the superimposable EFS and OS, it is abundantly clear, from the experience of several centers worldwide, that MUD-HSCT is still hampered by an increased risk of aGVHD and cGVHD in comparison with MSD, which accounts for a significant part of the morbidity occurring after allo-HSCT.[51,52,57,58]

Several immunogenetic variables, such as a donor-recipient HLA-Cw ligand group for killer immunoglobulin-like receptors (KIR), KIR genotypes, the HLA-G 14-bp polymorphism have been shown to affect the incidence and/or severity of aGVHD after MUD HSCT in TM.[46,59–61] Among other relevant immunogenetic factors, the presence of nonpermissive HLA-DPB1 mismatches in the host-versus-graft (HvG) direction, instead, has been associated with the risk of rejection in MUD HSCT for TM, regardless of the patient's class of risk.[62]

Umbilical cord blood transplant

In recent decades, related UCBT, where the stem cell derives from an HLA-identical sibling, or from unrelated CB, has also been evaluated as an alternative source of stem cells (see **Table 1**).

Although unrelated UCBT increases the potential donor pool for patients with TM, published data are limited. Ruggeri and colleagues[63] reported the outcomes of 35 patients undergoing unrelated UCBT, showing OS and TFS estimates of 62% and 21%, respectively, with a cumulative incidence of grade II to IV aGVHD and cGvHD of 23% and 16%, respectively. The cumulative graft failure rate was 52%. Better results have been published by Jiang and colleagues[64] in 35 patients with TM given unrelated UCBT after a BU/CY plus ATG preparative regimen. The 5-year overall survival and TFS were 88.3 and 73.9%, respectively, and such good outcomes were attributed to the high cell dose infused (at least 2.5×10^7 TNC/kg in all patients).

Currently, beyond limited reports, unrelated UCBT should be considered with caution in hemoglobinopathy because of the risk of transplant failure and delayed hematopoietic recovery.[55,65,66] Recent evidence has underscored the importance of allele-level HLA matching at HLA-A, -B, -C, and -DRB1 when selecting UCB units for transplantation for non-malignant diseases.[67]

When considering UCBT for hemoglobinopathy; however, the recommendation is still to prioritize units with a total nucleated cell dose of 4 to 5×10^7/kg and, thereafter, consider the degree of allelic HLA match.[67]

HLA-haploidentical hemopoietic stem cell transplantation

Haploidentical-HSCT (haplo-HSCT) has the unquestionable advantage of offering an immediate transplant treatment to virtually all patients in need of an allograft and lacking a suitable HLA-matched donor, either related or unrelated. However, in the context of TM, this approach has been historically characterized by a higher risk of graft rejection, GvHD and TRM.[68] Disease-specific features, including the hyperplastic BM and HLA-alloimmunization due to multiple transfusions, reinforce the bi-directional immunological barrier between donor and recipients and render haplo-HSCT at high risk for GF, especially when T-cell depletion strategies are used. Anti-HLA antibodies have a high prevalence in Patients with TM, even with current leukoreduction standards.[69] In recent years, several studies have shown an association between donor-specific anti-HLA antibodies (DSAs) and the occurrence of GF following haplo-HSCT. The EBMT group now recommends routine evaluation for DSAs before haplo-HSCT and the selection of a donor without the corresponding HLA antigens. However, if there are no such donors available, recipients with DSAs should undergo desensitization treatment before transplantation to prevent GF.[70]

Selective depletion of TCRαβ+ T-cells and CD19+ B-lymphocytes represented a relevant refinement in graft manipulation strategies for T-cell depleted (TCD) haplo-HSCT. With this approach, it is possible to transfer to the recipient not only donor HSCs but also committed hematopoietic progenitors, as well as high numbers of mature natural killer (NK) and γδ T cells, which are capable of exerting a first line of defense against life-threatening infections without increasing the risk of both acute and cGvHD.[71–75] This approach has shown safety and efficacy in several non-malignant disorders. A small cohort of patients with TM who received a TCRαβ+/CD19+ cell-depleted allograft was reported in 2018 by the group of the Mediterranean Institute of Hematology (IME) in Rome. Eleven patients with TM and 3 with Sickle Cell Disease (SCD) received a preparative regimen with BU/TT/CY/ATG preceded by a pre-conditioning phase with FLU/HU/azathioprine. Post-transplant immunosuppression consisted of CSA and methylprednisolone until day +60. With a median follow-up of 3.9 years, the OS and 5-year TFS were 84% and 69%. Grade II-IV aGvHD occurred in 28% of cases.[76] The results obtained with TCRαβ+/CD19+ depletion compared favorably with a historical group of 40 patients with hemoglobinopathies who received CD34+-selected grafts, in particular because of a significantly lower incidence of GF (14% in TCRαβ+/CD19+ TCD vs 45% with CD34+ selection, $P = .048$). Despite that, the incidence of GF in TM receiving a TCRαβ+/CD19+ TCD haplo-HSCT remains relatively high, as documented in a large cohort of patients with nonmalignant disorders.[77] In this regard, interferon-γ neutralization may represent a promising strategy to improve engraftment in patients at high risk of GF receiving TCD haplo-HSCT.[78,79] Since the recovery of adaptive immunity is suboptimal even with this refined method of T-cell depletion, the incidence of viral infections and reactivation still represent a relevant drawback.[77] To further improve immunological reconstitution, our group has investigated the adoptive post-transplant infusion of titrated numbers of donor T lymphocytes transduced with the inducible Caspase 9 suicide gene.[73] Among 24 patients with the erythroid disorder who were treated with this approach after a TCRαβ+/CD19+ cell depleted haplo-HSCT (20 with TM, 3 with Diamond-Blackfan Anemia, and one with SCD), the reported EFS probability was 82.6% (counting GF as an event), whereas, as 2 of the 3 subjects experiencing GF were successfully re-transplanted, the TFS was 95.7%.[80]

An alternative platform for haplo-HSCT is based on the use of T-cell repleted grafts followed by post-transplant cyclophosphamide (PT-CY) administration. The use of un-manipulated grafts from haploidentical donors and induction of tolerance with PT-CY was initially evaluated in hematologic malignancies, whereas early studies in patients with hemoglobinopathies were limited by high rates of acute and chronic GvHD of 58% and 18%, respectively.[81] In a study of 14 patients with SCD who received post-CY haplo-HSCT after an RIC regimen, a high rate of transplant failure (43%) was reported.[82] In the setting of TM, Anurathapan and colleagues[41] achieved promising results by intensive pre-conditioning immunoablation followed by a myeloablative preparative regimen and unmanipulated PBSC haplo-HSCT with PT-CY administration and multidrug pharmacological GvHD prophylaxis. In the first report, involving 31 Patients with TM, OS and TFS were estimated to be 95% and 94%, respectively. More recently, the same group refined the preconditioning strategy and reported the outcome of 83 children and young adults with TM, obtaining a predicted 3-year OS and EFS of more than 96%; although no GF was reported in the cohort who received intensified pre-conditioning, the incidence of both acute and chronic GvHD remained relatively high.[41] Another strategy, developed by a Chinese group, is based on a preparative regimen combining FLU, BU, CY, and ATG followed by unmanipulated haplo-HSCT and post-transplant GvHD prophylaxis with CSA and short-course MTX. Among the 8 TM children treated with this approach, all achieved stable donor engraftment.[83]

Life after Thalassemia

Mixed chimerism

The condition of mixed chimerism (MC), characterized by the co-existence of residual host cells and donor cells in the post-transplant period, can be observed in up to 35% to 45% of patients transplanted for hemoglobinopathies.[84,85] Evolution of MC over time in TM may be variable. A significant proportion of patients evolve toward complete donor chimerism or develop a stable status, defined as persistent MC, in which donor- and host-derived cells coexist for long time after HSCT. Intriguingly, even patients with persistent low-level MC show normal hemoglobin values, without requiring any transfusion support, and absence of iron accumulation or clinically relevant erythroid hyperplasia.[86,87] It has been suggested that as low as 10% donor chimerism may be sufficient to achieve a long-term cure.[88,89] However, the development of MC is a well-known risk factor for graft rejection, especially if it occurs in the early posttransplant period. Several studies have investigated the trajectory of MC over time and the relationship between MC and graft rejection. An analysis conducted on a long-term follow-up of 295 transplanted patients with TM showed that MC evolves in most cases toward complete donor chimerism or into a stable MC state.[87] In the same study, graft rejection did not occur in any of the 200 individuals with full donor engraftment at 2 months, whereas 33 of the 95 patients (35 percent) with MC at the same interval eventually lost the graft. In addition, the authors reported a correlation between the percentage of residual host cells and graft loss, with rejection occurring in 18 of 19 (97%) who had >25% host cells versus only 4 of 55 (7%) who had <10% host cells. These results were confirmed by other studies that showed, although with different cut-offs, a greater likelihood of graft rejection in patients with earlier or high-level percentages of recipient-derived cells.[43,85] Significant effort has been made in understanding the immunological profile of patients experiencing MC, to identify biomarkers capable of predicting evolution. In this regard, it has been shown that the frequency T regulatory type 1 (Tr1) cells, characterized by the co-expression of CD49b and LAG-3 and by their ability to secrete IL-10, correlates with presence and maintenance of persistent MC in beta-thalassemia patients after HSCT.[24]

Long-term complications

Thanks to the improvement in the outcome of HSCT from both HLA-identical siblings and alternative donors, the number of Patients with TM who achieve a definitive cure is increasing each year. Successful allo-HSCT not only allows to achieve of transfusion independence and resolves ineffective erythropoiesis but also results in long-term quality of life similar to that of the general population.[90,91] However, since allo-HSCT carries a limited but not absent risk of morbidity and mortality and TM is nowadays a disease in which prolonged, even undefined, survival can be achieved with conventional medical therapy, data on long-term real-life complications are essential to properly estimate the risk-benefit ratio of transplantation.[92] In recent years, the importance of late effects after HSCT is increasingly being recognized and a number of studies reported on these much-needed data.[93,94] As expected, late complications are more frequently observed in patients with pretransplant organ function impairment and older age at transplant.[93] Impaired fertility and gonadal function are the most frequent complication encountered in transplanted patients with TM across different studies.[92–94] Azoospermia and secondary amenorrhea are reported in more than 50% of male and female subject, respectively.[93,94] Interestingly, although hypogonadism is observed in an even larger proportion of patients, a significant number of pregnancies have been documented in transplanted females or in partners of transplanted males in recent studies.[94] Despite that, strategies to preserve fertility before transplantation are highly encouraged. Thyroid dysfunction is the other major endocrine complication in transplanted TM subjects, being reported in 10% to 20% of cases. Other endocrinological abnormalities include growth retardation, obesity, diabetes mellitus, and bone health impairment.[93,94] Additional complications, such as heart, lung, or kidney dysfunction, are reported less frequently, mainly in a patient with preexisting organ damage.[92–94] A point of strength and, at the same time, of the weakness of all the studies on transplant-related late effects for TM is that they all involve patients transplanted after BU-based conditioning regimens, mainly reflecting the results of transplants performed more than 20 years ago. Today, less toxic preparative regimens have been developed, but longer follow-up is required to evaluate their impact on the occurrence of late complications and on fertility.

Nonetheless, this evidence underscores the importance of careful and dedicated posttransplant monitoring for this expanding population of long-term thalassemia-free survivors to ensure that late effects and complications can be prevented, whenever possible, or promptly recognized and treated. In this regard, complications related to iron overload can be effectively avoided after HSCT with appropriate iron reduction therapy, which may be performed by either regular phlebotomies or by temporary re-introducing iron chelation therapy. Duration of treatment is closely related to the magnitude of iron overload, and it ranges from a few months to several years.

CONCLUSIONS AND FUTURE PERSPECTIVES

In the era of disease-modifying agents and gene therapy/genome-editing approaches, allo-HSCT continues to represent the most consolidated, potentially curative therapy for TM. With modern transplant protocols and improvements in patient preparation and selection, TFS rates around or even exceeding 90% are routinely reported after MSD-HSCT.[15,45] For this reason, in subjects who have an available MSD, allo-HSCT should be offered at a young age, before the development of significant iron overload and disease-specific complications (see **Fig. 1**) For those lacking an MSD, transplantation from a MUD offers nowadays OS and TFS rates comparable to those obtained using MSD, although at the price of a higher incidence of acute and chronic GvHD.[32,51]

Despite that, in the presence of a suitable donor, fully matched at a high-resolution level, MUD-HSCT can represent a valid alternative, especially for young patients with heavy transfusion requirements and/or poor tolerance or compliance to iron chelators (see **Fig. 1**). For the same category of subjects, the use of HLA-haploidentical donors might overcome the barrier of limited availability of matched-donors by expanding the donor pool with parents or mismatched siblings. Although promising data have been recently reported with refined approaches of haplo-HSCT, this type of transplant should be performed in qualified centers with specific experience.[41,77] Since in high-income countries, the prognosis of TM is currently "open-ended", particular attention should be paid to avoid the occurrence of cGvHD, which does not determine any favorable graft-versus-leukemia effect, but, on the contrary, may eventually transform one chronic disease into another one, potentially even worse, and also contribute to the occurrence of post-transplantation malignancies. As investigational methods for performing allo-HSCT from alternative donors or in less-fit patients evolve, the indications may broaden, especially for adolescents and young adults. In western countries, the use of donors other than matched siblings is going to be challenged by the emergence of gene therapy and genome-editing approaches based on transplantation of gene-modified autologous HSCs, which eliminate the need for an allogeneic donor, abrogate the risk of GVHD, and expand the applicability of highly-effective curative options also beyond pediatric age.[11,12] However, widespread adoption of these approaches is still hindered by affordability problems and, so far, the only licensed gene-therapy product for transfusion-dependent Thalassemia is available only in the United States.[95] In developing countries, where access to innovative therapies, unfortunately, remains prohibitive, the risk benefit-ratio of allo-HSCT may be different from high-income countries, as challenges in providing safe transfusions, ensuring regular chelation therapy and adequate monitoring significantly affect the effectiveness of conservative treatments.[2,10] Studies from Asia have clearly shown that, nowadays, highly effective allo-HCST is widely available worldwide and not anymore the exclusive prerogative of western countries.[32,37,96]

As several studies showed that transplantation is cost-effective in comparison to life-long supportive therapy[10,97,98] it is not surprising that allo-HSCT is increasingly used in countries with limited resources to cure a growing number of individuals (not necessarily children). As the number of long-term thalassemia-free-survivors increases each year with a worldwide distribution, real-life data on long-term survival and complications of transplanted patients are highly warranted to properly compare the burden of allo-HSCT with respect to that of chronic transfusions and iron-chelation. These aspects are crucial to provide the most comprehensive counseling to patients and families. Indeed, although allo-HSCT has been used for more than 40 years to cure thousands of patients with TM, no definitive indication exists and, with the exception of general recommendations, the definitive decision to proceed with transplantation or continue on conservative management will likely remain personal and highly individualized.

CLINICS CARE POINTS

- In subjects who have an available MSD, allo-HSCT should be offered at a young age, before the development of significant iron overload and disease-specific complications.

- When a suitable donor unrelated donor, fully matched at a high-resolution level, is available, allo-HSCT can represent a valid potentially curative option, especially for young patients with heavy transfusion requirements and/or poor tolerance or compliance to iron chelators.

- Haplo-HSCT is a feasible alternative for patients with TM lacking a fully-matched donor, but it carries a higher risk of GF and GvHD and, therefore, should be performed in selected cases and in qualified, high-volume centers.
- As investigational methods for performing allo-HSCT from alternative donors or in less-fit patients evolve, the indications may broaden although, at least in western countries, the use of donors other than matched siblings will likely be challenged by gene-therapy/genome-editing approaches.
- Despite the wide availability of highly-effective curative options, no definitive indication exists and the decision to proceed with allo-HSCT in TM will remain personal and highly individualized.
- Careful and dedicated posttransplant monitoring for thalassemia-free survivors is crucial to ensure that late effects and complications can be prevented, when possible, or promptly recognized and treated.

DISCLOSURES

F. Locatelli: Amgen Speakers' Bureau and advisory board membership, Novartis Speakers' Bureau and advisory board membership, Bellicum Pharmaceuticals advisory board membership, Miltenyi Speakers' Bureau, Jazz Pharmaceutical Speakers' Bureau, Takeda Speakers' Bureau, Neovii advisory board membership, and Medac Speakers' Bureau outside the submitted work. M. Algeri: Vertex Pharmaceuticals advisory board and steering committee membership, outside the submitted work.

REFERENCES

1. Borgna-Pignatti C, Cappellini MD, De Stefano P, et al. Survival and complications in thalassemia. Ann N Y Acad Sci 2005;1054:40–7.
2. Kattamis A, Kwiatkowski JL, Aydinok Y. Thalassaemia. Lancet Lond Engl 2022; 399(10343):2310–24.
3. Taher AT, Musallam KM, Cappellini MD. β-Thalassemias. N Engl J Med 2021; 384(8):727–43.
4. Arian M, Mirmohammadkhani M, Ghorbani R, et al. Health-related quality of life (HRQoL) in beta-thalassemia major (β-TM) patients assessed by 36-item short form health survey (SF-36): a meta-analysis. Qual Life Res Int J Qual Life Asp Treat Care Rehabil 2019;28(2):321–34.
5. Sobota A, Yamashita R, Xu Y, et al. Quality of life in thalassemia: a comparison of SF-36 results from the thalassemia longitudinal cohort to reported literature and the US norms. Am J Hematol 2011;86(1):92–5.
6. Lal A. Challenges in chronic transfusion for patients with thalassemia. Hematol Am Soc Hematol Educ Program 2020;2020(1):160–6.
7. Taher AT, Cappellini MD. How I manage medical complications of β-thalassemia in adults. Blood 2018;132(17):1781–91.
8. Borgna-Pignatti C, Rugolotto S, De Stefano P, et al. Survival and complications in patients with thalassemia major treated with transfusion and deferoxamine. Haematologica 2004;89(10):1187–93.
9. Cappellini MD, Viprakasit V, Taher AT, et al. A Phase 3 Trial of Luspatercept in Patients with Transfusion-Dependent β-Thalassemia. N Engl J Med 2020;382(13): 1219–31.
10. Weatherall DJ. The inherited diseases of hemoglobin are an emerging global health burden. Blood 2010;115(22):4331–6.

11. Locatelli F, Thompson AA, Kwiatkowski JL, et al. Betibeglogene Autotemcel Gene Therapy for Non-β0/β0 Genotype β-Thalassemia. N Engl J Med 2022;386(5): 415–27.

12. Frangoul H, Altshuler D, Cappellini MD, et al. CRISPR-Cas9 Gene Editing for Sickle Cell Disease and β-Thalassemia. N Engl J Med 2021;384(3):252–60.

13. Locatelli F, Frangoul H, Corbacioglu S, et al. EFFICACY AND SAFETY OF A SINGLE DOSE OF CTX001 FOR TRANSFUSION-DEPENDENT BETA-THALASSEMIA AND SEVERE SICKLE CELL DISEASE. EHA Library. Available at: https://library.ehaweb.org/eha/2022/eha2022-congress/366210/franco.locatelli.efficacy.and.safety.of.a.single.dose.of.ctx001.for.html?f=listing%3D0%2Abrowseby%3D8%2Asortby%3D2%2Aspeaker%3D202682.

14. Baronciani D, Angelucci E, Potschger U, et al. Hemopoietic stem cell transplantation in thalassemia: a report from the European Society for Blood and Bone Marrow Transplantation Hemoglobinopathy Registry, 2000-2010. Bone Marrow Transplant 2016;51(4):536–41.

15. Li C, Mathews V, Kim S, et al. Related and unrelated donor transplantation for β-thalassemia major: results of an international survey. Blood Adv 2019;3(17): 2562–70.

16. Lucarelli G, Galimberti M, Polchi P, et al. Bone marrow transplantation in patients with thalassemia. N Engl J Med 1990;322(7):417–21.

17. Giardini C, Lucarelli G. Bone marrow transplantation for beta-thalassemia. Hematol Oncol Clin North Am 1999;13(5):1059–64, viii.

18. Lucarelli G, Galimberti M, Giardini C, et al. Bone marrow transplantation in thalassemia. The experience of Pesaro. Ann N Y Acad Sci 1998;850:270–5.

19. Lucarelli G, Clift RA, Galimberti M, et al. Bone marrow transplantation in adult thalassemic patients. Blood 1999;93(4):1164–7.

20. Angelucci E, Pilo F, Coates TD. Transplantation in thalassemia: Revisiting the Pesaro risk factors 25 years later. Am J Hematol 2017;92(5):411–3.

21. Hongeng S, Pakakasama S, Chuansumrit A, et al. Outcomes of transplantation with related- and unrelated-donor stem cells in children with severe thalassemia. Biol Blood Marrow Transplant J Am Soc Blood Marrow Transplant 2006;12(6): 683–7.

22. Fang J-P, Xu L-H. Hematopoietic stem cell transplantation for children with thalassemia major in China. Pediatr Blood Cancer 2010;55(6):1062–5.

23. Mathews V, George B, Deotare U, et al. A new stratification strategy that identifies a subset of class III patients with an adverse prognosis among children with beta thalassemia major undergoing a matched related allogeneic stem cell transplantation. Biol Blood Marrow Transplant J Am Soc Blood Marrow Transplant 2007; 13(8):889–94.

24. Andreani M, Testi M, Lucarelli G. Mixed chimerism in haemoglobinopathies: from risk of graft rejection to immune tolerance. Tissue Antigens 2014;83(3):137–46.

25. Angelucci E, Baronciani D. Allogeneic stem cell transplantation for thalassemia major. Haematologica 2008;93(12):1780–4.

26. Thompson AA, Cunningham MJ, Singer ST, et al. Red cell alloimmunization in a diverse population of transfused patients with thalassaemia. Br J Haematol 2011;153(1):121–8.

27. Centis F, Tabellini L, Lucarelli G, et al. The importance of erythroid expansion in determining the extent of apoptosis in erythroid precursors in patients with beta-thalassemia major. Blood 2000;96(10):3624–9.

28. Isidori A, Loscocco F, Visani G, et al. Iron Toxicity and Chelation Therapy in Hematopoietic Stem Cell Transplant. Transplant Cell Ther 2021;27(5):371–9.

29. Mathews V, Savani BN. Conditioning regimens in allo-SCT for thalassemia major. Bone Marrow Transplant 2014;49(5):607–10.
30. Lucarelli G, Clift RA, Galimberti M, et al. Marrow transplantation for patients with thalassemia: results in class 3 patients. Blood 1996;87(5):2082–8.
31. Bernardo ME, Piras E, Vacca A, et al. Allogeneic hematopoietic stem cell transplantation in thalassemia major: results of a reduced-toxicity conditioning regimen based on the use of treosulfan. Blood 2012;120(2):473–6.
32. Li C, Wu X, Feng X, et al. A novel conditioning regimen improves outcomes in β-thalassemia major patients using unrelated donor peripheral blood stem cell transplantation. Blood 2012;120(19):3875–81.
33. Bertaina A, Bernardo ME, Mastronuzzi A, et al. The role of reduced intensity preparative regimens in patients with thalassemia given hematopoietic transplantation. Ann N Y Acad Sci 2010;1202:141–8.
34. Danylesko I, Shimoni A, Nagler A. Treosulfan-based conditioning before hematopoietic SCT: more than a BU look-alike. Bone Marrow Transplant 2012;47(1):5–14.
35. Hilger RA, Harstrick A, Eberhardt W, et al. Clinical pharmacokinetics of intravenous treosulfan in patients with advanced solid tumors. Cancer Chemother Pharmacol 1998;42(2):99–104.
36. Główka FK, Karaźniewicz-Łada M, Grund G, et al. Pharmacokinetics of high-dose i.v. treosulfan in children undergoing treosulfan-based preparative regimen for allogeneic haematopoietic SCT. Bone Marrow Transplant 2008;42(Suppl 2): S67–70.
37. Mathews V, George B, Viswabandya A, et al. Improved clinical outcomes of high risk β thalassemia major patients undergoing a HLA matched related allogeneic stem cell transplant with a treosulfan based conditioning regimen and peripheral blood stem cell grafts. PLoS One 2013;8(4):e61637.
38. Lüftinger R, Zubarovskaya N, Galimard J-E, et al. Busulfan-fludarabine- or treosulfan-fludarabine-based myeloablative conditioning for children with thalassemia major. Ann Hematol 2022;101(3):655–65.
39. Shenoy S, Walters MC, Ngwube A, et al. Unrelated Donor Transplantation in Children with Thalassemia using Reduced-Intensity Conditioning: The URTH Trial. Biol Blood Marrow Transplant J Am Soc Blood Marrow Transplant 2018;24(6): 1216–22.
40. Gaziev J, Marziali M, Isgrò A, et al. Bone marrow transplantation for thalassemia from alternative related donors: improved outcomes with a new approach. Blood 2013;122(15):2751–6.
41. Anurathapan U, Hongeng S, Pakakasama S, et al. Hematopoietic Stem Cell Transplantation for Severe Thalassemia Patients from Haploidentical Donors Using a Novel Conditioning Regimen. Biol Blood Marrow Transplant J Am Soc Blood Marrow Transplant 2020;26(6):1106–12.
42. Anurathapan U, Pakakasama S, Mekjaruskul P, et al. Outcomes of thalassemia patients undergoing hematopoietic stem cell transplantation by using a standard myeloablative versus a novel reduced-toxicity conditioning regimen according to a new risk stratification. Biol Blood Marrow Transplant J Am Soc Blood Marrow Transplant 2014;20(12):2066–71.
43. Lucarelli G, Gaziev J. Advances in the allogeneic transplantation for thalassemia. Blood Rev 2008;22(2):53–63.
44. Isgrò A, Gaziev J, Sodani P, et al. Progress in hematopoietic stem cell transplantation as allogeneic cellular gene therapy in thalassemia. Ann N Y Acad Sci 2010; 1202:149–54.

45. Locatelli F, Kabbara N, Ruggeri A, et al. Outcome of patients with hemoglobinopathies given either cord blood or bone marrow transplantation from an HLA-identical sibling. Blood 2013;122(6):1072-8.
46. Locatelli F, Rocha V, Reed W, et al. Related umbilical cord blood transplantation in patients with thalassemia and sickle cell disease. Blood 2003;101(6):2137-43.
47. Tucunduva L, Volt F, Cunha R, et al. Combined cord blood and bone marrow transplantation from the same human leucocyte antigen-identical sibling donor for children with malignant and non-malignant diseases. Br J Haematol 2015; 169(1):103-10.
48. Iravani M, Tavakoli E, Babaie MH, et al. Comparison of peripheral blood stem cell transplant with bone marrow transplant in class 3 thalassemic patients. Exp Clin Transplant Off J Middle East Soc Organ Transplant 2010;8(1):66-73.
49. Ghavamzadeh A, Iravani M, Ashouri A, et al. Peripheral blood versus bone marrow as a source of hematopoietic stem cells for allogeneic transplantation in children with class I and II beta thalassemia major. Biol Blood Marrow Transplant J Am Soc Blood Marrow Transplant 2008;14(3):301-8.
50. Irfan M, Hashmi K, Adil S, et al. Beta-thalassaemia major: bone marrow versus peripheral blood stem cell transplantation. JPMA J Pak Med Assoc 2008;58(3): 107-10.
51. Baronciani D, Pilo F, Lyon-Caen S, et al. Hematopoietic Stem Cell Transplantation in Thalassemia Major. Report from the EBMT Hemoglobinopathy Registry. Blood 2011;118(21):905.
52. He Y, Jiang H, Li C, et al. Long-term results of the NF-08-TM protocol in stem cell transplant for patients with thalassemia major: A multi-center large-sample study. Am J Hematol 2020;95(11):E297-9.
53. Rocha V, Locatelli F. Searching for alternative hematopoietic stem cell donors for pediatric patients. Bone Marrow Transplant 2008;41(2):207-14.
54. Gragert L, Eapen M, Williams E, et al. HLA match likelihoods for hematopoietic stem-cell grafts in the U.S. registry. N Engl J Med 2014;371(4):339-48.
55. La Nasa G, Giardini C, Argiolu F, et al. Unrelated donor bone marrow transplantation for thalassemia: the effect of extended haplotypes. Blood 2002;99(12): 4350-6.
56. La Nasa G, Caocci G, Argiolu F, et al. Unrelated donor stem cell transplantation in adult patients with thalassemia. Bone Marrow Transplant 2005;36(11):971-5.
57. Sun L, Wang N, Chen Y, et al. Unrelated Donor Peripheral Blood Stem Cell Transplantation for Patients with β-Thalassemia Major Based on a Novel Conditioning Regimen. Biol Blood Marrow Transplant J Am Soc Blood Marrow Transplant 2019;25(8):1592-6.
58. Locatelli F, Littera R, Pagliara D, et al. Outcome of unrelated donor bone marrow transplantation for thalassemia major patients. Blood 2011;118(21):149.
59. La Nasa G, Littera R, Locatelli F, et al. Status of donor-recipient HLA class I ligands and not the KIR genotype is predictive for the outcome of unrelated hematopoietic stem cell transplantation in beta-thalassemia patients. Biol Blood Marrow Transplant J Am Soc Blood Marrow Transplant 2007;13(11):1358-68.
60. La Nasa G, Littera R, Locatelli F, et al. The human leucocyte antigen-G 14-base-pair polymorphism correlates with graft-versus-host disease in unrelated bone marrow transplantation for thalassaemia. Br J Haematol 2007;139(2):284-8.
61. Littera R, Orrù N, Vacca A, et al. The role of killer immunoglobulin-like receptor haplotypes on the outcome of unrelated donor haematopoietic SCT for thalassaemia. Bone Marrow Transplant 2010;45(11):1618-24.

62. Fleischhauer K, Locatelli F, Zecca M, et al. Graft rejection after unrelated donor hematopoietic stem cell transplantation for thalassemia is associated with nonpermissive HLA-DPB1 disparity in host-versus-graft direction. Blood 2006; 107(7):2984–92.

63. Ruggeri A, Eapen M, Scaravadou A, et al. Umbilical cord blood transplantation for children with thalassemia and sickle cell disease. Biol Blood Marrow Transplant J Am Soc Blood Marrow Transplant 2011;17(9):1375–82.

64. Jaing T-H, Hung I-J, Yang C-P, et al. Unrelated cord blood transplantation for thalassaemia: a single-institution experience of 35 patients. Bone Marrow Transplant 2012;47(1):33–9.

65. Gluckman E. Milestones in umbilical cord blood transplantation. Blood Rev 2011; 25(6):255–9.

66. Shah SA, Shah KM, Patel KA, et al. Unrelated Umbilical Cord Blood Transplant for Children with β-Thalassemia Major. Indian J Hematol Blood Transfus 2015; 31(1):9–13.

67. Eapen M, Wang T, Veys PA, et al. Allele-level HLA matching for umbilical cord blood transplantation for non-malignant diseases in children: a retrospective analysis. Lancet Haematol 2017;4(7):e325–33.

68. Sodani P, Isgrò A, Gaziev J, et al. Purified T-depleted, CD34+ peripheral blood and bone marrow cell transplantation from haploidentical mother to child with thalassemia. Blood 2010;115(6):1296–302.

69. Yee MEM, Shah A, Anderson AR, et al. Class I and II HLA antibodies in pediatric patients with thalassemia major. Transfusion (Paris) 2016;56(4):878–84.

70. Ciurea SO, Al Malki MM, Kongtim P, et al. The European Society for Blood and Marrow Transplantation (EBMT) consensus recommendations for donor selection in haploidentical hematopoietic cell transplantation. Bone Marrow Transplant 2020;55(1):12–24.

71. Handgretinger R. New approaches to graft engineering for haploidentical bone marrow transplantation. Semin Oncol 2012;39(6):664–73.

72. Schumm M, Lang P, Bethge W, et al. Depletion of T-cell receptor alpha/beta and CD19 positive cells from apheresis products with the CliniMACS device. Cytotherapy 2013;15(10):1253–8.

73. Bertaina A, Lucarelli B, Merli P, et al. Clinical Outcome after Adoptive Infusion of BPX-501 Cells (donor T cells transduced with iC9 suicide gene) in Children with Thalassemia Major (TM) Given Alfa/Beta T-Cell Depleted HLA-Haploidentical Stem Cell Transplantation (HSCT). Biol Blood Marrow Transplant 2016;22(3, Supplement):S306.

74. Farnault L, Gertner-Dardenne J, Gondois-Rey F, et al. Clinical evidence implicating gamma-delta T cells in EBV control following cord blood transplantation. Bone Marrow Transplant 2013;48(11):1478–9.

75. Airoldi I, Bertaina A, Prigione I, et al. γδ T-cell reconstitution after HLA-haploidentical hematopoietic transplantation depleted of TCR-αβ+/CD19+ lymphocytes. Blood 2015;125(15):2349–58.

76. Gaziev J, Isgrò A, Sodani P, et al. Haploidentical HSCT for hemoglobinopathies: improved outcomes with TCRαβ+/CD19+-depleted grafts. Blood Adv 2018;2(3): 263–70.

77. Merli P, Pagliara D, Galaverna F, et al. TCRαβ/CD19 depleted HSCT from an HLA-haploidentical relative to treat children with different nonmalignant disorders. Blood Adv 2022;6(1):281–92.

78. Merli P, Caruana I, De Vito R, et al. Role of interferon-γ in immune-mediated graft failure after allogeneic hematopoietic stem cell transplantation. Haematologica 2019;104(11):2314–23.

79. Sabulski A, Myers KC, Bleesing JJ, et al. Graft rejection markers in children undergoing hematopoietic cell transplant for bone marrow failure. Blood Adv 2021; 5(22):4594–604.

80. Galaverna F, Li Pira G, Algeri M, et al. Alpha/beta T-cell depleted Haploidentical HSCT followed by infusion of donor lymphocytes transduced with inducible caspase9 gene is safe and effective for patients with erythroid disorders. Abstract 0039. The 44th Annual Meeting of the European Society for Blood and Marrow Transplantation: Physicians Oral Session. Bone Marrow Transplant 2019; 53(Suppl 1):19.

81. Luznik L, Fuchs EJ. High-dose, posttransplantation cyclophosphamide to promote graft-host tolerance after allogeneic hematopoietic stem cell transplantation. Immunol Res 2010;47(1–3):65–77.

82. Bolaños-Meade J, Fuchs EJ, Luznik L, et al. HLA-haploidentical bone marrow transplantation with posttransplant cyclophosphamide expands the donor pool for patients with sickle cell disease. Blood 2012;120(22):4285–91.

83. Sun Q, Wu B, Lan H, et al. Haploidentical haematopoietic stem cell transplantation for thalassaemia major based on an FBCA conditioning regimen. Br J Haematol 2018;182(4):554–8.

84. Andreani M, Gregori S. The study of engraftment after hematopoietic stem cell transplantation: From the presence of mixed chimerism to the development of immunological tolerance. HLA 2018;92(Suppl 2):57–9.

85. Fouzia NA, Edison ES, Lakshmi KM, et al. Long-term outcome of mixed chimerism after stem cell transplantation for thalassemia major conditioned with busulfan and cyclophosphamide. Bone Marrow Transplant 2018;53(2):169–74.

86. Andreani M, Manna M, Lucarelli G, et al. Persistence of mixed chimerism in patients transplanted for the treatment of thalassemia. Blood 1996;87(8):3494–9.

87. Andreani M, Nesci S, Lucarelli G, et al. Long-term survival of ex-thalassemic patients with persistent mixed chimerism after bone marrow transplantation. Bone Marrow Transplant 2000;25(4):401–4.

88. Andreani M, Testi M, Gaziev J, et al. Quantitatively different red cell/nucleated cell chimerism in patients with long-term, persistent hematopoietic mixed chimerism after bone marrow transplantation for thalassemia major or sickle cell disease. Haematologica 2011;96(1):128–33.

89. Alfred A, Vora AJ. What is the minimum level of donor chimerism necessary to sustain transfusion independence in thalassaemia? Bone Marrow Transplant 2011;46(5):769–70.

90. Caocci G, Orofino MG, Vacca A, et al. Long-term survival of beta thalassemia major patients treated with hematopoietic stem cell transplantation compared with survival with conventional treatment. Am J Hematol 2017;92(12):1303–10.

91. La Nasa G, Caocci G, Efficace F, et al. Long-term health-related quality of life evaluated more than 20 years after hematopoietic stem cell transplantation for thalassemia. Blood 2013;122(13):2262–70.

92. Shenoy S, Gaziev J, Angelucci E, et al. Late Effects Screening Guidelines after Hematopoietic Cell Transplantation (HCT) for Hemoglobinopathy: Consensus Statement from the Second Pediatric Blood and Marrow Transplant Consortium International Conference on Late Effects after Pediatric HCT. Biol Blood Marrow Transplant J Am Soc Blood Marrow Transplant 2018;24(7):1313–21.

93. Chaudhury S, Ayas M, Rosen C, et al. A Multicenter Retrospective Analysis Stressing the Importance of Long-Term Follow-Up after Hematopoietic Cell Transplantation for β-Thalassemia. Biol Blood Marrow Transplant J Am Soc Blood Marrow Transplant 2017;23(10):1695–700.
94. Rahal I, Galambrun C, Bertrand Y, et al. Late effects after hematopoietic stem cell transplantation for β-thalassemia major: the French national experience. Haematologica 2018;103(7):1143–9.
95. Thuret I, Ruggeri A, Angelucci E, et al. Hurdles to the Adoption of Gene Therapy as a Curative Option for Transfusion-Dependent Thalassemia. Stem Cells Transl Med 2022;11(4):407–14.
96. Mathews V, Srivastava A, Chandy M. Allogeneic stem cell transplantation for thalassemia major. Hematol Oncol Clin North Am 2014;28(6):1187–200.
97. Scalone L, Mantovani LG, Krol M, et al. Costs, quality of life, treatment satisfaction and compliance in patients with beta-thalassemia major undergoing iron chelation therapy: the ITHACA study. Curr Med Res Opin 2008;24(7):1905–17.
98. John MJ, Jyani G, Jindal A, et al. Cost Effectiveness of Hematopoietic Stem Cell Transplantation Compared with Transfusion Chelation for Treatment of Thalassemia Major. Biol Blood Marrow Transplant J Am Soc Blood Marrow Transplant 2018;24(10):2119–26.

Gene Therapy and Gene Editing for β-Thalassemia

Georgios E. Christakopoulos, MD[a], Rahul Telange, MS[b], Jonathan Yen, PhD[b], Mitchell J. Weiss, MD, PhD[b],*

KEYWORDS

- β-thalassemia • Gene editing • Gene therapy

KEY POINTS

- β-thalassemia is a common, frequently devastating hemoglobinopathy caused by *HBB* gene mutations that reduce or eliminate β-globin synthesis.
- Allogenic hematopoietic stem cell transplantation (HSCT) can cure transfusion-dependent β-thalassemia (TDT) but has several major problems, including a lack of human leukocyte antigen (HLA)-matched donors for most patients and immune complications.
- Genetic manipulation of patient hematopoietic stem cells (HSCs) to restore β-globin gene expression or induce fetal hemoglobin expression can potentially cure β-thalassemia while circumventing some problems associated with allogeneic HSCT.
- Methods for therapeutic manipulation of HSCs include lentiviral vectors, genome-editing nucleases, and base editors.
- Technical complexity and high costs associated with gene therapies threaten to restrict their commercialization and availability.

INTRODUCTION

β-thalassemia is one of the world's most common genetic anemias, affecting millions of individuals worldwide (Chapter 2).[1,2] The disease is caused by more than 300 different mutations in the *β*-globin gene (*HBB*), all of which cause quantitative deficiencies of β-globin protein and adult-type hemoglobin (HbA, α2β2) (Chapters 3, 4). Concomitantly, the accumulation of free α-globin forms toxic intracellular inclusions resulting in hemolysis and ineffective erythropoiesis (IE) (Chapters 8, 9). The clinical consequences are anemia, bone disease, extramedullary IE resulting organomegaly and soft tissue masses, and iron overload (Chapter 10). Medical theraies include red blood cell (RBC) transfusions and iron chelation, both of which cause major toxicities (Chapters 10-12).

[a] Department of Oncology, St. Jude Children's Research Hospital, 262 Danny Thomas Place, MS #355, Memphis, TN 38105, USA; [b] Department of Hematology, St. Jude Children's Research Hospital, 262 Danny Thomas Place, MS #355, Memphis, TN 38105, USA
* Corresponding author.
E-mail address: mitch.weiss@stjude.org

Hematol Oncol Clin N Am 37 (2023) 433–447
https://doi.org/10.1016/j.hoc.2022.12.012
0889-8588/23/© 2022 Elsevier Inc. All rights reserved.

Allogeneic hematopoietic stem cell transplantation (HSCT) is an effective cure for β-thalassemia, although not all patients have ideal donors and the procedure is associated with serious immune complications including, graft versus host disease, and graft rejection (Chapter 14).[3] These problems may be circumvented by experimental therapies in which autologous hematopoietic stem cells (HSCs) are isolated, genetically altered *ex vivo*, and reintroduced into the patient after the administration of myelotoxic bone marrow conditioning to facilitate engraftment of modified cells. Current methods for genetic modification, referred to collectively here as "gene therapy", include lentiviral transduction, genome editing, and base editing, aim to either restore normal levels of β-globin or to reactivate the production of fetal γ-globin, which binds α-globin to form fetal hemoglobin (HbF, α2γ2), which can replace HbA. Here we provide a succinct review of ongoing preclinical and clinical studies, problems, and future directions related to gene therapy for transfusion-dependent β-thalassemia (TDT). Most aspects of the field have been summarized in recently published review articles and in other chapters in this volume. Owing to word limitations, we refer to these reviews and other chapters rather than citing all original research publications.

Gene Manipulation Strategies for β-Thalassemia

Fig. 1 shows the overall strategy for current autologous HSC gene therapy. Gene manipulation strategies for treating TDT are shown in **Fig. 2**; similar strategies are being used to treat sickle cell disease (SCD). The field is advancing rapidly as new and improved tools for autologous HSCT and HSC gene manipulation become available.[4]

β-Globin Replacement Therapy with Lentiviral Vectors

Lentiviral vectors (LVVs) mediate the semirandom integration of a therapeutic transgene and linked regulatory elements into the genomic DNA of dividing and nondividing cells, the latter feature being important for manipulating quiescent HSCs.[5,6] Compared to γ-retroviral vectors that were used in early autologous HSC gene therapy protocols, LVVs have less propensity to cause insertional activation of oncogenes and resultant malignant transformation. Historically, the development of LVVs capable

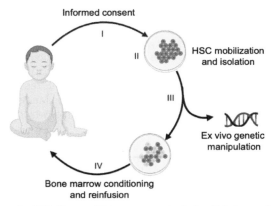

Fig. 1. Gene therapy for TDT. The multistep process includes (I) informed consent, including patient/family education and written consent; (II) mobilization, apheresis collection and enrichment of patient (autologous) HSCs; (III) ex vivo genetic manipulation of HSCs to restore erythroid expression of β-globin or induce HbF expression; and (IV) administration of bone marrow conditioning followed by infusion of the modified HSCs.

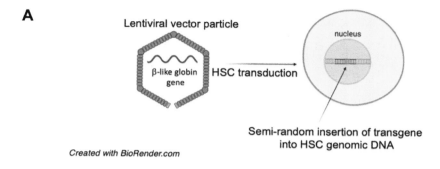

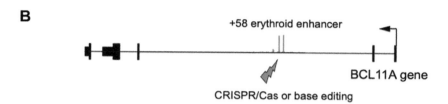

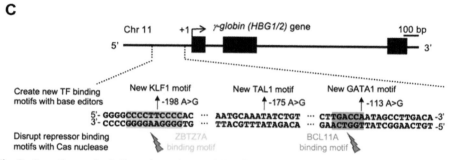

Fig. 2. Genetic manipulation of autologous HSCs for TDT gene therapy. (*A*) Patient HSCs are transduced with lentiviral vector (LVV) particles encoding a β-like globin gene. (*B*) Induction of fetal hemoglobin (HbF, α2γ2) by disrupting the +58 erythroid enhancer in intron 2 of the *BCL11A* gene by CRISPR/Cas genome-editing nuclease mediated non-homologous end joining (NHEJ) or base editing. (*C*) Induction of HbF by altering the γ-globin promoter. Bottom shows disruption of BCL11A or ZBTZ7A repressor binding motifs via genome-editing nuclease-mediated NHEJ to create insertion-deletion (indel) mutations. Top shows the installation of new binding motifs for one of several erythroid transcriptional activators with adenine base editors.

of driving sustained, high-level erythroid-specific expression of a β-like-globin transgene was a major challenge that was overcome by rational vector design and trial and error. Most current LVVs used to treat β-thalassemia and SCD include a β-like globin gene and promoter linked to a modified locus control region (LCR), a powerful enhancer in the β-like globin gene cluster. Another major challenge was to attain efficient transduction of HSCs with post-therapy vector copy numbers > 1 per diploid genome, which has been achieved by improved process development, including the use of transduction-enhancing reagents.[7,8] In November 2022, 10 clinical trials using LVV gene therapy to treat TDT were registered on clinicaltrials.gov/ (**Table 1**).

Table 1
Gene therapy and genome-editing clinical trials for transfusion-dependent β-thalassemia

Strategy	Modality	Sponsoring Agent	Clinical Trial ID Status	Estimated Participants	Results/Notes
β-Like globin gene replacement	Lentiviral vector (LVV) TNS9.3.55 LVV/β^A	Memorial Sloan Kettering Cancer Center (MSKCC)	NCT01639690 Phase I	10	4 participants followed for 90 months had stable engraftment. Transfusion requirements were reduced by 35–57% in 2 individuals. HSC transduction and LVV copy number were low.
	BB305 LVV/β^A-T87Q	bluebird bio	NCT01745120 Phase I, II	22	Reduced or eliminated RBC transfusions in 22 patients with TDT without LVV-related severe adverse events.
	BB305 LVV/β^A-T87Q	bluebird bio	NCT02151526 Phase I, II	7	4 patients followed for an approximately 4.5 years became transfusion independent with reductions in dyserythropoiesis and iron overload.
	OTL-300 GLOBE LVV/β^A	IRCCS San Raffaele & Orchard Therapeutics	NCT02453477 Phase I/II	10	Modified cell product administered into bone marrow. All three adults treated showed reduced transfusion requirements. Three of 4 evaluable pediatric patients became transfusion-independent.

	Sponsor	NCT / Phase	N	Results
BB305 LVV/β^A-T87Q	bluebird bio	NCT02906202 Northstar-2 Phase III	23	23 individuals treated, including children (4–34 years old). 91% became transfusion-independent with median follow-up of 29.5 months.
BB305 LVV/β^A-T87Q	bluebird bio	NCT03207009 Northstar-3 Phase III	18	No results reported
LVV/Undisclosed	Shenzhen Geno-Immune Medical Institute China	NCT03351829 Phase I/II	20	No results reported
LVV/β^A	Nanfang Hospital of Southern Medical University China	NCT03276455 Phase I/II	10	No results reported
LVV/βA-T87Q	BGI-research & Shenzhen Children's Hospital China	NCT04592458 Phase I	10	No results reported
LVV/β^A-T87Q	Shanghai BDgene Co., Ltd	NCT05015920 Phase I	10	No results reported
Nuclease/Target				
HbF Induction				
Cas9 disruption of *BCL11A* erythroid enhancer via NHEJ	CRISPR Therapeutics; Vertex Pharmaceuticals	NCT03655678 Phase I, II, III	45	42 of 44 pts stopped RBC transfusions; 2 pts had 75% and 89% reductions in RBC transfusions
BCL11A -Targeted zinc finger disruption of *BCL11A* erythroid enhancer via NHEJ (ST-400)	Sangamo Therapeutics and Sanofi	NCT03432364 Phase I, II	6	5 patients had a transient elevation of that was not sustained. No long-term therapeutic benefit due to low HSC transduction efficiency.
	Editas Medicine Inc.	NCT05444894 Phase I, II	6	No results reported

(continued on next page)

Table 1
(continued)

Strategy	Modality	Sponsoring Agent	Clinical Trial ID Status	Estimated Participants	Results/Notes
	Cpf1 NHEJ mediated disruption of BCL11A binding site (EDIT-301)				
	Cas9 disruption of *BCL11A* erythroid enhancer (ET01)	Edigene & Institute of Hematology & Blood Disease Hospital, Tianjin. China.	NCT04390971 Phase I	8	No results reported
	γ-Globin reactivation using Glycosylate Base Editors (exact mechanism not specified)	Bioray Laboratories. Shanghai, China	NCT05442346 Phase I/II	5	No results reported
	Cas9 disruption of *BCL11A* erythroid enhancer via NHEJ	Bioray Laboratories Shanghai China	NCT04211480 Phase I, II	12	2 children with TDT achieved transfusion independence with normal hemoglobin levels after f > 18 months follow-up

Abbreviations: CRISPR, Clustered regularly interspaced short palindromic repeats; HbF, fetal hemoglobin; HDR, homology-directed repair; HSC, hematopoietic stem cell; LVV, Lentiviral vector; NHEJ, non-homologous end joining; TDT, transfusion-dependent β-thalassemia.
Current clinical trials for TDT on ClinicalTrials.gov as of November 2022.

The most extensive study of LVV gene therapy for treating TDT uses the cellular drug product LentiGlobin (betibeglogene autotemcel), generated by transfecting patient $CD34^+$ hematopoietic stem and progenitor cells (HSPCs) with an LVV encoding a modified β-globin gene ($β^{A-T87Q}$) that inhibits polymerization of sickle hemoglobin.[5,9–13] Therefore, the same LVV and a similar manufacturing process are under investigation for treating SCD.[14] Two companion phase I/II clinical trials sponsored by bluebird bio (ClinicalTrials.gov: NCT01745120, HBG-204 NORTHSTAR and NCT02151526, HBG-205) treated 22 patients (12 to 35 years old) with TDT genotypes including $β^0/β^0$ or IVS1-110, which produces very low levels of β-globin (n = 9), $β^E/β^0$ (n = 9) or other ($n = 4$).[13] Of the nine individuals with $β^0/β^0$ or IVS1-110 genotypes, three became transfusion-independent, and six experienced reductions (median 73%) in RBC transfusion requirements. Of the remaining 13 patients with less severe genotypes (mainly $β^E/β^0$), 12 became RBC transfusion independent. In general, the clinical efficacy correlated with vector copy number in peripheral blood mononuclear cells at 6 months, which reflects LVV transduction efficiency of HSCs. The adverse events were due to myeloablative busulfan conditioning and not attributed to the drug product.

More recently, a completed phase III study sponsored by bluebird bio evaluated Lentiglobin therapy in 23 individuals (4 to 34 years old) with non-$β^0/β^0$ TDT (NCT02906202, HGB207, NORTHSTAR-2).[9] Transfusion independence and normal or near-normal blood hemoglobin levels occurred in 91% of individuals with up to 4 years follow-up. The improved clinical efficacy compared with the previous phase I/II studies was largely due to manufacturing improvements that resulted in more efficient transduction of HSCs and higher post-therapy vector copy numbers. Another phase III study for TDT, Northstar-3 (HGB-212; NCT03207009), is ongoing.

The GLOBE phase I/II clinical trial (NCT02453477) used an LVV harboring wild-type $β^A$-globin.[15] Three adult participants experienced reduced transfusion requirements and three of four pediatric participants achieved transfusion independence (4 to 13 years old) over 1 to 28 months follow-up. The MSKCC phase I clinical trial (NCT01639690) examined the β-globin LVV TNS9.3.55 and reduced intensity busulfan conditioning in four individuals with TDT.[16] After 6 to 8 years of follow-up, RBC transfusion requirements were reduced by approximately 50% in two individuals. The modest therapeutic response was associated with low post-therapy vector copy number, which most likely resulted from inefficient transduction of patient HSCs rather than reduced-intensity conditioning. Several LVV gene therapy trials for severe β-thalassemia have opened recently in China, where the disease is relatively common (see **Table 1**).

In August 2022, the US Food and Drug Administration approved betibeglogene autotemcel (Zynteglo) for treating patients with TDT.[17] This represents a major milestone and a culmination of more than a decade of intensive research. Updated information on clinical trials for Zynteglo and its regulatory approval process can be found on the FDA website [https://www.fda.gov/vaccines-blood-biologics/zynteglo].

Genome Editing for β-Thalassemia

Genome-editing nucleases

Genome-editing strategies use targeted nucleases to introduce sequence-specific double-stranded DNA breaks (DSBs) into the genome of live cells. The first genome editors to be developed were zinc finger nucleases, followed by transcription activator-like effector nucleases (TALENs); both require sophisticated protein engineering for DNA targeting.[18,19] The field was revolutionized by the discovery and adaptation of bacterial-derived CRISPR/Cas nucleases, which are rapidly and easily programmed by a single guide RNA (sgRNA) that directs the nuclease to a specified DNA target site via nucleotide sequence complementarity.[20,21] For current clinical applications, a ribonucleic acid-protein complex consisting of targeting sgRNA bound to a CRISPR/Cas nuclease are delivered into HSCs ex vivo by electroporation.

Two major cellular mechanisms exist to repair DSBs, including those that are created by genome editing nucleases: (1) error-prone non-homologous end joining (NHEJ), which introduces small insertions or deletions (indels) and (2) homology-directed repair (HDR), which employs a exogenous donor DNA template to introduce precise genomic alterations. Of the two cellular repair pathways, NHEJ occurs more readily in HSCs, with on-target efficiencies that can exceed 90%. Genome-edited-mediated NHEJ is being used to induce HbF for treating TDT and SCD. This versatile approach can be applied to most severe β-thalassemia mutations. In principle, HDR can be used to treat β-thalassemia by correcting individual mutations or by introducing a β-globin transgene into an α-globin locus (*HBA1*),[22] although this occurs at lower efficiency than NHEJ, typically less than 20%.

Genetic activation of fetal hemoglobin expression for β-thalassemia

Hereditary persistence of fetal hemoglobin (HPFH), a benign, naturally occurring genetic condition associated with high HbF levels throughout life, alleviates the symptoms of co-inherited SCD or β-thalassemia.[23] Hence, considerable research has been dedicated to understanding and manipulating the perinatal γ-to-β globin switch that causes the replacement of HbF with HbA.[24] This switch is mediated by repressor proteins BCL11A and ZBTB7A, which bind distinct cognate motifs in the γ-globin promoter to inhibit gene transcription.[25,26] Details of this process and the regulation of HbF are discussed in Chapters 4 and 5.

The CLIMB THAL-111 study (NCT03655678), sponsored by Vertex Pharmaceuticals and CRISPR Therapeutics, induces HbF by using CRISPR/Cas9 to disrupt an erythroid-specific enhancer in the *BCL11A* gene.[27] In a recent meeting abstract, the authors reported that 44 individuals with TDT who received the gene-modified cellular drug product CTX001 achieved either transfusion independence ($n = 42$) or reduced transfusion needs ($n = 2$) over 0.8 to 36.2 months follow-up.[28] Shanghai Bioray Laboratories Inc. used a very similar approach to treat two pediatric patients with TDT (7 and 8 years old) who achieved transfusion independence and normal hemoglobin levels at 18 months follow-up.[29] The THALES trial (NCT03432364, ST-400) sponsored by Sangamo Therapeutics & Sanofi, used a zinc finger nuclease to disrupt the *BCL11A* erythroid enhancer in five individuals with TDT.[30] Fetal hemoglobin levels rose transiently, but fell to near baseline after approximately one year with no long-term clinical improvement, reflecting the failure to achieve genetic modification of long-term bone marrow-repopulating HSCs.

Some HPFH variants disrupt the BCL11A or ZBTB7A binding motifs in the γ-globin promoter, indicating that disruption of the same motifs by genome-editing-mediated NHEJ could induce HbF therapeutically without eliminating expression of the erythroid repressor.[31–36] This is particularly important for ZBTB7A, which acts through non-globin target genes to prevent apoptosis of erythroid precursors.[37] The EDITHAL study sponsored by Editas Medicine (NCT05444894), uses the autologous HSPC drug product EDIT-301 generated by using Cas12a to disrupt the BCL11A binding motif in the γ-globin promoter.

Base editing

Base editors (BEs) consist of catalytically impaired Cas9 fused to a deaminase domain that generates A-to-G (Adenine Base Editors, ABEs) or C-to-T (Cytidine Base Editors,

CBEs) at precise positions in the genome.[38–40] Unlike Cas9 nuclease, BEs do not act through DSBs that can cause potentially deleterious chromosome-scale abnormalities or DNA damage responses. BEs can be used to correct some common β-thalassemia mutations, although these approaches have not yet been adapted for clinical application.[41]

BEs can induce HbF by generating point mutations in the γ-globin promoter that either disrupt BCL11A or ZBTB7A binding, or create new binding motifs for transcriptional activators, such as KLF1, TAL1, or GATA1.[42–45] Preliminary studies indicate that creation of new binding motifs, which cannot be achieved easily by Cas9-mediated NHEJ, induces HbF more potently than disruption of repressor binding motifs or interfering with BCL11A expression by targeting its erythroid enhancer. A recently opened clinical trial sponsored by Beam Therapeutics seeks to induce HbF in individuals with SCD by using an adenine BE to modify the γ-globin promoter at an undisclosed site (NCT05456880, BEACON study). If successful, this approach could be adapted for β-thalassemia.

Gene therapy genotoxicities

All gene therapy strategies cause genotoxicities with theoretical risks. Pre-HSCT myeloablative conditioning, usually with the alkylating agent busulfan, is common to most gene therapy approaches and predisposes to myelodysplastic syndrome (MDS) and acute myeloid leukemia (AML).[46]

LVVs insert semi-randomly into the genome and can potentially activate oncogenes or inactivate tumor suppressor genes, although this occurs less frequently than with γ-retroviral vectors.[47,48] No individuals with β-thalassemia have been reported to develop MDS or AML after LVV gene therapy, although concerning events have occurred. One individual with β-thalassemia developed a dominant HSC clone caused by LVV insertional activation of *HMGA2*, a transcription factor that has been linked to tumorigenesis.[49,50] This was detected at year 2 and resolved by year 8.[12] In 44 individuals with SCD who underwent LVV β-globin replacement gene therapy, two developed acute myeloid leukemia (AML) after 3 and 5.5 years.[14] These cases are believed to not be caused by LVV insertion.[51,52] The etiology remains uncertain, but may be related to SCD-specific predisposing factors.[53] Current research on LVV safety includes defining the integration profile of specific vectors in biologically relevant cell types, developing preclinical assays to detect oncogenicity, and tracking hematopoietic clones *in vivo* post-gene therapy by analyzing LVV integration sites.[54]

Genome-editing nucleases cause several genotoxicities that carry theoretical risks.[38–40,55–59] Unintended "off-target" DSBs, usually in genomic regions with partial homology to the sgRNA, can potentially interfere with normal gene function. Additionally, DSBs at on- or off-target sites can cause large chromosomal deletions, rearrangements, aneuploidy, or chromothripsis with TP53 activation.[60–65] Compared with Cas9 nuclease, BEs produce substantially lower rates of DSBs, which reduces certain genotoxicities.[38–40] However, BEs cause unique genotoxicities, including bystander mutations that occur at nucleotides adjacent to the target site, and Cas9/sgRNA independent deamination of DNA and/or RNA.[66–68]

Current research is focused on developing sensitive assays to detect genome-editing genotoxicities and designing modified versions of nucleases and BEs with enhanced specificity.[55,56,59,68–76] Available methods can detect off-target genome-editing activities or DSB-induced chromosomal rearrangements at a sensitivity of 0.1% genome-wide. Most genotoxic events are likely to be benign or result in cell death. However, rare unintended genetic events could predispose to malignancy by activating oncogenes or inactivating tumor suppressors. Such theoretical events are likely to be specific to the genome editor and sgRNA used and may be difficult to predict in advance of genome-editing therapy. For this reason, informed consent of clinical gene therapy studies require participants and long-term follow-up for the development of clonal hematopoiesis, MDS, or AML.

Perspectives and Future

Despite considerable advances in the treatment of severe β-thalassemia, life expectancy and quality of life remain lower than population norms.[77] Less than 25% of patients have access to an HLA-matched donor for allogeneic HSCT, the only approved cure until very recently. The emerging prospect of new curative approaches has generated considerable excitement and the FDA approval of betibeglogene autotemcel/Zynteglo LVV gene therapy for TDT in August 2022 represents "the end of the beginning" for gene therapy. Genome-editing/base-editing approaches are not far behind, and the field is advancing at lightning speed.

Newer, more versatile technologies, such as advanced generation BEs, prime editing, and adapted transposases will enhance further our ability to manipulate the genome.[40,41] Other components of the gene therapy process (see **Fig. 1**) are being refined to improve safety and efficacy. This includes new drugs to enhance the collection of autologous HSCs for gene correction,[78,79] and antibody-based approaches for bone marrow conditioning that are less toxic than current myeloablative protocols.[80,81] The development of "in vivo gene therapies" that can be administered parentally via modified viral vectors or lipid nanoparticles promises to simplify administration and increase access to curative therapies in low- and middle-income countries where β-thalassemia is prevalent.[82,83] Most likely, the whole HSC gene therapy process (see **Fig. 1**) will continue to be refined and improved over time as new technologies are adapted to clinical use. The best approaches are not yet known. Ideal HSC gene therapies for TDT and other blood disorders will show long-term safety and efficacy over at least 5 years and be relatively straightforward to manufacture and administer so as to be accessible for all patients.

Although the science and technology of gene therapy for β-thalassemia and other blood disorders have made exciting strides in the past few years, there have been recent setbacks in delivering these new medicines to patients.[84] This year, bluebird bio closed its operations in Europe due to difficulties in negotiating with payors for pricing of gene therapies for β-thalassemia and adrenoleukodystrophy, a rare neurodegenerative disorder. Orchard Therapeutics will discontinue gene therapy for three rare immunodeficiencies. Reasons for these disinvestments include the high costs of developing, manufacturing, and administering autologous cell-based therapies, regulatory and reimbursement complexities that vary across different countries,[77] and commercialization by companies whose survival may depend on short-term profits. Solving these problems for the benefit of all patients will require close collaboration between many stakeholders. Ultimately, society will profit from one-treatment cures for chronic diseases such as TDT by eliminating the cost of therapy over the whole lifespan, reducing depletion of donor RBCs, and improving lives.

SUMMARY

After many years of painstaking research, the potential of gene therapy to cure severe β-thalassemia is now becoming evident through recent clinical trials. Therapeutic protocols will continue to evolve and improve as new innovations are incorporated over time. Establishing the most safe and effective approaches will require long-term comparative studies. Ideally, pharmaceutical companies, governments, payors, and health care reimbursement systems will collaborate and adapt to optimize the delivery of these new personalized medicines.

CLINICS CARE POINTS

- Lentiviral vector-mediated β-globin replacement gene therapy for severe β-thalassemia was recently approved by the US Food and Drug Administration.
- Additional gene therapy approaches for β-thalassemia are emerging.
- Potential toxicities of hematopoietic stem cell gene therapy can result from myeloablative busulfan conditioning and/or unintended effects of genetic manipulation.
- Hematopoietic cell gene therapy requires long term clinical follow-up that includes monitoring for the development of clonal hematopoiesis, myelodysplastic syndrome and acute myeloid leukemia.
- Gene therapy has great promise for curing severe β-thalassemia; the best approaches are not yet known.

ACKNOWLEDGEMENTS

Our work on β-thalassemia is supported by the American Society of Hematology Research Training Award for Fellows (GC), and funding to MJW from the NIH (P01HL053749, R01HL156647, R01HL165798), Doris Duke Foundation (grant 2021054), the Assisi Foundation and ALSAC.

CONFLICT OF INTEREST

MJW is a consultant for Novartis, Graphite Bio, GlaxoSmithKline, Cellarity Inc. and Dyne Therapeutics and owns equity in Cellarity Inc.

REFERENCES

1. Taher AT, Musallam KM, Cappellini MD. β-Thalassemias. N Engl J Med 2021; 384(8):727–43.
2. Weatherall DJ. The inherited diseases of hemoglobin are an emerging global health burden. Blood 2010;115(22):4331–6.
3. Strocchio L, Locatelli F. Hematopoietic stem cell transplantation in thalassemia. Hematol Oncol Clin North Am 2018;32(2):317–28.
4. Leonard A, Tisdale JF, Bonner M. Gene therapy for hemoglobinopathies: beta-thalassemia, sickle cell disease. Hematol Oncol Clin North Am 2022;36(4): 769–95.
5. Magrin E, Miccio A, Cavazzana M. Lentiviral and genome-editing strategies for the treatment of β-hemoglobinopathies. Blood 2019;134(15):1203–13.
6. Naldini L. Genetic engineering of hematopoiesis: current stage of clinical translation and future perspectives. EMBO Mol Med 2019;11(3). https://doi.org/10.15252/emmm.201809958.
7. Delville M, Soheili T, Bellier F, et al. a nontoxic transduction enhancer enables highly efficient lentiviral transduction of primary murine T cells and hematopoietic stem cells. Mol Ther Methods Clin Dev 2018;10:341–7.
8. Hauber I, Beschorner N, Schrödel S, et al. Improving lentiviral transduction of CD34. Hum Gene Ther Methods 2018;29(2):104–13.

9. Locatelli F, Thompson AA, Kwiatkowski JL, et al. Betibeglogene autotemcel gene therapy for non-beta(0)/beta(0) genotype beta-thalassemia. N Engl J Med 2022; 386(5):415–27.

10. Magrin E, Semeraro M, Hebert N, et al. Long-term outcomes of lentiviral gene therapy for the beta-hemoglobinopathies: the HGB-205 trial. Nat Med 2022; 28(1):81–8.

11. Negre O, Eggimann AV, Beuzard Y, et al. Gene therapy of the beta-hemoglobinopathies by lentiviral transfer of the beta(A(T87Q))-globin gene. Hum Gene Ther 2016;27(2):148–65.

12. Pawliuk R, Westerman KA, Fabry ME, et al. Correction of sickle cell disease in transgenic mouse models by gene therapy. Science 2001;294(5550):2368–71.

13. Thompson AA, Walters MC, Kwiatkowski J, et al. Gene therapy in patients with transfusion-dependent β-thalassemia. N Engl J Med 2018;378(16):1479–93.

14. Kanter J, Walters MC, Krishnamurti L, et al. Biologic and clinical efficacy of lenti-globin for sickle cell disease. N Engl J Med 2022;386(7):617–28.

15. Marktel S, Scaramuzza S, Cicalese MP, et al. Intrabone hematopoietic stem cell gene therapy for adult and pediatric patients affected by transfusion-dependent ß-thalassemia. Nat Med 2019;25(2):234–41.

16. Boulad F, Maggio A, Wang X, et al. Lentiviral globin gene therapy with reduced-intensity conditioning in adults with β-thalassemia: a phase 1 trial. Nat Med 2022; 28(1):63–70.

17. Rubin R. New Gene Therapy for β-Thalassemia. JAMA 2022;328(11):1030.

18. Ochiai H, Yamamoto T. Construction and evaluation of zinc finger nucleases. Methods Mol Biol 2017;1630:1–24.

19. Hensel G, Kumlehn J. Genome engineering using TALENs. Methods Mol Biol 2019;1900:195–215.

20. Doudna JA, Charpentier E. Genome editing. The new frontier of genome engineering with CRISPR-Cas9. Science 2014;346(6213):1258096.

21. Doudna JA. The promise and challenge of therapeutic genome editing. Nature 2020;578(7794):229–36.

22. Cromer MK, Camarena J, Martin RM, et al. Gene replacement of α-globin with β-globin restores hemoglobin balance in β-thalassemia-derived hematopoietic stem and progenitor cells. Nat Med 2021;27(4):677–87.

23. Forget BG. Molecular basis of hereditary persistence of fetal hemoglobin. Ann N Y Acad Sci 1998;850:38–44.

24. Vinjamur DS, Bauer DE, Orkin SH. Recent progress in understanding and manipulating haemoglobin switching for the haemoglobinopathies. Br J Haematol 2018; 180(5):630–43.

25. Martyn GE, Wienert B, Yang L, et al. Natural regulatory mutations elevate the fetal globin gene via disruption of BCL11A or ZBTB7A binding. Nat Genet 2018;50(4): 498–503.

26. Masuda T, Wang X, Maeda M, et al. Transcription factors LRF and BCL11A independently repress expression of fetal hemoglobin. Science 2016;351(6270): 285–9.

27. Frangoul H, Altshuler D, Cappellini MD, et al. CRISPR-Cas9 gene editing for sickle cell disease and β-thalassemia. N Engl J Med 2021;384(3):252–60.

28. Locatelli F, Frangoul H, Corbacioglu S, et al. Efficacy and safety of a single dose of CTX for transfusion-dependent beta-thalassemia and severe sickle cell disease. HemaSphere 2022;6:S3.

29. Fu B, Liao J, Chen S, et al. CRISPR-Cas9-mediated gene editing of the BCL11A enhancer for pediatric beta(0)/beta(0) transfusion-dependent beta-thalassemia. Nat Med 2022;28(8):1573–80.

30. Walters MC, Smith AR, Schiller GC, et al. Updated Results of a Phase 1/2 Clinical Study of Zinc Finger Nuclease-Mediated Editing of BCL11A in Autologous Hematopoietic Stem Cells for Transfusion-Dependent Beta Thalassemia. Blood 2021;138(Suppl 1):3974.

31. Métais JY, Doerfler PA, Mayuranathan T, et al. Genome editing of HBG1 and HBG2 to induce fetal hemoglobin. Blood Adv 2019;3(21):3379–92.

32. Weber L, Frati G, Felix T, et al. Editing a γ-globin repressor binding site restores fetal hemoglobin synthesis and corrects the sickle cell disease phenotype. Sci Adv 2020;6(7). https://doi.org/10.1126/sciadv.aay9392.

33. Humbert O, Radtke S, Samuelson C, et al. Therapeutically relevant engraftment of a CRISPR-Cas9-edited HSC-enriched population with HbF reactivation in nonhuman primates. Sci Transl Med 2019;11(503). https://doi.org/10.1126/scitranslmed.aaw3768.

34. Traxler EA, Yao Y, Wang YD, et al. A genome-editing strategy to treat β-hemoglobinopathies that recapitulates a mutation associated with a benign genetic condition. Nat Med 2016;22(9):987–90.

35. Ye L, Wang J, Tan Y, et al. Genome editing using CRISPR-Cas9 to create the HPFH genotype in HSPCs: An approach for treating sickle cell disease and β-thalassemia. Proc Natl Acad Sci U S A 2016;113(38):10661–5.

36. Lux CT, Pattabhi S, Berger M, et al. TALEN-Mediated Gene Editing of. Mol Ther Methods Clin Dev 2019;12:175–83.

37. Maeda T, Ito K, Merghoub T, et al. LRF is an essential downstream target of GATA1 in erythroid development and regulates BIM-dependent apoptosis. Dev Cell 2009;17(4):527–40.

38. Gaudelli NM, Komor AC, Rees HA, et al. Programmable base editing of A•T to G•C in genomic DNA without DNA cleavage. Nature 2017;551(7681):464–71.

39. Komor AC, Kim YB, Packer MS, et al. Programmable editing of a target base in genomic DNA without double-stranded DNA cleavage. Nature 2016;533(7603):420–4.

40. Anzalone AV, Koblan LW, Liu DR. Genome editing with CRISPR-Cas nucleases, base editors, transposases and prime editors. Nat Biotechnol 2020;38(7):824–44.

41. Antoniou P, Miccio A, Brusson M. Base and Prime Editing Technologies for Blood Disorders. Front Genome Ed 2021;3:618406.

42. Wang L, Li L, Ma Y, et al. Reactivation of γ-globin expression through Cas9 or base editor to treat β-hemoglobinopathies. Cell Res 2020;30(3):276–8.

43. Li C, Georgakopoulou A, Mishra A, et al. In vivo HSPC gene therapy with base editors allows for efficient reactivation of fetal γ-globin in β-YAC mice. Blood Adv 2021;5(4):1122–35.

44. Ravi NS, Wienert B, Wyman SK, et al. Identification of novel HPFH-like mutations by CRISPR base editing that elevate the expression of fetal hemoglobin. Elife 2022;11. https://doi.org/10.7554/eLife.65421.

45. Antoniou P, Hardouin G, Martinucci P, et al. Base-editing-mediated dissection of a gamma-globin cis-regulatory element for the therapeutic reactivation of fetal hemoglobin expression. Nat Commun 2022;13(1):6618.

46. Bhatia S. Therapy-related myelodysplasia and acute myeloid leukemia. Semin Oncol 2013;40(6):666–75.

47. Cesana D, Ranzani M, Volpin M, et al. Uncovering and dissecting the genotoxicity of self-inactivating lentiviral vectors in vivo. Mol Ther 2014;22(4):774–85.

48. Baum C, Kustikova O, Modlich U, et al. Mutagenesis and oncogenesis by chromosomal insertion of gene transfer vectors. Hum Gene Ther 2006;17(3):253–63.

49. Cavazzana-Calvo M, Payen E, Negre O, et al. Transfusion independence and HMGA2 activation after gene therapy of human beta-thalassaemia. Nature 2010;467(7313):318–22.

50. Bonner MA, Morales-Hernandez A, Zhou S, et al. 3' UTR-truncated HMGA2 overexpression induces non-malignant in vivo expansion of hematopoietic stem cells in non-human primates. Mol Ther Methods Clin Dev 2021;21:693–701.

51. Hsieh MM, Bonner M, Pierciey FJ, et al. Myelodysplastic syndrome unrelated to lentiviral vector in a patient treated with gene therapy for sickle cell disease. Blood Adv 2020;4(9):2058–63.

52. Goyal S, Tisdale J, Schmidt M, et al. Acute myeloid leukemia case after gene therapy for sickle cell disease. N Engl J Med 2022;386(2):138–47.

53. Jones RJ, DeBaun MR. Leukemia after gene therapy for sickle cell disease: insertional mutagenesis, busulfan, both, or neither. Blood 2021;138(11):942–7.

54. Lidonnici MR, Paleari Y, Tiboni F, et al. Multiple Integrated Non-clinical Studies Predict the Safety of Lentivirus-Mediated Gene Therapy for β-Thalassemia. Mol Ther Methods Clin Dev 2018;11:9–28.

55. Kim D, Lim K, Kim ST, et al. Genome-wide target specificities of CRISPR RNA-guided programmable deaminases. Nat Biotechnol 2017;35(5):475–80.

56. Kim D, Luk K, Wolfe SA, et al. Evaluating and Enhancing Target Specificity of Gene-Editing Nucleases and Deaminases. Annu Rev Biochem 2019;88:191–220.

57. Kim DY, Moon SB, Ko J-H, et al. Unbiased investigation of specificities of prime editing systems in human cells. Nucleic Acids Res 2020;48(18):10576–89.

58. Tsai SQ, Joung JK. Defining and improving the genome-wide specificities of CRISPR-Cas9 nucleases. Nat Rev Genet 2016;17(5):300–12.

59. Cheng Y, Tsai SQ. Illuminating the genome-wide activity of genome editors for safe and effective therapeutics. Genome Biol 2018;19(1):226.

60. Leibowitz ML, Papathanasiou S, Doerfler PA, et al. Chromothripsis as an on-target consequence of CRISPR-Cas9 genome editing. Nat Genet 2021;53(6):895–905.

61. Enache OM, Rendo V, Abdusamad M, et al. Cas9 activates the p53 pathway and selects for p53-inactivating mutations. Nat Genet 2020;52(7):662–8.

62. Haapaniemi E, Botla S, Persson J, et al. CRISPR-Cas9 genome editing induces a p53-mediated DNA damage response. Nat Med 2018;24(7):927–30.

63. Ihry RJ, Worringer KA, Salick MR, et al. p53 inhibits CRISPR–Cas9 engineering in human pluripotent stem cells. Nat Med 2018;24(7):939–46.

64. Kosicki M, Tomberg K, Bradley A. Repair of double-strand breaks induced by CRISPR–Cas9 leads to large deletions and complex rearrangements. Nat Biotechnol 2018;36(8):765–71.

65. Blattner G, Cavazza A, Thrasher AJ, et al. Gene editing and genotoxicity: targeting the off-targets. Front Genome Ed 2020;2:613252.

66. Grünewald J, Zhou R, Garcia SP, et al. Transcriptome-wide off-target RNA editing induced by CRISPR-guided DNA base editors. Nature 2019;569(7756):433–7.

67. Zhou C, Sun Y, Yan R, et al. Off-target RNA mutation induced by DNA base editing and its elimination by mutagenesis. Nature 2019;571(7764):275–8.

68. Doman JL, Raguram A, Newby GA, et al. Evaluation and minimization of Cas9-independent off-target DNA editing by cytosine base editors. Nat Biotechnol 2020;38(5):620–8.

69. Jeong YK, Song B, Bae S. Current Status and Challenges of DNA Base Editing Tools. Mol Ther 2020;28(9):1938–52.

70. Kim D, Kim DE, Lee G, et al. Genome-wide target specificity of CRISPR RNA-guided adenine base editors. Nat Biotechnol 2019;37(4):430–5.

71. Yu Y, Leete TC, Born DA, et al. Cytosine base editors with minimized unguided DNA and RNA off-target events and high on-target activity. Nat Commun 2020; 11(1). https://doi.org/10.1038/s41467-020-15887-5.

72. Zuo E, Sun Y, Yuan T, et al. A rationally engineered cytosine base editor retains high on-target activity while reducing both DNA and RNA off-target effects. Nat Methods 2020;17(6):600–4.

73. Liang M, Sui T, Liu Z, et al. AcrIIA5 suppresses base editors and reduces their off-target effects. Cells 2020;9(8):1786.

74. Coelho MA, De Braekeleer E, Firth M, et al. CRISPR GUARD protects off-target sites from Cas9 nuclease activity using short guide RNAs. Nat Commun 2020; 11(1):4132.

75. Naeem M, Majeed S, Hoque MZ, et al. Latest Developed Strategies to Minimize the Off-Target Effects in CRISPR-Cas-Mediated Genome Editing. Cells 2020;9(7): 1608.

76. Richter MF, Zhao KT, Eton E, et al. Phage-assisted evolution of an adenine base editor with improved Cas domain compatibility and activity. Nat Biotechnol 2020; 38(7):883–91.

77. Beaudoin FL, Richardson M, Synnott PG, et al. Betibeglogene Autotemcel for Beta Thalassemia: Effectiveness and Value; Evidence Report. Institute for Clinical and Economic Review; 2022. Available at: https://icer.org/beta-thalassemia-2022/#timeline. Accessed June 2, 2022.

78. Fukuda S, Bian H, King AG, et al. The chemokine GROβ mobilizes early hematopoietic stem cells characterized by enhanced homing and engraftment. Blood 2007;110(3):860–9.

79. Hoggatt J, Singh P, Tate TA, et al. Rapid Mobilization Reveals a Highly Engraftable Hematopoietic. Stem Cell. Cell 2018;172(1–2):191–204.e10.

80. Czechowicz A, Palchaudhuri R, Scheck A, et al. Selective hematopoietic stem cell ablation using CD117-antibody-drug-conjugates enables safe and effective transplantation with immunity preservation. Nat Commun 2019;10(1):617.

81. Palchaudhuri R, Saez B, Hoggatt J, et al. Non-genotoxic conditioning for hematopoietic stem cell transplantation using a hematopoietic-cell-specific internalizing immunotoxin. Nat Biotechnol 2016;34(7):738–45.

82. Cullis PR, Hope MJ. Lipid Nanoparticle Systems for Enabling Gene Therapies. Mol Ther 2017;25(7):1467–75.

83. Raguram A, Banskota S, Liu DR. Therapeutic in vivo delivery of gene editing agents. Cell 2022;185(15):2806–27.

84. Aiuti A, Pasinelli F, Naldini L. Ensuring a future for gene therapy for rare diseases. Nat Med 2022;28(10):1985–8.

Emerging Therapies in β-Thalassemia

Rayan Bou-Fakhredin, MSc[a], Kevin H.M. Kuo, MD, MSc[b], Ali T. Taher, MD, PhD[c],*

KEYWORDS

- β-Thalassemia • Novel therapies • Quality of life • Advancement of care
- Transfusion burden • Clinical trial

KEY POINTS

- Unmet needs in the treatment of β-thalassemia remain.
- Several novel approaches to correct the resulting α/β-globin chain imbalance, treat ineffective erythropoiesis, and improve iron overload are currently being developed.
- The aim of all these emerging therapies is to improve outcomes for β-thalassemia patients and their overall quality of life.

INTRODUCTION

Major advancements in transfusion programs and iron chelation therapy (ICT) administration strategies have increased the life expectancy of β-thalassemia patients and improved their overall quality of life. These advances have also aided both clinicians and scientists to further optimize their disease management approaches and construct a plan for the development of novel therapeutic agents, with the ultimate goals of prolonging longevity, reducing symptom burden, and improving patient compliance and adherence.[1–4] These can be classified into three major categories based on their ability to target different features of the underlying disease pathophysiology: correction of the α/β globin chain imbalance, targeting ineffective erythropoiesis (IE), and targeting iron dysregulation (**Fig. 1**). This article provides an overview of these different emerging therapies that are currently in development for β-thalassemia.

[a] Department of Clinical Sciences and Community Health, University of Milan, Milan, Italy; [b] Division of Hematology, University of Toronto, Toronto, ON, Canada; [c] Division of Hematology-Oncology, Department of Internal Medicine, American University of Beirut Medical Center, Beirut, Lebanon
* Corresponding author.
E-mail address: ataher@aub.edu.lb

Hematol Oncol Clin N Am 37 (2023) 449–462
https://doi.org/10.1016/j.hoc.2022.12.010
0889-8588/23/© 2022 Elsevier Inc. All rights reserved.

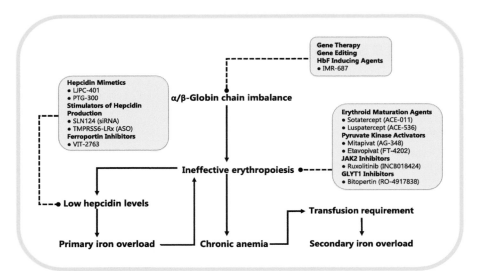

Fig. 1. Summary of novel agents that have been or that currently are being evaluated in clinical trials of β-thalassemia.

CORRECTION OF THE α/β-GLOBIN CHAIN IMBALANCE
Gene Therapy and Genome Editing Strategies

Lentiviral and genome-editing strategies for the treatment of β-thalassemia are now possible. Multiple clinical trials are currently underway globally to improve overall outcomes for patients using these genetic approaches. Further information on this subject is available in Georgios E. Christakopoulos and colleagues' article, "Gene Therapy and Gene Editing For β Thalassemia," in this issue.

Fetal Hemoglobin Inducing Agents

Advancements in the use of current pharmacologic agents for fetal hemoglobin (HbF) induction in β-thalassemia and the identification of novel experimental therapeutic strategies for HbF induction have been made possible as a result of a better understanding of the mechanism of γ-globin regulation. Several of these agents have been evaluated in β-thalassemia, mostly off-label, as monotherapy or in combination. A summary of all these approaches has been previously described thoroughly by our group.[5] Data on agents such as hydroxyurea (NCT03183375), benserazide (NCT04432623), thalidomide (NCT0651102, and NCT02995707), and sirolimus (NCT04247750) come from small clinical trials and are often limited to patients from single centers or specific regions of the world. One agent of interest is IMR-687 or Tovinontrine. This is a potent, specific, and highly selective small molecule inhibitor of phosphodiesterase-9 (PDE-9) that increases intracellular cyclic guanosine monophosphate levels and reactivation of HbF.[6] The Forte trial, a phase 2b, study, was established and initiated to evaluate the safety, tolerability, pharmacokinetics, and pharmacodynamics of IMR-687, administered once daily orally for 36 weeks in a cohort of β-thalassemia patients (NCT04411082). The primary objective of this study was to assess the safety and tolerability of IMR-687 in adult subjects with transfusion-dependent thalassemia (TDT) and nontransfusion-dependent thalassemia (NTDT). Secondary objectives in patients with TDT include reduction in red blood cell (RBC) transfusion burden, iron load rate, the mean number of transfusion events, and mean change in ICT dose and serum ferritin (SF) levels. Secondary objectives in patients with NTDT include the change in hemoglobin (Hb), mean change in HbF levels, and mean change in ICT dose and SF levels. On April 5, 2022, however, this trial was terminated as interim results showed no meaningful benefit in transfusion burden or improvement in most disease-related biomarkers[7] (**Table 1**).

TARGETING INEFFECTIVE ERYTHROPOIESIS
Erythroid Maturation Agents

Sotatercept (ACE-011), a ligand-trap fusion protein containing the modified extracellular domain of activin receptor type IIA, has been shown to correct IE by acting as a ligand trap to inhibit negative regulators of late-stage erythropoiesis in the transforming growth factor-β superfamily. Sotatercept was evaluated in a phase 2 trial on adult β-thalassemia patients (NCT01571635).[8] Patients with TDT treated with higher doses of sotatercept achieved notable reductions in transfusion requirements. Most of the patients with NTDT on the other hand achieved sustained increases in Hb level. Although sotatercept was efficacious, exhibited an overall good safety profile, and was tolerated by most patients, a decision was made not to advance sotatercept to phase 3 trial.

Luspatercept (ACE-536), on the other hand, is a recombinant fusion protein that is made of a modified extracellular domain of the human activin receptor type IIB fused to the Fc domain of human IgG1.[9,10] This protein inhibits the SMAD2/SMAD3 signaling and promotes late-stage erythropoiesis.[11,12] Initially, the murine analog of this agent, RAP-536, showed beneficial effects by decreasing IE, splenomegaly, and iron overload (IOL).[12,13] Then, a phase 2 study showed that luspatercept at 0.2 to 1.25 mg/kg subcutaneously every 3 weeks for at least five cycles was effective and well tolerated in adult patients with β-thalassemia (NCT01749540, NCT02268409).[14]

This paved the way for the phase III BELIEVE trial (NCT02604433). A total of 336 adult patients with either TDT or Hb E/β-thalassemia were enrolled. The patients had no transfusion-free period of >35 days within the 24 weeks before randomization. These patients were then randomized 2:1 to receive luspatercept or placebo subcutaneously every 3 weeks for ≥48 weeks.[15] The starting dose of luspatercept was 1.0 mg/kg of body weight with titration up to 1.25 mg/kg. A significantly greater percentage of patients receiving luspatercept achieved the primary endpoint of a ≥33% reduction in

Table 1
Summary of the fetal hemoglobin-inducing agents for correcting the α/β globin chain imbalance

Agent	National Clinical Number (NCT)	Design	Enrollment	Locations	Status[a]
IMR-687	NCT04411082 (IMR-BTL-201)	Phase 2	122 participants (TDT, NTDT) aged 18–65 years	Denmark, France, Georgia, Greece, Israel, Italy, Lebanon, Malaysia, Morocco, Netherlands, Tunisia, Turkey, and United Kingdom	Terminated

[a] Status per clinicaltrials.gov on October 1, 2022.

transfusion burden from baseline during any rolling 12-week interval or any 24-week interval, with a reduction of ≥ 2 RBC units compared with placebo. The percentage of patients achieving a $\geq 50\%$ reduction in transfusion burden vs baseline was greater in the luspatercept group at all examined time points. During any 8-week interval, transfusion independence was achieved by 11% of the patients in the luspatercept group.[15] All patient subgroups in the study showed a benefit from luspatercept treatment, including those with the β^0/β^0 genotype.[15] Clinically meaningful improvements in HRQoL and physical functions were also observed, particularly in patients responding to luspatercept, as measured by the TranQoL and SF-36 questionnaires.[16]

Initial data from 5-year open-label extension phase of the BELIEVE trial showed that luspatercept-treated patients continued to show meaningful reductions in transfusion burden over two years of therapy.[17] In addition, a higher proportion of luspatercept-treated patients shifted to lower SF levels, liver iron concentration (LIC), and myocardial iron levels during the first 48 weeks, indicative of lower risk of IOL complications.[18] Luspatercept was eventually approved for the treatment of anemia in adult patients with TDT by the US Food and Drug Administration in November 2019 and by the EMA in June 2020.[19,20]

Most recently in 2022, a long-term analysis of the efficacy of luspatercept treatment (for over 3 years) on transfusion burden and LIC showed that in luspatercept-treated patients with TDT, RBC units transfused decreased over the longer-term treatment period and the time between transfusions increased compared with baseline for $\geq 50\%$ of responders.[21] More patients with TDT experienced RBC-TI ≥ 8 weeks and in addition to a decreasing trend in LIC.[21] A long-term safety study showed that treatment discontinuations due to treatment-emergent adverse events (TEAEs) were more common in the luspatercept arm compared with placebo, as expected due to longer treatment exposure. Yet no new safety concerns were reported, and results were consistent with the safety profile of luspatercept.[22] As a result of all these positive findings, the efficacy and safety of luspatercept is currently being evaluated in a phase 2 study in pediatric patients with TDT (NCT04143724).

BEYOND is a phase 2 trial evaluating the efficacy and safety of luspatercept in 145 adult patients with NTDT and a Hb level ≤ 10 g/dL (NCT03342404).[23] The study met its primary endpoint: 74 (77%) of 96 patients in the luspatercept group and none in the placebo group had an increase of at least 1.0 g/dL in Hb concentration.[23] The key secondary endpoint was also met, with improvements in the patient-reported outcome measure of tiredness/weakness (NTDT-PRO T/W) being more pronounced in NTDT patients with longer luspatercept treatment. The proportion of patients with serious adverse events (AEs) was lower in the luspatercept group than in the placebo group (11 [12%] vs 12 [25%]). TEAEs most commonly reported with luspatercept were bone pain (35 [37%]), headache (29 [30%]), and arthralgia (28 [29%]). No thromboembolic events or deaths were reported during the study.[23] Long-term data from the BEYOND trial are awaited.

Pyruvate Kinase Activators

In patients with either α or β thalassemia, imbalance in α/β globin chain leads to globin precipitation and aggregation, and oxidative damage, leading to IE, reduced red cell lifespan, hemolysis, and anemia. Pyruvate kinase-R (PKR) catalyzes the final step in glycolysis in the RBC to generate pyruvate and adenosine triphosphate (ATP). ATP is deficient in thalassemia.

Mitapivat (AG-348) is an oral, small-molecule activator of wild-type and mutant forms of PKR.[24] In studies of adult patients with pyruvate kinase (PK) deficiency, twice daily dosing with mitapivat reduced hemolysis and improved anemia.[25–28]

Mitapivat increased PKR activity ex vivo in RBCs from patients with beta-thalassemia, and was shown to ameliorate IE, IOL, and anemia in a mouse model of beta-thalassemia intermedia.[29,30] These preclinical findings led to the phase 2, open-label, multicenter study of mitapivat in nontransfusion-dependent α- and β-thalassemia.[31] Twenty patients with β-thalassemia with or without α-globin gene mutations, HbE/β-thalassemia, or α-thalassemia with Hb < 10 g/dL, and nontransfusion dependency (defined as < 6 RBC units transfused in the preceding 24 weeks and none in the 8 weeks before study drug) were enrolled in the study. Patients initially received mitapivat 50 mg BID orally, followed by a dose increase to 100 mg BID at week 6 based on safety and tolerability, for a total of 24 weeks in the core period. Patients who completed the core period have the option of enrolling in the 10-year extension period. Sixteen of 20 patients (80%) met the primary endpoint, defined as an increase of Hb by at least 1 g/dL from baseline between weeks 4 and 12. Fifteen of the 20 patients were with β-thalassemia, of which 11 met the primary endpoint, despite the heterogeneity in the participants' genotype. The secondary endpoint of sustained Hb response (defined as meeting the primary response and at least 1 g/dL increase in Hb in at least two readings between weeks 12 and 24) was met in 65% of the 20 patients. An increase in Hb was seen as early as 4 weeks of dosing on the drug, with a mean change in Hb from baseline between weeks 12 and 24 at 1.3 g/dL. An increase in Hb was sustained over the 24-week core period and into the extension period, with a mean Hb increase of 1.7 g/dL at week 72. A trend in decreasing markers of hemolysis and erythropoiesis, including total bilirubin, lactate dehydrogenase, and erythropoietin, were observed as early as week 2, and maintained over the core and extension period up to week 72. The most commonly reported TEAEs were initial insomnia ($n = 10$ [50%]), dizziness ($n = 6$ [30%]), and headache ($n = 5$ [25%]), consistent with prior studies of mitapivat in healthy volunteers and patients with PK deficiency. Of note, initial insomnia was observed in the core period but not in the extension period. No trends in decreases were observed in bone mineral density up to week 72. On the basis of these results, two phase-3 trials in α- and β-thalassemia, one in patients who are nontransfusion-dependent (ENERGIZE; NCT04770753) and one in patients who are transfusion-dependent (ENERGIZE-T; NCT04770779), are enrolling.

Etavopivat (FT-4202) is another oral private kinase activator currently under evaluation. In phase 1 randomized, placebo-controlled, double-blinded study of etavopivat, 90 healthy adults were enrolled in four single-ascending dose cohorts (8 subjects per cohort) and four 14-day multiple ascending dose cohorts (12 subjects per cohort). Results from the pharmacokinetic/pharmacodynamic analysis indicate that maximal PKR activation is achieved at a dose of ≥ 400 mg once daily. Most TEAEs were grade 1 and none led to discontinuation. On the basis of the results of phase 1 study, a phase 2, an open-label study examining the safety and efficacy of etavopivat in TDT, NTDT, and sickle cell disease is currently enrolling.[32,33]

Janus Kinase 2 Inhibitors

Janus Kinase 2 (JAK2), a signaling molecule that regulates proliferation, differentiation, and survival of erythroid progenitors in response to erythropoietin, has also emerged as a therapeutic target in β-thalassemia. Preclinical studies have shown that JAK2 inhibition not only improved IE but also reversed splenomegaly.[34,35] These encouraging findings paved the way for a phase 2a study to evaluate the efficacy and safety of ruxolitinib (JAK2 inhibitor) administered orally at a starting dose of 10 mg twice daily in adult TDT patients with splenomegaly (NCT02049450).[36] A decrease in spleen size from baseline was observed in ruxolitinib-treated patients. There was also a mean change in spleen volume from baseline to week 12 ($n = 26$) and week 30 ($n = 25$).[36] At week 30, one patient who initially had a 15% decrease in spleen volume at week 12 showed an increase in spleen volume.[36] However, there were no clinically significant improvements in pretransfusion Hb, and thus no related reduction in transfusion needs. Moreover, although hepcidin levels increased in the ruxolitinib treatment group, no significant changes in iron parameters were observed over time.[36] For all the aforementioned reasons, the study did not further proceed into Phase 3.[36]

A recent study looked at the efficacy and safety of ruxolitinib in IE suppression as a pretransplantation treatment in 10 pediatric patients with TDT. After 3 months of treatment with ruxolitinib, spleen volume decreased in 9 of 10 cases by 9.1% to 67.5% ($M = 35.4\%$) compared with the initial size ($p = 0.003$), with AEs successfully managed through dose reductions.[37] The outcomes of hematopoietic stem cell transplantation (HSCT) post-ruxolitinib treatment were favorable in seven of eight cases. Ruxolitinib could potentially be a promising agent as a short-term pre-HSCT treatment of pediatric TDT patients with pronounced IE.[37]

Glycine Transporter 1 Inhibitors

Bitopertin (RO-4917838), a small-molecule selective inhibitor of glycine transporter 1 (GlyT1), also gained significant interest as an emerging therapy for β-thalassemia. The oral administration of bitopertin in β-thalassemia mice resulted in reduced anemia and hemolysis, enhanced in vivo survival of erythrocytes, and diminished IE.[38] A phase 2 study investigating the hematological effects of oral bitopertin in 12 adults with NTDT (NCT03271541) was conducted. Patients received oral bitopertin 30, 60, and then 90 mg/day during a 6-week intrapatient dose escalation phase, followed by $\leq$ 10 weeks at the target dose of 90 mg.[39] The first eight patients assessed at an 8-week preliminary efficacy analysis showed a mean total Hb reduction. Other selected hematological and chemical biomarkers of disease activity did not show clinically meaningful improvement. For these reasons, the trial was prematurely terminated.[39]

Table 2 provides a comprehensive summary of all novel agents aimed at targeting IE.

TARGETING IRON DYSREGULATION
Hepcidin Mimetics

Preclinical studies have proposed that minihepcidins, or synthetic long-acting hepcidin analogs, can restrict iron absorption with favorable effects as well on IE, anemia, and splenomegaly.[40–42] Their use was thus considered as a possible novel therapeutic startegy for β-thalassemia. Several studies have assessed the efficacy and safety of minihepcidin. The first is a phase 2 with LJPC-401 for the treatment of myocardial IOL in adult patients with TDT (NCT03381833). The primary objective of the study was to evaluate the effect of LJPC-401 on iron levels in adult patients with TDT that suffer from myocardial IOL. This trial, however, was prematurely terminated, as an interim analysis on the safety and efficacy data showed an absence of efficacy with the protocol treatment regimen, thus indicating an unfavorable risk-benefit profile for patients. Another phase 2 study evaluating an injectable hepcidin mimetic, PTG-300, was also conducted (TRANSCEND trial) (NCT03802201). Primary outcome measures of this study include: (a) NTDT subjects who achieve an increase in Hb without transfusion and (b) TDT subjects who achieve a decrease in RBC units required over an 8-week period. This study was stopped, however, due to efficacy issues of the drug.

Table 2
Summary of emerging therapies targeting ineffective erythropoiesis

Agent	National Clinical Number (NCT)	Design	Enrollment	Locations	Status[a]
Sotatercept (ACE-011)	NCT01571635	Phase 2	46 participants (TDT, NTDT) aged ≥18 years	France, Greece, Italy, and United Kingdom	Completed
Luspatercept (ACE-536)	NCT01749540	Phase 2	64 participants (TDT, NTDT) aged ≥18 years	Greece and Italy	Completed
Luspatercept (ACE-536)	NCT02268409	Phase 2 (extension)	51 participants (TDT, NTDT) aged ≥18 years	Greece and Italy	Completed
Luspatercept (ACE-536)	NCT02604433 (BELIEVE)	Phase 3	336 participants (TDT) aged ≥18 years	Australia, Bulgaria, Canada, France, Greece, Israel, Italy, Lebanon, Malaysia, Taiwan, Thailand, Tunisia, Turkey, United Kingdom, and United States	Completed
Luspatercept (ACE-536)	NCT04143724	Phase 2	54 participants (TDT), aged 6 months to 18 years[b]	Germany, Greece, Italy, Thailand, Turkey, and United States	Recruiting
Luspatercept (ACE-536)	NCT03342404 (BEYOND)	Phase 2	145 participants (NTDT) aged ≥18 years	Greece, Italy, Lebanon, Thailand, United Kingdom, and United States	Active, not recruiting
Mitapivat (AG-348)	NCT03692052	Phase 2	20 participants (NTDT) aged ≥18 years	Canada, United Kingdom, and United States	Active, not recruiting
Mitapivat (AG-348)	NCT04770779 (ENERGIZE-T)	Phase 3	240 participants (TDT, including	Bulgaria, Canada, France, Germany,	Recruiting

(continued on next page)

Table 2
(continued)

Agent	National Clinical Number (NCT)	Design	Enrollment	Locations	Status[a]
			α-thalassemia) aged ≥18 years[b]	Greece, Italy, Lebanon, Malaysia, Netherlands, Spain, Taiwan, Thailand, United Kingdom, and United States	
Mitapivat (AG-348)	NCT04770753 (ENERGIZE)	Phase 3	171 participants (NTDT, including α-thalassemia) aged ≥18 years[b]	Bulgaria, Canada, France, Germany, Greece, Italy, Lebanon, Malaysia, Netherlands, Spain, Taiwan, Thailand, United Kingdom, and United States	Recruiting
Etavopivat (FT-4202)	NCT04987489	Phase 2	60 participants (Thalassemia or SCD) aged 12 to 65 years[b]	United States	Recruiting
Ruxolitinib	NCT02049450	Phase 2	30 participants (TDT) aged ≥18 years	Greece, Italy, Lebanon, Thailand, and Turkey	Completed
Bitopertin (RO-4917838)	NCT03271541	Phase 2	12 participants (NTDT) aged 18 to 55 years	Italy, Lebanon, and Thailand	Completed (prematurely terminated)

[a] Status per clinicaltrials.gov on October 1, 2022.
[b] Estimated enrollment.

Stimulators of Hepcidin Production

Other novel therapeutic approaches to target iron dysregulation include suppressing the TMPRSS6 gene, thus increasing the hepatic synthesis of hepcidin. The inactivation of TMPRSS6 with small interfering RNA (siRNA) or antisense oligonucleotides (ASO) in preclinical studies led to increased hepcidin levels, ameliorated IOL, and improved IE.[43–46] Two major currently ongoing clinical trials are looking at stimulators of hepcidin production. The first is a phase 1 study (GEMINI II) investigating the safety, tolerability, pharmacokinetic, and pharmacodynamic response of SLN124, a GalNAc conjugated double-stranded fully modified siRNA that targets TMPRSS6 messenger RNA, in adult patients with NTDT and MDS (NCT04718844). The second is phase 2a study in adult patients with NTDT who will be administered with TMPRSS6-LRx (a generation 2+ ligand-conjugated ASO targeting TMPRSS6) (NCT04059406). Interim data from both of these clinical are awaited.

Ferroportin Inhibitors

Direct inhibition of the ferroportin receptor represents a novel approach to targeting the hepcidin–ferroportin axis.[47] VIT-2763 is an oral ferroportin inhibitor that has been specifically designed to target the hepcidin–ferroportin axis and ameliorate IE. Preclinical data from NTDT mouse models showed that VIT-2763 decreased organ iron levels and improved hematological parameters, showing amelioration of anemia and improved erythropoiesis.[48] In addition, the use of ICT in combination with VIT-2763 revealed no negative impact on the efficacy of either agent.[49] On the basis of this, a Phase 1 study was conducted on healthy subjects and showed that VIT-2763 administered at single oral doses up to 240 mg or multiple oral doses up to 120 mg twice daily was well tolerated compared with placebo. There were no serious or severe AEs or discontinuations due to AEs.[50]

A Phase 2a trial to evaluate the safety and tolerability of Vamifeport (given once [QD] or twice [BID] daily) over a 12-week treatment period in patients with NTDT is currently ongoing (NCT04364269). This study assesses improvements in hematological parameters, iron-related markers, and biomarkers for hemopoietic/erythropoietic activity. Initial preliminary data from 25 patients (vamifeport QD $n = 9$, vamifeport BID $n = 12$, placebo $n = 4$) showed that this study met its primary endpoint by showing a favorable safety and tolerability profile in adults with NTDT over the 12-week treatment period.[51] Vamifeport also met its secondary endpoints by demonstrating promising target engagement and pharmacodynamic effects on serum iron and transferrin saturation levels. All TEAEs were mild or moderate intensity, and each was reported only once. There were no deaths or serious AEs.[51] Further exploratory analyses from this study are ongoing. A Phase 2, multiple-dose, double-blind, randomized, placebo-controlled, parallel-group, multicenter trial in adult patients with TDT will also soon be initiated (VIT-2763-Thal-203). It will comprise a 24-week treatment phase with vamifeport. This planned clinical trial will also asses and observe changes in Hb and RBC indices, iron metabolism parameters, and markers of erythropoietic activity.[47] A summary of all novel agents targeting iron dysregulation is provided in **Table 3**.

SUMMARY

A new era of novel therapies is emerging with the aim of advancing care and improving outcomes for β-thalassemia patients. For some of these agents, the efficacy and safety has been established, whereas for others more data are awaited. More importantly, reports on the use of these novel therapies in the real world outside clinical trials and subsequent outcomes are awaited. This ultimate test will determine whether

Table 3
Summary of emerging therapies targeting iron dysregulation

Agent	National Clinical Number (NCT)	Design	Enrollment	Locations	Status[a]
LJPC-401	NCT03381833	Phase 2	100 participants (TDT) aged ≥18 years	Australia, Greece, Italy, Lebanon, Thailand, Turkey, United Kingdom, and United States	Terminated
PTG-300	NCT03802201 (TRANSCEND)	Phase 2	63 participants (TDT, NTDT) aged 12 to 65 years	Greece, Italy, Lebanon, Malaysia, Thailand, Tunisia, Turkey, United Kingdom, and United States	Completed
SLN124 (siRNA)	NCT04718844 (GEMINI II)	Phase 1	112 participants (NTDT including α-thalassemia or very low/low-risk MDS) aged ≥18 years[b]	Germany, Israel, Italy, Jordan, Malaysia, Thailand, and United Kingdom	Recruiting
TMPRSS6-LRx (ASO)	NCT04059406	Phase 2	36 participants (NTDT) aged 18 to 65 years	Australia, Greece, Lebanon, Thailand, and Turkey	Active, not recruiting
VIT-2763	NCT04364269 (VITHAL)	Phase 2	36 participants (NTDT) aged 12 to 65 years	Greece, Israel, Italy, Lebanon, and Thailand	Completed

[a] Status per clinicaltrials.gov on October 1, 2022.
[b] Estimated enrollment.

these agents can be integrated into the standard care of β-thalassemia and used as monotherapy or in combination with other established/conventional therapeutic approaches.

DISCLOSURE

R.B. reports no conflicts of interest. K.H.M. Kuo reports receiving fees for consultancy work from Agios Pharmaceuticals, Alexion, Apellis, bluebird bio, Celgene, Pfizer, United States, and Novartis; honoraria from Alexion and Novartis; research funding from Pfizer; and membership on an entity's Board of Directors or advisory committees from Bioverativ/Sanofi/Sangamo. A.T. Taher reports receiving consultancy from Novartis, Bristol Myers Squibb/Celgene, Vifor Pharma, Ionis Pharmaceuticals, Imara and Agios Pharmaceuticals, and research funding from Novartis, Switzerland, Bristol Myers Squibb, Canada/Celgene, United States, Vifor Pharma, Switzerland, Imara, Ionis Pharmaceuticals, United States and Agios Pharmaceuticals, United States.

CLINICS CARE POINTS

- Reports on the use of these novel therapies in the real world outside clinical trials and subsequent outcomes are awaited.
- As more of these novel agents become approved and available to β-thalassemia patients, it will be important to determine whether they can be used as monotherapy or in combination with other novel or conventional therapeutic approaches.
- Accessibility and availability to these novel therapeutic agents in resource-limited countries is pivotal, especially in areas around the world where disease prevalence is high.

REFERENCES

1. Bou-Fakhredin R, Motta I, Cappellini MD. Advancing the care of beta-thalassaemia patients with novel therapies. Blood Transfus 2022;20(1):78–88.
2. Musallam KM, Bou-Fakhredin R, Cappellini MD, et al. 2021 update on clinical trials in beta-thalassemia. Am J Hematol 2021;96(11):1518–31.
3. Bou-Fakhredin R, Tabbikha R, Daadaa H, et al. Emerging therapies in beta-thalassemia: toward a new era in management. Expert Opin Emerg Drugs 2020;25(2):113–22.
4. Motta I, Bou-Fakhredin R, Taher AT, et al. beta thalassemia: new therapeutic options beyond transfusion and iron chelation. Drugs 2020;80(11):1053–63.
5. Bou-Fakhredin R, De Franceschi L, Motta I, et al. Pharmacological Induction of Fetal Hemoglobin in beta-Thalassemia and Sickle Cell Disease: An Updated Perspective. Pharmaceuticals (Basel) 2022;15(6):753.
6. McArthur JG, Svenstrup N, Chen C, et al. A novel, highly potent and selective phosphodiesterase-9 inhibitor for the treatment of sickle cell disease. Haematologica 2020;105(3):623–31.
7. Imara announces results of interim analyses of Tovinontrine (IMR-687) Phase 2B clinical trials in Sickle Cell Disease and Beta-Thalassemia. Press Release. 2022. Available at: https://imaratx.gcs-web.com/news-releases/news-release-details/imara-announces-results-interim-analyses-tovinontrine-imr-687. Accessed October 1, 2022.

8. Cappellini MD, Porter J, Origa R, et al. Sotatercept, a novel transforming growth factor beta ligand trap, improves anemia in beta-thalassemia: a phase II, open-label, dose-finding study. Haematologica 2019;104(3):477–84.

9. Cappellini MD, Taher AT. The use of luspatercept for thalassemia in adults. Blood Adv 2021;5(1):326–33.

10. Taher AT, Cappellini MD. Luspatercept for beta-thalassemia: beyond red blood cell transfusions. Expert Opin Biol Ther 2021;21(11):1363–71.

11. Suragani RN, Cadena SM, Cawley SM, et al. Transforming growth factor-beta superfamily ligand trap ACE-536 corrects anemia by promoting late-stage erythropoiesis. Nat Med 2014;20(4):408–14.

12. Suragani RN, Cawley SM, Li R, et al. Modified activin receptor IIB ligand trap mitigates ineffective erythropoiesis and disease complications in murine β-thalassemia. Blood 2014;123(25):3864–72.

13. Martinez PA, Li R, Ramanathan HN, et al. Smad2/3-pathway ligand trap luspatercept enhances erythroid differentiation in murine beta-thalassaemia by increasing GATA-1 availability. J Cell Mol Med 2020;24(11):6162–77.

14. Piga A, Perrotta S, Gamberini MR, et al. Luspatercept improves hemoglobin levels and blood transfusion requirements in a study of patients with β-thalassemia. Blood 2019;133(12):1279–89.

15. Cappellini MD, Viprakasit V, Taher AT, et al. A Phase 3 Trial of Luspatercept in Patients with Transfusion-Dependent beta-Thalassemia. N Engl J Med 2020; 382(13):1219–31.

16. Cappellini MD, Taher AT, Piga A, et al. Health-Related Quality of Life Outcomes for Patients with Transfusion-Dependent Beta-Thalassemia Treated with Luspatercept in the Believe Trial [abstract]. Blood 2020;136(Supplement 1):8–9.

17. Taher AT, Viprakasit V, Hermine O, et al. Sustained Reductions in Red Blood Cell (RBC) Transfusion Burden and Events in β-Thalassemia with Luspatercept: Longitudinal Results of the Believe Trial [abstract]. Blood 2020;136(Supplement 1):45–6.

18. Hermine O, Cappellini MD, Taher AT, et al. Longitudinal effect of luspatercept treatment on iron overload and iron chelation therapy (ICT) in adult patients (pts) with β-thalassemia in the BELIEVE trial [abstract]. Blood 2020; 136(Supplement 1):47–8.

19. REBLOZYL FDA. label. Silver Spring, MD: FDA. 2019. Available at: https://www.accessdata.fda.gov/drugsatfda_docs/label/2019/761136lbl.pdf.   Accessed October 1, 2022.

20. European Medicines Agency (EMA). Meeting highlights from the Committee for Medicinal Products for Human Use (CHMP) 28-30 April 2020. Amsterdam: EMA. 2020. Available at: https://www.ema.europa.eu/en/news/meeting-highlights-committee-medicinal-products-human-use-chmp-28-30-april-2020. Accessed October 1, 2022.

21. Cappellini MD, Taher AT, Porter JB, et al. S270: Longer-term analysis of efficacy of luspatercept versus placebo in patients with transfusion-dependent beta-thalassemia enrolled in the BELIEVE study. HemaSphere 2022;6:171–2.

22. Viprakasit V, Cappellini MD, Porter JB, et al. P1518: Long-term safety results of the BELIEVE study of Luspatercept in adults with Beta-Thalassemia. HemaSphere 2022;6:1399–400.

23. Taher AT, Cappellini MD, Kattamis A, et al. Luspatercept for the treatment of anaemia in non-transfusion-dependent beta-thalassaemia (BEYOND): a phase 2, randomised, double-blind, multicentre, placebo-controlled trial. Lancet Haematol 2022;9(10):e733–44.

24. Yang H, Merica E, Chen Y, et al. Phase 1 Single- and Multiple-Ascending-Dose Randomized Studies of the Safety, Pharmacokinetics, and Pharmacodynamics of AG-348, a First-in-Class Allosteric Activator of Pyruvate Kinase R, in Healthy Volunteers. Clin Pharmacol Drug Dev 2019;8(2):246–59.

25. Grace RF, Rose C, Layton DM, et al. Safety and Efficacy of Mitapivat in Pyruvate Kinase Deficiency. N Engl J Med 2019;381(10):933–44.

26. Al-Samkari H, Galacteros F, Glenthoj A, et al. Mitapivat versus Placebo for Pyruvate Kinase Deficiency. N Engl J Med 2022;386(15):1432–42.

27. Glenthøj A, Van Beers E, Al-Samkari H. ACTIVATE-T: a phase 3, open-label, multicenter study of mitapivat in adults with pyruvate kinase deficiency who are regularly transfused. Eur Hematol Assoc 2021;9:17.

28. Xu JZ, Conrey A, Frey I, et al. Phase 1 multiple ascending dose study of safety, tolerability, and pharmacokinetics/pharmacodynamics of Mitapivat (AG-348) in subjects with sickle cell disease. Blood 2020;136:21–2.

29. Rab MA, van Oirschot BA, van Straaten S, et al. Decreased activity and stability of pyruvate kinase in hereditary hemolytic anemia: a potential target for therapy by AG-348 (Mitapivat), an allosteric activator of red blood cell pyruvate kinase. Blood 2019;134:3506.

30. Matte A, Federti E, Kung C, et al. The pyruvate kinase activator mitapivat reduces hemolysis and improves anemia in a beta-thalassemia mouse model. J Clin Invest 2021;131(10):e144206.

31. Kuo KHM, Layton DM, Lal A, et al. Safety and efficacy of mitapivat, an oral pyruvate kinase activator, in adults with non-transfusion dependent alpha-thalassaemia or beta-thalassaemia: an open-label, multicentre, phase 2 study. Lancet 2022;400(10351):493–501.

32. Lal A, Brown C, Coates T, et al. S103: trial in progress: a phase 2, open-label study evaluating the safety and efficacy of the pkr activator etavopivat (ft-4202) in patients with thalassemia or sickle cell disease. HemaSphere 2022;6:2.

33. Lal A, Brown RCC, Coates TD, et al. Trial in Progress: A Phase 2, Open-Label Study Evaluating the Safety and Efficacy of the PKR Activator Etavopivat (FT-4202) in Patients with Thalassemia or Sickle Cell Disease. Blood 2021;138:4162.

34. Libani IV, Guy EC, Melchiori L, et al. Decreased differentiation of erythroid cells exacerbates ineffective erythropoiesis in beta-thalassemia. Blood 2008;112(3): 875–85.

35. Casu C, Presti VL, Oikonomidou PR, et al. Short-term administration of JAK2 inhibitors reduces splenomegaly in mouse models of beta-thalassemia intermedia and major. Haematologica 2018;103(2):e46–9.

36. Taher AT, Karakas Z, Cassinerio E, et al. Efficacy and safety of ruxolitinib in regularly transfused patients with thalassemia: results from a phase 2a study. Blood 2018;131(2):263–5.

37. Ovsyannikova G, Balashov D, Demina I, et al. Efficacy and safety of ruxolitinib in ineffective erythropoiesis suppression as a pretransplantation treatment for pediatric patients with beta-thalassemia major. Pediatr Blood Cancer 2021;68(11): e29338.

38. Matte A, Federti E, Winter M, et al. Bitopertin, a selective oral GLYT1 inhibitor, improves anemia in a mouse model of β-thalassemia. JCI Insight 2019;4(22): e130111.

39. Taher AT, Viprakasit V, Cappellini MD, et al. Haematological effects of oral administration of bitopertin, a glycine transport inhibitor, in patients with non-transfusion-dependent beta-thalassaemia. Br J Haematol 2021;194(2):474–7.

40. Preza GC, Ruchala P, Pinon R, et al. Minihepcidins are rationally designed small peptides that mimic hepcidin activity in mice and may be useful for the treatment of iron overload. J Clin Invest 2011;121(12):4880–8.

41. Casu C, Oikonomidou PR, Chen H, et al. Minihepcidin peptides as disease modifiers in mice affected by beta-thalassemia and polycythemia vera. Blood 2016; 128(2):265–76.

42. Casu C, Chessa R, Liu A, et al. Minihepcidins improve ineffective erythropoiesis and splenomegaly in a new mouse model of adult beta-thalassemia major. Haematologica 2020;105(7):1835–44.

43. Nai A, Pagani A, Mandelli G, et al. Deletion of TMPRSS6 attenuates the phenotype in a mouse model of beta-thalassemia. Blood 2012;119(21):5021–9.

44. Nai A, Rubio A, Campanella A, et al. Limiting hepatic Bmp-Smad signaling by matriptase-2 is required for erythropoietin-mediated hepcidin suppression in mice. Blood 2016;127(19):2327–36.

45. Guo S, Casu C, Gardenghi S, et al. Reducing TMPRSS6 ameliorates hemochromatosis and beta-thalassemia in mice. J Clin Invest 2013;123(4):1531–41.

46. Schmidt PJ, Toudjarska I, Sendamarai AK, et al. An RNAi therapeutic targeting Tmprss6 decreases iron overload in Hfe(-/-) mice and ameliorates anemia and iron overload in murine beta-thalassemia intermedia. Blood 2013;121(7):1200–8.

47. Porter J, Taher A, Viprakasit V, et al. Oral ferroportin inhibitor vamifeport for improving iron homeostasis and erythropoiesis in beta-thalassemia: current evidence and future clinical development. Expert Rev Hematol 2021;14(7):633–44.

48. Manolova V, Nyffenegger N, Flace A, et al. Oral ferroportin inhibitor ameliorates ineffective erythropoiesis in a model of beta-thalassemia. J Clin Invest 2019; 130(1):491–506.

49. Nyffenegger N, Flace A, Doucerain C, et al. The Oral Ferroportin Inhibitor VIT-2763 Improves Erythropoiesis without Interfering with Iron Chelation Therapy in a Mouse Model of beta-Thalassemia. Int J Mol Sci 2021;22(2).

50. Richard F, van Lier JJ, Roubert B, et al. Oral ferroportin inhibitor VIT-2763: First-in-human, phase 1 study in healthy volunteers. Am J Hematol 2020;95(1):68–77.

51. Taher A, Kourakli-Symeonidis A, Tantiworawit A, et al. S272: safety and preliminary pharmacodynamic effects of the ferroportin inhibitor vamifeport (VIT-2763) in patients with non-transfusion-dependent beta thalassemia (NTDT): results from a phase 2A study. HemaSphere 2022;6:173–4.

Printed and bound by CPI Group (UK) Ltd, Croydon, CR0 4YY

08/05/2025

01864749-0005